Controlling Stress and Tension

EIGHTH EDITION

Controlling Stress and Tension

EIGHTH EDITION

Daniel A. Girdano, Ph.D.

Dorothy E. Dusek, Ph.D.

George S. Everly, Jr., Ph.D.

PEARSON

Benjamin Cummings

San Francisco   Boston   New York
Cape Town   Hong Kong   London   Madrid   Mexico City
Montreal   Munich   Paris   Singapore   Sydney   Tokyo   Toronto

Acquisitions Editor: *Sandra Lindelof*
Project Editor: *Anne Scanlan-Rohrer*
Editorial Assistants: *Joanna Nasar, Jacob Evans*
Managing Editor: *Deborah Cogan*
Production Supervisor: *Mary O'Connell*
Production Management and Composition: *Pre-Press PMG*
Interior Design: *Hespenheide Design*
Cover Designer: *Yvo Riezebos, Riezebos Holzbaur Design Group*
Director, Image Resource Center: *Melinda Patelli*
Image Rights and Permissions Manager: *Zina Arabia*
Manufacturing Buyer: *Dorothy Cox*
Marketing Manager: *Neena Bali*
Text Printer: *RR Donnelley*
Cover Printer: *Phoenix Color*
Cover Photo Credit: *Morgan David de Lossy/Corbis*

Library of Congress Cataloging-in-Publication Data

Girdano, Daniel A.
    Controlling stress and tension/Daniel A. Girdano, Dorothy E. Dusek, George S. Everly, Jr. —
        8th ed.
        p. cm.
Includes bibliographical references and index.
ISBN 0-321-53702-5
1. Stress management. 2. Stress (Psychology)
I. Dusek, Dorothy. II. Everly, George S., 1950- III. Title.
    RA785.G57 2008 (2009)
    616.9'8–dc22

ISBN-10: 0-321-53702-5   2007032069
ISBN-13: 978-0-321-53702-7

Many of the designations used by manufacturers and sellers to distinguish their products are
claimed as trademarks. Where those designations appear in this book, and the publisher was
aware of trademark claim, the designations have been printed in initial caps or all caps.

1 2 3 4 5 6 7—RRD—12 11 10 09 08
www.aw-bc.com

Contents

Preface

A major factor in the maintenance of health is the ability to live in harmony within society while keeping to a minimum the detrimental effects of one pervasive by-product of modern society—*excess stress and tension.*

This, of course, is the object of the book. We feel that this goal is best accomplished through a multifaceted and holistic approach to the control of stress and tension. This approach operates on many levels, encompassing self and environment and incorporating the physical, emotional, mental, social, and spiritual facets of life. Stress management is not just academic information; it is an active pursuit. The academic part takes the form of knowledge about psychophysical process, sociological situations, and statistics on the behavior of humans in general and our peers in particular. The active part appears in the form of dozens of stress management exercises—some developed from our research, but most adapted from tried-and-true techniques, some centuries old, some based on more recent clinical trials.

Our teaching philosophy and by extension our writing is largely based on natural curiosity, the desire to understand why. Knowing the logical association among various parts of the whole usually increases motivation; and as we will mention over and over, motivation is the key ingredient in any behavior change program. In service of this philosophy, the first part of the book discusses the stress problem and our potential for achieving a solution, examining the relationship between mind and body, the nature of stress and the stress response, the mind-body theory of disease, and the psychoneuroimmunological mechanisms that link stress and illness. A thought-provoking look at stress and the human spirit is followed by an in-depth look at emotions, thoughts, and beliefs that forms a foundation for the next section of the book.

The next several chapters examine a number of specific categories of potential stress-producing elements in everyday life. Examples of these categories are patterns of behavior; demands and expectations; environmental relationships; human relationships; crisis, violence, and trauma; and job stress. Through self-assessment exercises in each category, readers are given the opportunity to determine the stressful factors in their own lives. The self-assessment techniques culminate in the construction of a personal stress profile. Stress management techniques, many original and others popular, time-tested relaxation methods and exercises, are presented for each stress problem and combined into a complete stress management system.

The remainder of the book consists of techniques used to alleviate stress and tension. Some are specific to the causes of stress mentioned above, whereas others are general techniques for reducing stress reactions, such as deep breathing and meditation.

Detailed instructions are provided along with discussion of the basic mechanism underlying each technique.

It may be logical to wonder why so many different stress management techniques exist and why so many are presented. The answer can be seen in the philosophy of different strokes for different folks. While all the techniques presented have been shown to be effective, it is impossible to know which ones will work in any given situation, with specific personalities. The best advice is to try them on and feel what fits. Stress is not like other health problems, such as gaining weight, for instance. There you know it when your pants no longer fit. Thus much of the book is intended to be a journey of self-discovery, which is why there are so many self-assessment diagnostic tools presented. The development of awareness of stress and stressful situations is a large part of the process of stress management.

In addition to numerous and varied techniques found within the chapters, larger, more inclusive exercises referred to as "Journal Entries" are presented at the end of each chapter. When these Journal Entries are viewed together, a complete picture of your strengths and weaknesses in dealing with life and stress will emerge. These insights help you complete the final chapter, which guides you through a step-by-step procedure to build your own holistic stress management program, based on your personal insights, needs, and abilities.

Stress is a multidimensional phenomenon. Reducing the detrimental effects of stress is best accomplished by modifying many varied aspects of your lifestyle. This modification involves reducing the stressfulness of interactions with other people and the environment. An often unspoken, yet very important aspect of stress is that it is a by-product of your belief system, which is an outgrowth of your personal philosophy. Aligning your behavior with your philosophy may be the ultimate stress-reduction technique. Behavior is dependent on becoming aware of your emotional response system and learning how to balance your feelings with appropriate social behaviors. Finally, becoming aware of the connection between mind and body as it applies to both arousal and relaxation, as well as mastering techniques of relaxation both provide a healthy means of perceiving the inner and outer world. Incorporating nutritional and exercise patterns completes the stress management package.

Acknowledgments

We would like to thank the following reviewers: Nicholas DiCicco, Camden County College; Barbara Funke, Georgia College; Earl Goldberg, La Salle University; Brian Hickey, Florida A&M University; Terry Lawton, Los Angeles Harbor College; Jon Peters, Indiana University–Bloomington; Gretchen Reevy, California State University–East Bay; and Bill Thompson, Belmont University.

Introduction

Life is a journey with a purpose. All of the people, places, things, and events we encounter along the way help us learn what we need to learn to reach our ultimate goal. Stress is a gift we give ourselves to remind us that we have temporarily lost our way, and the discomfort we feel provides us with the motivation to get back on track. When we are experiencing the signs and symptoms of excess stress, it is a sign that the people, places, things, and events have become the focus of our lives instead of ourselves and our purposeful journey. Stress is not about what the world does to us; stress is about how we interact with the world. Our stress is determined by our relationship to the people, places, things, and events in our world.

If life's journey is about learning, then the people, places, things, and events of our lives are our teachers, classmates, and books. As you work through the Journal Entries in this book, hopefully you will come to see these learning tools as part of your learning journey. Take the time to stop and reflect on the people you have met along the way, especially those who have impacted your life. Take the time to analyze the paths you have taken and not taken and how each has influenced you to be who you are now.

Physics teaches us that energy cannot be created or destroyed, only transformed. The energy you give off will be picked up and used by some other life form, and theirs will be used by you. The teaching energy put into this book is among the millions of teaching instruments you will encounter in your life. However, you will ultimately teach yourself. You will accept the teacher and the lesson when you are ready. You will learn when you embrace the value of the lesson, when you believe in your ability to succeed, and when you are sufficiently motivated to do that which is necessary to accomplish the goal. Stress is a gift of motivation and a compass to remind us we are off course. However, your whole life is your journey, so there is no need to hurry—if you miss this bus (or lesson) or if this bus takes you only part of the way, there will be another along shortly.

The purpose of this journal is to help you stay on track or find your way back to the feelings of peace and tranquility, and health and happiness, which are the signs that you are sailing smoothly along on your life's journey. Hopefully, it will help you add positive energy to the universe, and motivate you to help your fellow travelers along their journey. The important thing is to keep a journal of your journey lest you forget what you have learned. From the beginning of time, people have recorded the events of their journey for a record and for later contemplation. A journal has been and remains one of the most useful therapeutic tools and is one of the key elements of this stress management program.

Introduction to Journaling

Here are the keys to how to use the Journal Entries:

 This symbol appears when there is information or knowledge that is important to the exercise. Read through that information before doing anything else.

 Next, there is the writing or journaling phase. Each exercise provides space for you to write down your immediate or past experiences, sometimes even what you expect to happen in the future.

 Probably the richest experience you can have with the workbook is discovering the insights about you and your life that your journaling has evoked.

 At the end of each exercise, you will see this icon and a reminder to write down a brief word or phrase that you can use as a tool in the future as a sort of affirmation—a way to remind yourself how to manage a stressful situation. The last exercise in the book helps you put these tools together into a meaningful stress management toolbox.

Now, get to "work."

Journaling

Writing down your feelings about stressful experiences is a way of releasing the emotions that might stay inside and fester into stress-related conditions that lead to illness. Not everyone has another person that they can (or are willing to) tell their deepest feelings. A journal can be one of the best friends that you've ever had.

Later on in the book you will learn that when you become stressed, the part of your brain that processes emotion is instantly stimulated and in nanoseconds your autonomic nervous system begins the stress response. What *does not* happen automatically in your brain is giving conscious, rational response to the stress. In fact, the emotion-perceiving part that has just been stimulated is not directly connected to speech or dominant-hand writing. So in order to know what/how you feel, you must consciously apply yourself to the task . . . and by so doing, not only can you bring up the emotion, you can air it, see it, think about it, deal with it.

We know from scientific research that people who have the opportunity to write down their negative experiences keep less residual tension from those experiences. At the University of North Dakota, patients with asthma or rheumatoid arthritis who wrote about traumatic moments had greater health gains than students who made notes on emotionally neutral topics. Students at Southern Methodist University who wrote about one specific stressful experience for fifteen minutes on several days in a row were later found to visit university health services less than controls who had written about nonstressful topics. Further research has found that the immune systems of those who journal stressful emotional experiences are healthier than in those who diary nonemotional events.

Emotions are held within the body until their messages are delivered or played out. If there is no resolution to the original traumatic event, the initial hurt or sadness is buried and turns into anger. Buried anger turns into guilt and eventually into depression.

Isn't it better to work with the hurt and sadness? What easier and more cost-effective way than with a journal?

The pages of the Journal Entries are on tear sheets so that with the completion of each one, you can remove it and collate all of them into one convenient, accessible Diary for future use. Put some extra blank pages in your Diary and continue to write your thoughts when stressful events fill your life.

For further study:

Ira Progoff, *At a Journal Workshop* (New York: Dialogue House, 1975). Progoff is the acknowledged "Father of Journaling."

Ira Progoff, *The Practice of Process Meditation* (New York: Dialogue House, 1980).

Louise Desalvo, *Writing as a Way of Healing* (San Francisco: HarperSanFrancisco, 1999).

James Pennebaker, *Opening Up the Healing Power of Expressing Emotions* (New York: Guilford Press, 1997). Pennebaker has done decades of academic study regarding the effects of journaling.

Philipp Keel, *All about Me* (New York: Broadway Books, 1999).

Christina Baldwin, *Life's Companion: Writing as a Spiritual Quest* (New York: Bantam, 1998).

This exercise is an introduction to journaling. If you already keep a journal, humor us and try this method. It can't hurt you, and may even give you a new direction from which to approach your emotional hurts of the day.

First, think of a recent emotional event that is still tugging at you. It might be ongoing grief over losing something or someone dear to you, or it might be the argument that didn't turn out very good for you, or the thought that you didn't do something quickly enough or well enough or intelligently enough for someone who expected it of you. When you have a negative emotion in mind and the story that goes along with it . . .

Then, in the left-hand column of the space provided on the next page, write a brutally honest account of that stressful situation. Write about how it hurt you, how it made you sad, mad, or afraid. Write down who said what to you, what you said to yourself, what you felt like saying but didn't.

Third, after you have written the events and your feelings in the left-hand column, go back over what you wrote. Slowly read it, and as you do, write down in the right-hand column any insights that come to you. Have you had these feelings before? When? Do any childhood feeling-memories come back? Who else was involved in similar situations? What is the symbolic thing going on here? What is the gift in what you experienced? What hits you as important and that may pertain to other parts of your life?

The concept of journaling is to (1) write down your feelings about an experience and (2) look for and write down the insights from the experience. This may be done in a vertical format as shown here, or in a horizontal manner as in some of the other exercises in this book. Your descriptions do not have to be exhaustive. A few honest words or sentences about your feelings are often sufficient. Don't put off writing in your journal because you feel you don't have enough time to write a thesis. You will find various forms of journaling throughout this book.

The Journal

Events	Insights
_____	_____
_____	_____
_____	_____
_____	_____
_____	_____
_____	_____
_____	_____
_____	_____

 Write a positive word or short phrase about journaling that will be useful to you in future situations.

CHAPTER 1

Stress, Stressors, and Stress Management

Stress is a mind-body arousal that can, on the one hand, save our lives and, on the other, fatigue body systems to the point of malfunction and disease. Stress is both a physical response that protects us and a natural defense mechanism that has allowed our species to survive. We need stress and would not want to eradicate our capacity for the stress response even if this were possible. Stress can be motivating, energizing, exciting, and fun; it can challenge us to greater endeavor. At the same time, stress arousal is thought to be in some way related to or responsible for most illnesses that plague modern society. A review of hundreds of studies over the last three decades has shown that stress arousal is implicated in 70 to 80 percent of all the visits to physicians and at least 50 percent of all illnesses in general (Young and Walsh 2005). In this first chapter, we lay the foundation for understanding the concepts and issues relevant to the relationship between stress arousal and disease. We also will generally introduce the methods and techniques that have been shown to reduce the negative impact of stress and that will be covered in depth in subsequent chapters in the book.

Stressors in Life

A **stressor** is any condition or event that causes a stress response. Stressors can be physical, emotional, intellectual, social, economic, or spiritual. A stressor may be real or imagined; however, the response to the stressor (i.e., the human stress response) is always real.

Look at your surroundings, your situation, and your life in general. Opportunities to be stressed are everywhere, from minor annoyances, such as not being able to find a parking spot, to major fears, such as getting fired or failing to get into grad school.

The challenge to your serenity is not only next week's test or finding the right employment—more often and more intensely it is human relationships: intimate partners, friends, children, parents, employers, coworkers, teachers, siblings, even campus police and store clerks. Imagine a circus juggler tossing knives up in the air and fretfully managing to keep them safely in motion. Such is the stress of relationships—trying to balance your needs with those of others and still be loved, cared for, admired, and rewarded. The stress of relationships may be summed up in one word: expectations. Stress in human relationships comes from a combination of failure to meet the expectations of others and failure to get your needs met. On the positive side, relationships pressure us to grow and change, and they ground us when they are loving.

Intimate relationships bring up issues such as loyalty, values, morals, defending lifestyle choices, competition, rivalry, compatibility, jealousy, and control. These same issues follow us into the workplace: trying to please, get noticed, get promoted, and get a raise. The workplace has great potential for satisfaction, yet it also has potential for disappointment, frustration, and discrimination.

Personal safety is becoming a greater concern for everyone. Terrible incidents such as school shootings and the events of September 11, 2001, make us wonder whether any place is safe. Conflict is a universal stressor with profound implications for health and well-being. Fear, worry, anger, and revenge are emotions that are directly related to stress. Posttraumatic stress and its treatment have become a given for those who have survived (or for many who have even observed) traumatic experiences such as rape, murder, bombings, natural disasters, and combat.

Underlying all of our short- and long-term stressors is the inner conflict of matching our behaviors with our personal code of ethics. Most of us struggle with an inner conflict, a clash of values, a war waged on a philosophical/spiritual level for control of our behavior. We struggle between what we know is right and what is convenient or economical or feels good at the moment. We practice self-deception with rationalization, denial, and other psychological defense mechanisms. "Everyone else is doing it." "I'll suck it up now, make big money, and straighten out my life after I'm at the top." How many are brave enough to follow their personal code of ethics? How many even know what their personal code of ethics is?

Much of this book is about psychology, that is, what we think and how we think. All stress relates to how we think or we perceive the world—in other words, our philosophy of life, our ideals, and our beliefs. Philosophy has many aspects, and one is the belief that there is order to the universe and our place in it. This order dictates that a right way and a wrong way, a loving way and a fearful way all exist. Inner peace, which comes from a more joyful and less stressed life, is the result of living closer to what we believe is right and loving. Both Eastern and Western philosophers agree that our spiritual path transforms our consciousness and that the forces that create suffering and stress in ourselves and in the world, such as greed, hatred, ignorance, fear, envy, and jealousy, originate in our hearts.

Frequency, Intensity, and Duration

In physical terms, stress means strain, pressure, or force on a system. In the context of the human experience, it is the body's reacting to the environment through the buildup of internal pressure and the strain of muscles tensing for action. If prolonged, this physical pressure and strain can fatigue or damage the body. W. B. Cannon (1939) first defined stress as the **fight-or-flight** syndrome: When one becomes stressed, the proper use of that stress is either to fight off the threat or to run from it. To do either, the body prepares itself through the psychological mechanisms of coping and cognition and the motor act (behavior) that alleviates the stressor. The goal is to manage stress by diminishing the excess stress in our lives, the stress that is inappropriate for accomplishing our objectives.

Three aspects that help frame an understanding of stress are:

- frequency—how often does one trigger a physical stress response
- intensity—how severe is the stress response
- duration—how long is the body's physiology altered

The most important of these is the duration of the stress response. Even stress that is not particularly severe can, if prolonged, fatigue and damage the body to the point of malfunction and disease. Disease is not the only focus. A more immediate consequence is that excess stress robs us of joy in our lives. If we are worried about money, success, or image, if we are pressured by expectations and work demands, if we are angry and looking for ways to get revenge, we eventually lose our ability to feel the happiness, joy, and love that represent the core of the human experience. When we are under stress, our attention focuses on survival, and we retreat to escapist daydreams of a better tomorrow instead of finding ways to live each moment with joy and enthusiasm. Most philosophers and religious leaders teach that the purpose of life is to increase our enlightenment and to perfect our spirit. This becomes difficult to accomplish when our stressed lives do not allow for the silence so necessary for introspection. Stress can be a thief that robs us of not only our health but also our happiness.

The stress response of modern man and woman is often inappropriate both to the situation and in its level of intensity. Although physical stressors still exist, most of the stressors of modern society are primarily social or ego related. When a stressor is ego related or is a response to a social situation, it cannot be solved by a physical response. In addition, it may not be alleviated for a long period. If the threat is imagined and the stress response is stimulated, we cannot physically run from it. Pressure builds up, and part of us wants to strike out while the other part strains to hold back. Externally, nothing happens. Internally, the body is trapped in the tension.

Stressors occur daily; they are part of life. However, we must examine the valence of the stressor when we talk about its effect on health. Stress is negative when it exceeds our ability to cope, fatigues body systems, and causes behavioral or physical problems. Stress is positive when it forces us to adapt and thus to increase the strength of our adaptation mechanisms. Stress is also positive when it warns us that we are not coping well and that a lifestyle change is warranted if we are to maintain optimal health. When the body tolerates stress and uses it to overcome lethargy or enhance performance, the stress is positive, healthy, and challenging. Hans Selye (1956), one of the pioneers of the modern study of stress, termed this **eustress**. Eustress is action-enhancing stress that gives the athlete the competitive edge and the public speaker the enthusiasm to project optimally. Selye termed negative, debilitating, or harmful stress **distress**. Distress produces overreaction, confusion, poor concentration, and performance anxiety, and usually results in subpar performance. An individual in distress cannot cope competently. Prolonged distress moves the organism into the health danger zone. Somewhere

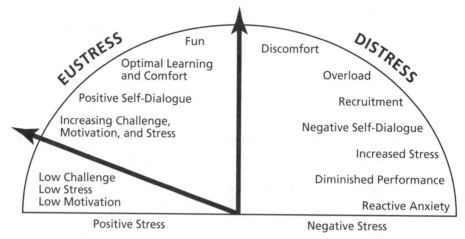

Figure 1.1 Stress and performance: the area of optimal performance

between eustress and distress is a level of stress that can promote optimal performance. **Figure 1.1** illustrates this concept.

The best way to find and use our optimal stress level is to develop the ability to recognize the signs and symptoms of distress. That sounds simple enough, but in actuality is not, because the body's sensitivity to the awareness of stress arousal tends to wane. The human organism characteristically becomes accustomed to its level of arousal, which often becomes the body's normal state. In other words, people become conditioned to their level of stress arousal if it lasts for a few weeks to the point they do not realize they are distressed.

Stress and Disease

Stress may be thought of as a response that links a stressor stimulus to any stress-related disease, symptom, or dysfunction.

All too often our interest in health begins when it deteriorates and when pain and dysfunction begin to dictate a lifestyle of diminished capacity. Virtually everyone knows disease. It is a condition of the body that presents symptoms peculiar to it. Disease or the fear of diminished capacity has prompted the study of stress, now a well-documented cause of illness. The primary vehicle and unifying thread in this research is the mind-body concept, which simply means the mind and the body working in harmony and with mutual influence and effect.

The mind-body concept of illness explains how our environment and social interactions, our perception of our environment, and our personal choices and emotional states produce a physical stress response. Moreover, it explains how stress arousal can eventually lead to illness and reveals a map of the interrelations among our mind, body, and social environment.

The mind-body influence on illness is not a new concept, as written accounts appeared in earliest Greek literature and reemerged in relation to modern medicine around

1927 with the teachings of Felix Deutsch (later published in 1959) and with the writings of Helen Dunbar (1935). Mind-body disease refers to any condition thought to be the result of excess emotional arousal, maladaptive coping, and chronic distress. The basis for this concept is that emotional disturbances such as anxiety, anger, fear, and frustration can increase the body's susceptibility to organic diseases.

In 1965, René Dubos noted that even infectious organic diseases do not commonly occur simply from pathogenic (disease-causing) microbes entering the body. Dubos studied the role of what we are calling the mind-body phenomenon. The sciences concerned with microbial diseases, he explained, developed almost exclusively from the study of acute or semiacute infections caused by virulent microorganisms acquired through exposure to an external agent.

In contrast, the microbial diseases most common in our communities today arise from microorganisms that are always present in the environment. These organisms remain in the body and under normal conditions do not cause obvious harm; they have pathological effects only when a person is weakened, often due to excess stress arousal. In this type of microbial disease, the event of infection is less important than the hidden manifestation of the smoldering infectious process. The stressful disturbance that converts latent infection into overt pathology is all-important. Stress appears to lower the body's resistance or immunity to disease. Dubos pointed out that being infected or having some organ system begin to degenerate is not the critical factor in the course of the illness. The critical factor is the body's ability to defend itself against these common infectious and degenerative processes, which are part of everyday life. We now know that distress impedes the body's ability to defend itself against all diseases.

Thus, stress may act as a catalyst for an organic disease already present by (1) allowing the disease to establish a foothold in the body from which to spread destruction or (2) accelerating the spread of the disease throughout the body. In short, almost any organic disease may have a mind-body or psychosomatic component, depending, of course, on an individual's psychological makeup.

Disorders of Arousal

Research has substantially increased our understanding of how stress arousal can be precipitated by a wide variety of environmental stimuli. In addition, stress arousal can result in an equally wide variety of disorders whose only common characteristic is that they occur in response to the arousal. Therefore, diseases caused or characterized by excessive stress arousal are commonly called disorders of arousal. They can be psychological disorders, such as those caused by anxiety, or very definable stress-related syndromes, such as cardiovascular or gastrointestinal diseases.

Research on the physiology of arousal is centered in the areas of the brain below the thinking cortex within the limbic, hypothalamic, and reticular activation centers (these areas are illustrated in Chapter 2). These "hardwired" centers communicate with the cells of the entire body through informational substances that interact with receptor sites throughout the various systems, especially the gut, spinal column, endocrine glands, and immune system (Pert 1999). Involved in sensory stimulation and emotional expression, these brain structures are also responsible for integration of the nerve stimuli sent from the brain to the body and thus have a profound impact on physical and mental health.

These same brain structures contribute to states of hyperalertness, hypersensitivity, and nervous-system hyperactivity in association with worry, threat, and the avoidance behavior of flight. Limbic-system arousal and sensitization have been implicated in a variety of anxiety disorders, personality disorders, posttraumatic reactions, addictive disorders, and withdrawal syndromes (Pert 1995).

One of the most substantial advances in the study of mind-body interaction is the theory that various disorders of the informational substance network that includes neurohormones, steroid hormones, peptides, growth factors, and polypeptides (what Pert calls the "molecules of emotion") are involved in disease. This theory implicates stress in the development of diseases ranging from the common cold to cancer. There is little doubt that information received from the environment, the way it is perceived and evaluated, and its influence on thought processes and muscle activity contribute to disease. The pathway from the social environment to ill health is a complex one that involves the interaction of mind and body (see **Figure 1.2**). Even positive events can produce stress when they demand distressing change and adaptation, but most stress begins with the negative, painful, and unpleasant events of our lives. An inseparable aspect of environmental stress is our varied and complex social interaction, fraught with feelings, expectations, and often frustration.

Figure 1.2 Stress and disease

Different pathways, two of which are represented in Figure 1.2, process the information from the environment. One pathway is thought to be largely subconscious and is thus named the subconscious-appraisal pathway. If this pathway is stimulated, coping action may eventually be required, in which case the pathway's innate physical and emotional reflexes prepare the body for action. It is important to note that this system only prepares the body for action and that this preparation, which we term background action, is independent of the final action. It is the second, or voluntary, pathway that determines whether this background arousal is necessary and used.

The voluntary pathway controls perception, evaluation, and decision making and is responsible for voluntary action. How you perceive an event largely depends on your concept of self, ego strengths, value system, mood, temperament, and even heredity. The emotions aroused are tempered by your psychological defenses, which are gained from experience, especially childhood responses. These lead to physical arousal, and you feel a need to act. Action itself is also complex; as a result of the consequences of a possible action, the reaction to a stressor is often no action at all. (For example, you may hold back a harsh comment after you realize it may hurt someone's feelings.)

Background action is very important here—it is arousal that is not conscious or noticed by the individual. It supports any potential action that may follow. The idea of background action is intriguing because it probably developed from the superior intelligence of humans and their capacity to perform several activities simultaneously. Sport offers a good example. Novice basketball players must concentrate very intensely when learning to dribble, just as novice ice skaters must work very hard to remain balanced in an upright position on their skates. As people learn a sport, they establish the neural pathways that allow the most efficient transmission of messages between the brain and the muscles. They develop the necessary muscles and build the confidence to perform the activity. Day by day, the activity becomes more automatic until the accomplished basketball player can dribble the length of the court while remembering the coach's selection of plays in any situation. Now apply this example to stress behaviors. If we live stressful lives, the body learns how to position itself for action very efficiently. Imagine a boxer having to think about tensing his muscles or concentrate on getting his heart to pump more blood to his muscles while he tries to defend himself.

When we are frightened by a situation or hurt because of the way people talked or looked at us, our bodies are affected by stress responses that have become automatic. We behave in a stressful or defensive manner without knowing it because we respond to the stressful situation on that automatic or subconscious level that allows us to do two or more things at once. The groundbreaking research of neurophysiologist Candice Pert (1999), who believes that the subconscious is the body and those body cells hold a memory pattern, reveals that a person who has a low threshold for frustration and is quick to become defensive might have developed a predisposition to be reactive. This predisposition is often referred to as **tone** and is analogous to muscle tone. The person who is highly toned is conditioned to react in a stressful manner when any number of situational triggers is present. Often the triggers are unknown on a conscious level or are forgotten if a certain memory is too painful to think about. Victims of childhood physical, emotional, and/or sexual abuses often bury the memory of the actual abuse. However, the body remembers the feeling and responds to triggers in a stressful manner even when no conscious appraisal is apparent. Thus, our emotions exert an all-important measure of background control over our thoughts and behaviors.

To summarize this point, we become very efficient at being aroused even when we are not conscious of the arousal (the triggering situation). We often feel stressed and do not know why. Not until we consciously interpret the stress arousal can we begin to deal with the stress, for at this point our emotions are integrated with our thoughts, and we interpret the experience in light of our knowledge and the situation. If we appraise the threat and no solution is forthcoming, then our stress arousal may be compounded by additional stress arising from fear of failure or harm. If a solution is forthcoming and involves an angry attack on the stressor, then the stress may be likewise compounded. If a solution is planned and then inhibited, stress arousal might be compounded by numerous psycho-physiological factors. If a solution is forthcoming, stress arousal can begin to dissipate; however, the physiological resolution may take as long as twenty-four hours.

As Figure 1.2 illustrates, both the subconscious and voluntary pathways can lead to physical arousal; arousal is not totally dependent on voluntary action. If the body prepares for action (for example, by bracing itself in a defensive posture) but then finds the action thwarted, the person is often left with chronic low-to-moderate tension. Prolonged physical arousal can go unheeded when its symptoms are not overt and do not produce noticeable pain or discomfort. However, if fatigue of an organ system ensues or if the system malfunctions, noticeable symptoms will appear.

Physical or behavioral signs and symptoms of stress arousal may appear when a body system is excessively stimulated. These signs may include feelings such as moodiness, irritability, depression, and anxiety, and behavior such as withdrawal, drug and alcohol abuse, and various forms of hostile and aggressive actions.

To be optimally healthy, we should be able to cope with life's trials and tribulations while minimizing the detrimental effects of excess stress. **Coping** is any attempt to neutralize stress arousal. Coping systems include behaviors, physiological reactions, cognitions, perceptions, and motor acts. Coping can be healthy and growth producing (competent) or can be unhealthy and cause additional problems that persist long after stress arousal has diminished (incompetent). **Competent coping** results in retaining optimal health and maintaining control while meeting life's demands. **Incompetent coping** results in the sacrifice of health and control and the inability to meet demands.

People characterized by incompetent coping are drawn to unhealthy physical or psychological means in order to cope. The psychological term for this is **recruitment.** There are numerous examples of recruitment. Bradshaw's (1990) examples of classic ego defenses people use when reality becomes intolerable include the following: conversion ("I eat, drink alcohol, or take drugs when I can't cope with reality"), denial ("It didn't happen," or "It's not really happening to me"), dissociation ("I can't remember what happened"), minimizing ("Oh, it wasn't really that bad"), projection ("It's your reaction, not mine"), repression (force oneself not to think about it), and withdrawal from the world. These are all examples of incompetent coping.

We orient ourselves, what we know, what we feel, and what we value by banking it off the outside world. We learn the fear of rejection, the anger of being thwarted, and the guilt of unacceptable behavior, and we experience the anxiety of struggling between needs and what we have to do to fulfill them. Stress can change minds and mold bodies. It influences the length and quality of life. It determines the amount of peace we enjoy or struggle we endure. Interactions with other people are not only the stimulus for our stress, but how we deal with relationships determines the amount of stress we experience. Until each person releases the tension between what they are and what they are experiencing, and what they think they should be, anxiety and discomfort of stress will be their companions. Releasing this tension is the goal of stress management.

Stress Management

Stress operates in many dimensions and is not always predictable. How stressfully we react to our environment is determined to a large extent by such factors as our attitudes, values, personality, and emotional development as well as by our ability to relax, our diet and physical activity patterns, and our ability to modify our lifestyles. If these stress-determining factors were points plotted on a stressor-stress-disease continuum, one might view stress management as intervention at each of these points, specifically related to each of the factors. In other words, stress management intervention points are techniques specific to each factor, but really only become effective when they consider the whole person from numerous and varied perspectives, incorporating mental, physical, philosophical or spiritual, social, and environmental interactions.

Choices

Like everything in life, stress management is about making choices. All of the techniques that are typically learned in a stress management course fit under a large "umbrella" that can be conceptualized as having the free will to make choices. "Make the wise and healthy choice" is easy to say, but the pressures promoting stressful choices are substantial, starting with a stressor-filled environment. The action or behavior of each individual or institution in the world becomes the input for other individuals. As we go about our daily activities, each individual with whom we interact presents some manner of stimulation. All of life's pursuits create potential stressors—from noise and pollution to competition for a seat on the bus, a place on the highway, or a position with a company or a seat in a popular class. Generally speaking, more people mean more complexity in social as well as in institutional organizations.

One of the easiest and most effective techniques of stress management is to identify stress-promoting activities and develop a lifestyle that modifies or avoids these stressors. These activities are designed to quiet the external environment in order to reduce the stressors in life. They should prompt a cognitive awareness of life events and then be utilized in restructuring your environment, thought patterns, and behavior.

Quieting the external environment to reduce stimulation of the individual produces the following effects:

- a cognitive awareness of life events and lifestyle
- a cognitive restructuring of the environment, one's thought patterns, and one's behavior

The next set of choices involves your internal world. The choice here is whether to learn techniques designed to allow you to better control your thoughts or to allow stressful, irrational thoughts and out-of-control emotions to dictate your behavior and to permit the chatter of your mind about worry, fear, "what ifs," and "should be's" to rob you of your ability to concentrate and to be quiet.

To a large degree, the amount of stress that society and the environment create depends on what information you take in and what you block; how you perceive, evaluate, and give meaning to that information; and what effect this whole process has on mental and physical activity. Attitude, which is the meaning and value you give to various events in life in combination with characteristic ways of behaving (behavioral patterns), has the awesome capacity to transform a normally neutral aspect of life into a psychosocial stressor. Few events are innately stressful, but we make them stressful by the way in which we perceive them. A person may alter stress-causing attitudes by learning how these attitudes are formed and then working to change that process. If this is effective, you will change the way in which you perceive a particular event to the point that there will be little or no physical arousal.

The stress response, which is physical arousal, can be elicited by conscious, voluntary action or by subconscious, involuntary (autonomic) activation, which keeps the body in a state of readiness. The constant state of readiness to respond with the fight-or-flight reaction when such a response is unwarranted is called "emotional reactivity." If the body remains in this state for long periods, organ systems become fatigued, and the result is often organ-system malfunction. Relaxation training can help reduce emotional reactivity. It promotes voluntary and autonomic control over some central-nervous-system activities associated with arousal and promotes a quiet sense of control that eventually influences attitudes, perception, and behavior. Relaxation training fosters interaction with your inner self, and you will learn by actual feeling (visceral learning) that what you are thinking influences your body processes and that your body processes in turn influence your thoughts. You will come to know your feelings and emotions as part of your thinking experience; your behavior will come more from what is within you rather than from how you feel you should respond to people and your environment. Primary therapeutic benefits of this phase of relaxation include learning to focus concentration on one thing at a time (especially on what is happening and what is being felt at the moment) and to quiet internal chatter that often comes from worrying about the future or feeling guilty about the past. When you have learned to stay in the present, to focus on what is happening right now and spend less time in needless worry and fantasy, you become more peaceful.

Quieting the internal environment in order to reduce sensory stimulation of the central nervous system has the following effects:

- decreased stimulation
- a calming or relaxation response
- a greater relaxation response

Yet another basic choice involves how your body handles stress once it occurs. You have the choice of sitting and stewing or getting rid of it by learning techniques to appropriately utilize the by-products of excessive stress arousal. The primary stress response is the fight-or-flight response, which has always helped ensure human survival and continues to do so today. In fact, no amount of relaxation training can diminish the intensity of this innate reflex. Stress is physical and is intended to enable a physical response to a physical threat. However, any threat, whether physical or symbolic, can evoke this response. Once the stimulation of the event penetrates the psychological defenses, the body prepares for action. Increased hormonal secretion, energy supply, and cardiovascular activity signify a state of stress, a state of extreme readiness to act as soon as the voluntary control centers decide what action to take. Usually the threat is not physical and holds only symbolic significance; our lives are not in danger—only our egos. Physical action is not warranted and must be subdued, but for the body organs it is too late: What took only minutes to start will take hours to undo. The stress products are flowing through the system and will activate various organs until these by-products are reabsorbed into storage or gradually used by the body. While this gradual process is taking place, the body organs suffer.

The simple solution is to use the physical stress arousal for its intended purpose—physical movement. The increased energy intended for fight or flight can be used for running, swimming, or bicycling. In this way, one can accelerate the dissipation of the stress products, and, if the activity is vigorous enough, it can cause a rebound or overshoot after exercise into a state of deep relaxation.

Utilizing the stress by-products through physical exercise has the following effects:

- decreased arousal
- a sense of well-being and a feeling of imperturbability

Finally, there is a choice that involves conditioning and learning to prevent future stress problems from developing. The choice is to be at the mercy of your environment or to build up your immunity to stress and decrease your susceptibility to future stressors by conditioning the mind to reduce stress-arousing thoughts and conditioning the body to be less reactive to stress. Stress arousal is a mind-and-body response to a social event. Throughout the day, each new stress situation leaves a residual amount of tension in the body, the accumulation of which cannot all be dissipated. The longer you practice relaxation exercises, the more you dissipate your residual tension and increase your general state of relaxation. Gradually, the relaxed state becomes a stable part of your personal choice and lifestyle. Representative techniques include many varieties of meditations. These activities are designed to train the mind to reduce arousing thoughts. They reduce stress-arousing memories and anticipations and instead direct thoughts to produce a peaceful and tranquil state. Meditation training yields the following effects:

- reduced mind chatter; fewer arousing memories and anticipations
- thoughts that produce peace and tranquility
- increased philosophical awareness

SUMMARY

This initial chapter is an introduction to the concepts in stress and is an overview of the stress management techniques that will be discussed throughout the book. Some of the key points to remember are:

- The stress response is a natural physical response that accelerates the body's defenses when threatened.

- The stress response is a natural, positive reaction programmed into our DNA for the purpose of saving our lives in an emergency.

- Stress is positive when it helps us "rise to the occasion" and negative when it debilitates or causes harm.

- Stress is supposed to be of short duration, again to help in an emergency. As such, the long-term protection programmed into most of our physical process is overridden; therefore, prolonged stress can be harmful.

- Duration of the stress response is more indicative of ill health than are the intensity and frequency of the stressor(s).

- Stress is a response to a stressor, which can be an actual physical threat or a perceived threat.

- Actual threats usually are of short duration; perceived threats can be of long duration.

- Prolonged arousal can damage organs, causing exhaustion and system failure (disease). These diseases are known as disorders of arousal.

- Stressors can be physical, mental (thought based), imaginary (perceived), or social.

- Human relationships are life's greatest stressors.

- Stress management is an organized system of activities and techniques designed to immediately reduce the impact of various stressors or be a conditioning process that promotes preventive resistance to stress.

- Conditioning to resist stress usually begins with a mindful series of choices that consider an awareness of life events and lifestyle and a conscious restructuring of one's environment when possible and, most important, one's behavior.

- The most effective stress management is holistic and multidimensional, and it includes activities that alter one's relationship with the environment, strengthens one's relationship with other people in the social milieu, mitigates stress-promoting personality characteristics and belief systems, and encourages relaxation.

SOURCES CITED

Bradshaw, J. (1990). *Homecoming*. New York: Bantam.
Cannon, W. B. (1939). *The wisdom of the body,* 2nd edition. New York: W. W. Norton.

Deutsch, F. (1959). *On the mysterious leap, from the mind to the body.* New York: International Universities Press.

Dubos, R. (1965). *Man adapting.* New Haven, CT: Yale University Press.

Dunbar, H. (1935). *Emotions and bodily changes.* New York: Columbia University Press.

Maslow, A. (1968). *Toward a psychology of being.* New York: Van Nostrand Reinhold.

Pert, C. (1995). Neuropeptides, AIDS, and the science of healing. *Alternative Therapies,* 1, no. 3 (July), 70–76.

Pert, C. (1999). *Molecules of emotion.* New York: Simon and Schuster.

Selye, H. (1956). *The stress of life.* New York: McGraw-Hill.

Young, R. C. and Walsh, C. J. (2005). Stress, health and disease. *Cellscience Reviews,* 2, no. 2 (October).

Journal Entry 1

Stress Is . . .

Stress Is Positive

- when it forces us to adapt, thus increasing our coping skills
- when it increases our awareness of problem areas

Stress Is Negative

- when it exceeds our ability to cope
- when it fatigues our systems
- when it results in behavior or physical problems

Stress is a mind-body arousal that, on one hand, can save your life and, on the other hand, can fatigue your body systems to the point of malfunction and disease. Stress is a physical response to protect your life. It is a natural defense mechanism that has allowed our species to survive. You need some stress and would not want to eradicate your capacity for the stress response, even if this were possible.

You are robbed of the joy in your life when you worry about money, success, or image; if you are pressured by expectations and work demands; if you are angry and looking for ways to get even; or if you fear tomorrow. When you are under stress, your attention becomes focused on survival, and you resort to unskillful responses and decisions in your daily work and relationships.

In this exercise, look for examples in your life where stress has motivated you and where stress has been a diminishing, negative, harmful factor in your life—perhaps even causing disease. Use the left-hand column in the space provided to write three personal examples of (1) when stress proved to be positive in your life and (2) when stress had a negative impact on your life.

In the right-hand column below, write your insights into the three situations you journaled in the left-hand column. You might examine your examples in terms of:

1. Themes—is there a common theme that runs through your positive stress events? Is there some special challenge or expected reward?

2. Are certain people involved in those events?

3. Were the events negative at first and then turned out positive?

4. What else do these events have in common that you could use for the future to make more of your experiences positive?

Personal Examples of Positive Stress Experiences	**Insights about Positive Stress**
1.	
2.	
3.	

Now repeat the instructions above with your negative stress experiences. How could you have made them positive?

Personal Examples of Negative Stress Experiences	**Insights about Negative Stress**
1.	

Personal Examples of Negative Stress Experiences	**Insights about Negative Stress**
2.	
3.	

 Write a word or short phrase about how stress can be positive that will be useful to you in future situations.

CHAPTER 2

Systems that Control Stress Arousal

The Purpose of the Stress Response

The purpose of this chapter is to promote an understanding of the alerting and arousal response we call stress. When one understands the mechanisms of stress, one can better see the relationship between the environment, the mind, and the body. Hopefully this understanding will eventually lead to the adoption of measures to prevent excess stress.

The body responds to new stimuli by preparing to take physical action in order to protect life. The stimulus (the stressor) alerts the body (the stress response), and as a result the body performs at a higher level. Early science liked to think that the brain was in charge of the stress response, yet the newer paradigm discovered through research in neurophysiology, endocrinology, and immunology allows us to suspect that the whole body is aware of stress at once (Pert 1999) and that the response occurs on many levels. The higher-brain centers, especially the frontal cortex, add perception and meaning to new information, and action may or may not be initiated. If there is perception that the new information is a threat to physical or psychological survival, the stress response is continued through additional outpouring of the informational substances. These substances in turn affect not only neurons but also cells throughout the body that have receptors for messenger molecules.

What are these receptors and molecules of communication? Virtually all cells contain many receptor sites whose function is to receive information from other cells of the body. They act somewhat like the scanners in a grocery store, except each scans for a specific molecule that has specific information for that cell. The information comes in the form of amino acid molecules (or **ligands**), which Pert (1999) breaks into three classifications. The smallest, simplest molecules are the **neurohormones**, such as norepinephrine and acetylcholine, which carry information across the synapse between nerve cells. The second category consists of **steroids** such as the sex hormones and the stress hormone cortisol. The third category, the **peptides**, is the largest, comprising perhaps 95 percent of all the ligands. They are involved in regulating practically all life processes.

Receptors are located on the surface membrane of a cell and have roots deep into the cell's interior. When a specific ligand communicates with the receptor, a message is sent to the interior of the cell that may initiate or halt production of an enzyme, cause the cell to become more or less permeable, or initiate any one of the myriad functions of that cell.

If the response to stress is physical action, the stress products within the body are utilized and dissipated. This is what nature intended. If the stress is not resolved and the products of the alarm reaction are not used for their intended purpose (action), all the systems of the body continue to react and over time will show the adverse effects of the stress response. As will be discussed further in Chapter 3, those adverse effects are seen as system malfunction, fatigue, disease, and even death (Metcalfe 2005).

Neuroplasticity

Neuroplasticity: the idea that the brain continually changes as a result of our experience.

An exciting revolution in neuroscience is its supposition about the malleability of the brain. Does the brain respond to experience with new nerve connections and actual nerve growth? A mere decade ago, the dogma in neuroscience was that the brain contained all of its neurons at birth and was unchanged by life's experiences. It was only in 1998 that neuroscientists discovered that new neurons are continually being generated in the adult brain (Ericksson et al. 1998; McEwen 2000).

MRI (magnetic resonance imaging) studies find that in a violinist, the areas of the brain that control movements in the fingering hand grow in size. Of interest to those in stress management, we now find that through the use of a more sophisticated imaging technique (diffusion tensor imaging), scientists are studying how methods that transform emotion may be changing the connectivity of the brain. Likewise there seems to be an impact on the brain, mind, and body from extensive practice of meditation showing a dose-dependent relationship, the more total hours of practice producing the stronger changes. More specifically, they are studying which types of meditation can be used to change circuitry in the brain associated with different aspects of emotion, especially replacing destructive or afflicted emotion with constructive states. Davidson and colleagues (2000) have convincing data that meditation can shift the brain as well as the body.

The frontal lobes of the cortex are especially important to the study of stress management in that this is the location for all the higher cognitive functions, such as planning for the future, making decisions, and formulating intentions to change. The frontal cortex is the most newly evolved of the brain structures and the one that is most fully developed in human beings in comparison to other species. It enables humans to learn to control their emotions and act unselfishly. In humans, this part of the brain does not fully develop until some time in the early twenties, which gives us a developmental cue for understanding and patience with young people.

The Basic Systems of Control

Currently, scientific research supports the existence of three basic systems in the human body that are highly implicated in the control of the stress and disease process. These are as follows:

1. the central nervous system (CNS), particularly that portion of it that is called the autonomic nervous system (ANS);

2. the endocrine system, especially the pituitary and the adrenal glands; and

3. the immune system and its interaction with the rest of the body.

The informational substances, or **neuropeptide system,** connect these three systems and, indeed, all the systems of the body.

> **Neuropeptides:** short strings of amino acids produced by nerve cells. When neuropeptides lock into receptors attached to cells throughout the body, they cause physiological reactions. Neuropeptides and their receptors form an extensive network that the body uses to communicate with itself. This network is the biochemical substrate of emotions and provides a scientific explanation for mind-body healing.

Historically, the brain was the main focus of stress research. It could be scientifically demonstrated that stimulation of various brain structures brought about both immediate and delayed stress responses. Research found that the center of physical control was the hypothalamus, deep within the brain, which receives constant input from the limbic system. This concept of a limbic-hypothalamic center is sometimes extended to include the pituitary gland and referred to in the literature on mind-body disease and psychoneuroimmunology (PNI) as the limbic-hypothalamic-pituitary axis. **Figure 2.1** illustrates the portions of the central nervous system that this section discusses. Our intention in this discussion is to elaborate on the two central nervous systems highly implicated in the stress response.

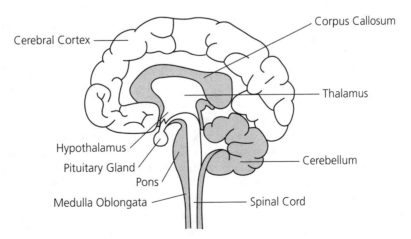

Figure 2.1 The Central Nervous System

The Autonomic Nervous System (ANS)

Actions of the central nervous system—the brain, brain stem, and spinal cord—can be classified as either autonomic or voluntary. Autonomic functioning is automatic or reflexive: It regulates heart rate, body temperature, respiration, and other vital functions without our having to think about doing so. The voluntary system allows us to think before we act.

There are two main classifications within the autonomic nervous system:

1. the sympathetic nervous system, which sets off the alarm response that in turn energizes the body to respond to stress; and

2. the parasympathetic nervous system, which reverts the energized systems to normal, more relaxed function.

The sympathetic system is best known for its lifesaving fight-or-flight capacities. When this system is stimulated, all its parts react with a mass neural discharge to accomplish a common purpose—enabling the body to act above and beyond its normal, everyday function. For example, in a fight-or-flight situation, the body needs more blood, more oxygen, and more energy. Therefore, the heart beats faster and pumps more blood per beat. At the same time, the body makes more efficient use of the available blood supply by constricting blood vessels in organs, such as the gastrointestinal tract, that are not essential to the stress response. This decreases the function of the unneeded organs and allows an increased flow of blood to essential organs such as the heart and skeletal muscles. In the lungs, the bronchials (which carry air) expand, and breathing becomes deeper, faster, and generally more efficient. The pupils of the eyes enlarge, improving visual sensitivity, and salivary secretion increases. The adrenal glands, sitting atop the kidneys, secrete adrenaline, which reinforces and prolongs the sympathetic effect and stimulates the liver to release more glucose to fuel the action. Adrenaline also stimulates the adipose tissue to release fatty acids to fuel the muscles. See **Table 2.1** for a summary of the effects on the body of the fight-or-flight response. In short, stimulation of the sympathetic system increases the activity of the organs needed for the fight-or-flight response and inhibits the organs that are not essential. Prolonged stimulation or inhibition of organs can cause malfunction and in turn promote stress-related illness.

The fight-or-flight response, mediated by epinephrine, norepinephrine, and dopamine (hormones of the sympathetic and adrenal systems), demands an integrated adjustment of many processes, as Table 2.1 shows. This response is facilitated by other hormones of the endocrine system, the central nervous system, and the various peptides.

The parasympathetic system, in contrast to the sympathetic system, does not exhibit a mass reaction to stimulation. It acts on specific organs, increasing the action of some while inhibiting that of others. Parasympathetic stimulation of the organ systems listed in Table 2.1 has the following effects: The heart slows down, most blood vessels expand, and the functions of the gastrointestinal system increase. The bronchials constrict, as do the pupils, and salivary secretion increases. After the arousal response, the parasympathetic system normalizes the functions of all the organs involved.

Most organs in the body respond to both the sympathetic and parasympathetic systems. Some organs, however, are stimulated by only one. In this case, the controlling system determines whether the organ is activated or inhibited.

Table 2.1 Physiological Changes in the Fight-or-Flight Response

Organ	Change
Fat tissue	Increased breakdown of stored fat, more fatty acids, and glycerol in the bloodstream
Brain	Increased blood flow, increased metabolism of glucose
Cardiovascular system	Increased heart rate and force of contraction, vasoconstriction of peripheral blood vessels
Lungs	Increased respiratory rate, dilation of bronchi, increased oxygen supply
Muscles	Increased breakdown of glycogen to glucose for immediate energy supply, increased contraction, decreased uptake of glucose, increased uptake of fatty acids for energy
Liver	Increased glucose production via gluconeogenesis
Skin	Decreased blood flow
Gastrointestinal tract	Decreased protein synthesis
Genitourinary tract	Decreased protein synthesis
Lymph tissue	Increased breakdown of protein

Source: Adapted from Martin et al. (1990).

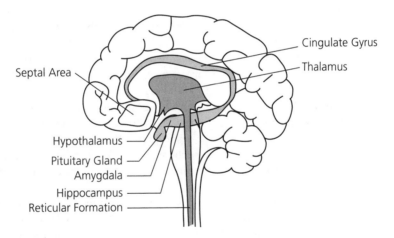

Figure 2.2 The Inner Brain

Structure and Function of the ANS The lower-brain structures of the autonomic nervous system respond to the physical world and are basically reflexive. These structures include the spinal cord, the cerebellum (the center of muscle coordination), the medulla oblongata (which controls heart rate, circulation of blood, respiration, coughing, and sneezing), the pons (a network that sends nerve impulses to various parts of the brain), the thalamus (the "switchboard" that sends incoming signals to proper brain areas), and the hypothalamus (see **Figure 2.2**). Throughout this area of the brain is a specialized system called the **reticular formation,** which we will discuss later.

If humans have any resemblance to other animal species, it is in the basic programs stored within these lower centers, which govern actions or behaviors that are natural, direct, and open without a great deal of learned inhibition. Activities centered in survival and reproduction (such as preparing a homesite, establishing and defending territory, hunting, homing, hoarding, mating, forming simple social groups, and doing routine daily activities) are instinctive and performed by lower animals as well as humans. But with their higher level of brain evolution, humans have shown the ability to override some of these basic responses for psychological and social survival.

The Hypothalamus   Located at the base of the forebrain, the hypothalamus is not so much a distinct, identifiable organ as it is a combination of tissues with a somewhat vague boundary. These tissues are made up of a number of nuclei, or nerve centers, that control the basic autonomic functions.

The hypothalamus is at the very center of the limbic system and has profuse communication pathways with all levels of this system (Ganong 1995). It sends neural signals in two major directions: (1) down through the brain stem, mainly to the reticular formation within the pons, medulla, hypothalamus, and thalamus; and (2) up to many areas of the cortex. The hypothalamus affects the cortex indirectly, but dramatically, through its control of the brain stem portion of the reticular activating system.

The hypothalamus is the major integrator of the body's regulatory systems (such as hunger, thirst, temperature, blood pressure, heart rate, and sex drive). Stimulation of appropriate areas of the hypothalamus can activate the sympathetic system strongly enough to increase arterial blood pressure by more than 100 percent. Other areas control temperature by allowing more or less blood to flow to the surface of the skin. Still others increase or decrease salivation, control sexual responses, and regulate the digestive process and other responses to physical threat.

The hypothalamus is a major part of the "physical" brain: It receives physical messages and responds on a basic, physical level. When it receives messages that are either threatening or new and unique, it responds with a sympathetically controlled alarm reaction. When the threat abates or the new message is somehow integrated, calming messages are sent through the parasympathetic system to the excited organs so that their function is normalized.

Consider, for example, the response to noise. A noise is first perceived by the lower centers before it is registered in the cortex. Once the hypothalamus is stimulated, it prepares for possible action by increasing the discharge of hormones, increasing the availability of energy, preparing the cardiovascular (heart and circulatory) system by shifting blood flow to essential organs, and at the same time tensing the muscles. The conscious cortex may ultimately prevent the action, but the body is prepared for any eventuality and is technically in a state of stress. So, now you know why parents or roommates may respond so adversely to loud, obnoxious music.

The hypothalamus, with its intimate relationship to the pituitary gland, links the nervous system with the endocrine system. The hypothalamic-controlled ANS communicates through **neurotransmitters,** or **neurohormones,** with the parts of the body it affects. The sympathetic-system nerve endings secrete the neurotransmitter norepinephrine to activate receptors on the cells of the organs that the nerve endings modulate, and parasympathetic-system nerve endings secrete acetylcholine. These neurotransmitters bind with receptors in the cell walls of the target organs, changing the permeability of the organ's cell wall and causing targeted internal events to occur. In addition to changing cell permeability, neurohormones, peptides, polypeptides, and other messenger substances may activate receptors on the cell membrane of the target organ, thereby causing enzymatic events to initiate the autonomic response characteristic of that organ.

The Limbic System   The limbic system offered its evolutionary predecessor, the physical brain, a measure of freedom from stereotyped behavior. Primarily, this newer system added the concept of feeling and emotion, which further ensured attendance to basic survival activities by making activities pleasurable or displeasurable. Feelings such as fear, anger, and love became attached to certain situations, guiding behavior toward that which protected and away from that which threatened. Understandably, two of our major neural pathways (those governing eating and reproduction) have intricate connections to the pleasure and unpleasure centers of the limbic system (Pert 1999). The concepts of reward or pleasure and punishment or displeasure are important to the concept of stress.

Because stress is an integrated response of the body, it must have an integrative conduit, and about seventy years ago that area was demonstrated to be the limbic system (MacLean 1949). The limbic system is the hub of the central nervous system and the human stress response as well. This system (particularly the septal, hippocampal, and hypothalamic areas) integrates cognitive appraisals from the prefrontal cortex with the higher-order emotions arising in the cingulate and amygdaloid areas. The result of this input is neuromuscular articulation and stress-related symptoms and signs (Glaser and Kiecolt-Glaser 1994).

The amygdala and hippocampus are particularly important areas of the limbic system as far as emotion is concerned. The amygdala is critical for certain kinds of negative emotions, particularly fear. It is activated by fear and is important to both the detection of signals of fear, such as being confronted by someone with an angry facial expression, and the generation of fear in the body. The amygdala is also involved in the anticipation of the negative consequences of rage.

The hippocampus has an important role in emotion in that it supplies, or is the background for, the context (specific situation or environmental circumstances) of events. It helps regulate emotional responses so that they are appropriate to the context. When a setting feels particularly secure to you, just the act of going into that environment is comforting. The appreciation of that environment involves the hippocampus. Some emotional disorders involve abnormalities in the hippocampus, particularly depression and posttraumatic stress disorder. It has been found that the hippocampus actually shrinks in both of these conditions (Goleman 2003). When depression is treated with antidepressant medication, it prevents the atrophy of the hippocampus that typically occurs if left untreated.

One of the most impressive discoveries in neuroscience over the last decade is that these areas of the brain change in response to experience. They are dramatically affected by repeated experience and the emotional environment in which one is raised. When raised in a nurturing environment, people show demonstrable, objective changes in gene expression; that is, there are genes for certain molecules that play an important role in regulating the emotions and that respond to nurturing (Davidson et al. 2000). This research shows that individuals brought up in a nurturing environment have a greater degree of ability to regulate their emotions.

The Cerebral Cortex   As biology has shown, the brain continued to develop with the addition of the cerebral cortex, also called the neocortex or forebrain (see **Figure 2.3**). The addition of a vast number of cortical cells allowed the development and storage of analytical skills, verbal communication, writing ability, fine motor control, additional emotion, memory, learning, and rational thought as well as more sophisticated problem-solving and survival abilities. New dimensions were added to oral and sexual behaviors, and vision replaced smell as the primary sense. Voluntary control of movement made reactions more than mere reflex responses. For better or worse, an individual's reality could be determined by his or her own perceptions. Behavior could be weighed against possible outcomes. Symbolism, goals, motivation, and anticipation became part of the functioning human being.

Even though the brain developed in three stages, its three areas do not function independently. Although the lower centers deal mainly with survival and the higher centers permit the existence of complex society, we cannot view the lower centers as primitive entities requiring control by the higher centers.

Recent study in neurophysiology (Goleman 2003) has found that the front medial portion of the left frontal lobe is more highly defined and/or more highly stimulated during times of happiness, joy, and contentment (more "positive" emotional states), whereas the opposite is true of the corresponding area of the right frontal lobe. That is, people feeling hostility, anger, fear, and so on, show higher activity in the latter area. Goleman (2003) notes that we probably have an emotional set point, a ratio between the right and left activity of these special areas in the frontal lobes, that gives background to our minute-to-minute emotions, hour-to-hour moods, and long-term temperament.

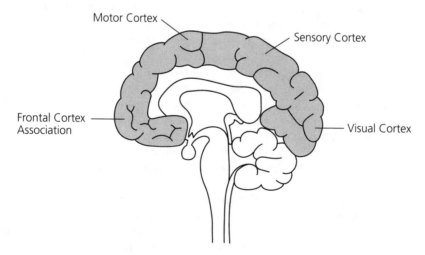

Figure 2.3 The Cerebral Cortex

Blood flow in these areas is closely regulated by emotional peptides, which signal receptors on blood vessel walls to constrict or dilate, and so influence the amount of nourishment to the cells. If emotions are blocked (e.g., due to denial or repression), blood flow can become constricted, depriving the frontal cortex of vital nourishment. This may be the basis for the refractory period that occurs between the time of a strong emotion and the time that we recover from the emotion. A strong emotion such as anger can leave you out of touch with reality and limited in your awareness, and thus can diminish your ability to intervene or make decisions that resolve the emotion. A long-term result may be that you become unable to respond to the world around you in a rational way, repeating old patterns of behavior and feelings that are responses to an outdated knowledge base (Ekman 2003).

By learning to bring awareness to past experiences and conditioning, functions of the frontal lobes, we can release ourselves from these old blocks.

It helps to understand the function of each of these specific nervous-system structures in order to understand stress and how to overcome it. At the same time, it is important to think of stress as the response of an integrated whole brain.

The Reward System   The reward system may help us to understand the drive to cope with our internal and external environments. Major reward areas are located at the limbic and hypothalamic levels and are involved with how easily we are aroused, our motivation, and our emotional memory.

Coping with adversity is an attempt to move our emotional, physical, mental, or spiritual being away from pain or toward pleasure and reward. CNS reward systems have developed over time, presumably to reinforce useful behaviors and extinguish harmful ones. In addition, these reward systems regulate the basic drives related to pleasure, pain, emotional comfort, sexual satisfaction, hunger, satiety, and thirst. If we learn to throw our reward systems off balance, we subsequently strive to bring them back into balance from a very deep subconscious level throughout the body up to an intentional conscious level in the brain.

The middle limbic area has a specialized area of intense reward, mediated by dopamine, the neurohormone that normally controls homeostasis. This area provides such intense reward that laboratory animals will stimulate themselves to death with intravenous psychomotor stimulants. Although scientific controversy exists as to whether there is one main reward pathway or many redundant pathways, it is accepted that the experiencing of pleasure most likely includes dopamine effects in the brain.

In recent years, the costs of cocaine, heroin, and other drug addictions (and the crime that accompanies them) have spurred research on the natural reward systems. It has been found that the body produces its own opiate-like substances (**endorphins**) to help alleviate pain and produce pleasure. Since then, receptors for nicotine, cocaine, marijuana, and other drugs have also been discovered. The relationship between drugs and stress management is not subtle—human beings seek pleasure and avoid pain. This is a driving principle of human behavior.

The Reticular Formation   The reticular formation is often referred to as the reticular activating system (RAS) or the ascending reticular activating system (ARAS). It is a network of nerve cells (or neurons) that extends from the spinal cord up through the thalamus.

The RAS itself is categorized as neither sensory (connected to the sense organs) nor motor (connected to the muscles), but it links sensory and motor impulses. It is a two-way street, carrying impulses from brain to body and from body to brain.

The RAS was discovered by Moruzzi and Magoun (1949), who noted that its nerve connections projected to the limbic system, the hypothalamus, the thalamus, and throughout the cortex in order to stimulate or alert the brain. The RAS receives information from all of the body's incoming nerves, filters this input, and then forwards to the brain only new or persistent information (Bloom, Lazerson, and Hofstadter 1995; Robinson 1996). When RAS centers in the pons area of the brain stem signal new stimuli, the message immediately heightens awareness both in the cortex and in the limbic-hypothalamic center, which integrates memory and houses reward or pleasure mechanisms. At the same time, neuropeptides may be carrying the message throughout the body. In the brain, perception is added to the stimuli, and we may consciously choose to either ignore or attend to the stimuli.

A unique feature of the messages that pass through the RAS is that they are general as well as specific. In hearing, for example, once a sound is perceived by the auditory mechanism, it sends both specific and general impulses through the appropriate parts of the RAS. The specific arousal alerts the brain for increased attention to the sound, while the alerting, or general, impulses cause a general arousal of the cortex. Even before the cortex appraises the potential threat of the sound, this general arousal stimulates the limbic system and the hypothalamus, which in turn prepare the body for potential action. Muscle tension and hormonal and metabolic action increase before the cortex identifies the source of the stimulus. These increases are sensed by, and further alert and arouse, the RAS. If action occurs, the arousal was purposeful, and the products of arousal are utilized. If the sound is never consciously appraised or if no action is pursued, the RAS has become aroused (stressed) for no reason, and the products of arousal must circulate until they can be reabsorbed or otherwise used up. **Figure 2.4** illustrates this process.

Of great importance in the study of stress and disease is the capacity of the RAS for reverberation (prolonged vibration) of an impulse, which will prolong a response. This means that the RAS can maintain a resting level of activity reflecting the general state of the other brain structures. A high level of resting activity increases and prolongs arousal, whereas a lower level of resting activity inhibits and shortens potential arousal. If you live a stressful life and find you are stressed many times during the day, the parts of your brain that become aroused to deal with that stress also affect the RAS, which adapts to frequent arousal by staying aroused. It is as though the RAS is saying, "Well, if you are going to be aroused so often, I might as well just stay aroused and save the time and energy of going up and down." The RAS also has the capacity to recruit impulses from other brain structures, and it will adapt to stimuli. Partly because of this ability to adapt, repeated situations cause less conscious stress than do novel experiences. For example, the noise of a city is less stressful for the permanent resident than it is for the visitor from a quieter environment.

The RAS is an essential part of the integrated limbic-hypothalamic-pituitary axis, which is responsible for an integrated physiological response to a life situation perceived as threatening. This response allows the organism to cope with the situation in a way that ensures its survival. However, when the response is chronically elicited, changes

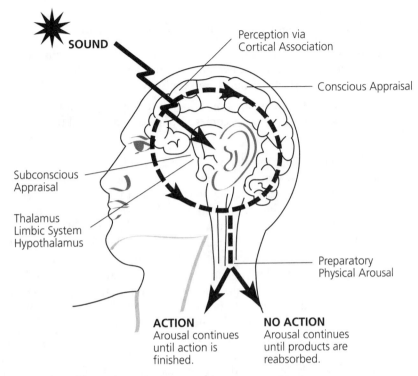

Figure 2.4 Specific and general arousal in response to stress

occur in the individual's normal physiological state. Under repeated stimulation (prolonged vibration) of the limbic-hypothalamic-pituitary axis, the transient elevations of activity become permanent. This phenomenon can be thought of as a hypersensitivity to stimulation or a lowered threshold for activation of emotional arousal. Gellhorn (1970) called it "tuning." With chronic stimulation, the level of tuning increases in the part of the sympathetic nervous system that involves activity; the increased tuning is thus described as work. Gellhorn noted that this sympathetic tuning serves as a nervous predisposition to stress arousal, anxiety, and related stress disorders such as were mentioned in Chapter 1.

As we have seen, however, the activity of body organs is controlled by the relative level of activity of the sympathetic and parasympathetic nervous systems (as well as by endocrine activity). Tuning may be thought of as a balance between these two parts of the nervous system. According to Gellhorn, tuning dominated by sympathetic stimulation is ergotropic tuning (meaning work or action related). As ergotropic activity or tone increases, a reciprocal decrease in tone in the opposing trophotropic system occurs, and vice versa. Increasing ergotropic tone through constant stimulation (thus decreasing the tone in the opposing trophotropic system) augments dysfunction and pathology in the enervated organ systems. Increasing the activity in the trophotropic system through relaxation training reduces the tone in the opposing ergotropic system. Thus, any relaxation activity, especially those involving skeletal muscles, can charge the trophotropic system and discharge the ergotropic tuning, providing protection against chronic arousal and significantly reducing anxiety and other conditions related to arousal.

> **Ergotropic tuning:** stress-response tuning governed by the sympathetic (fight-or-flight) nervous system. The nervous systems of a chronically irritable person or a dog trained to attack are tuned ergotropically.

> **Trophotropic tuning:** relaxation-response tuning governed by the parasympathetic nervous system. A person becomes trophotropically tuned through relaxation training.

John Weil (1974), another pioneer in the study of the neurophysiology of stress, elaborated on Gellhorn's tuning model by broadening the concept of sympathetic versus parasympathetic tuning. He wrote that aspects of both systems work in concert with various hypothalamic-limbic structures on the basis not so much of anatomical structure as of physiological activity that results in either arousal or tranquility. Weil suggested that the arousal system can be "charged" by high-intensity stimulation or by an increased rate of repeated low-intensity stimulation.

Once charged, the limbic-hypothalamic-reticular hub is capable of sustaining a high level of arousal through the discharge of impulses, providing general tonic activation. Gellhorn and Keily (1972), Benson (1992), and Weil (1974) suggest that decreases in proprioceptive input to the RAS and the limbic-hypothalamic-pituitary axis may be the underlying mechanism in relaxation training that charges or tunes the trophotropic system.

Pert (1999) also explains that when receptors are flooded with a particular ligand (neuropeptide), the cell membrane changes so that the probability of an electrical impulse crossing the membrane at the point is facilitated or inhibited, thus defining the bioelectric circuitry in that area. We become more easily stressed when we have this wiring.

Autonomic Control of the Stress Response

The autonomic nervous system ultimately controls how the body responds to new information. When the senses (sight, sound, touch, smell, and taste) and neuropeptides bring new information into the brain, the lower brain stem areas orchestrate an immediate low-level physical arousal. The conductor of this orchestration is the hypothalamus, which immediately prepares the body with the arousal response. Background theme is added by the limbic system, which lends a feeling of pleasure or unpleasure. The intensity of response depends on the tone that has been set by the firing of RAS neurons. The cortex then assesses the physical arousal and tone and either enhances or inhibits them with conscious thought, tapping both conscious and subconscious memories. If the new information triggers a feeling of threat or a need for increased sensitivity, the stress response is heightened; if it triggers a feeling of safety, the stress response is allowed to diminish.

The fight-or-flight response is by no means the only contributor to the stress response. Actually, many emotional situations can alter the body's function, and different emotions evoke different physical states. When we feel anger, we become flushed, excited, and full of energy. Wolf and Wolff first reported in 1947 that in anger situations, the mucous membranes of the nose and stomach redden, swell, and become congested to the point of hemorrhage. Often gastritis can be traced to this cause. Fear also has its own symptoms. When we are afraid, we tremble, our knees feel weak, and we often have difficulty speaking. Here, the mucous membranes of the nose and stomach become pale and shrunken.

It is difficult to generalize about how the nervous system affects stress-related disorders, for both stimulation and inhibition of the organ systems involved in the stress response can lead to body malfunction. Moreover, the nervous system both controls and is influenced by another major system that controls the stress response of the body— the endocrine system. It is particularly harmful when these two systems get caught in a positive-feedback cycle, with each exciting the other and thereby increasing the stress response initially. Prolonged exposure, however, may fatigue the system, resulting in system depression and eventual disease as is suspected in some diabetes (Chan et al. 2002).

The Endocrine System

The endocrine system consists of glands that secrete substances called hormones into the bloodstream. These various hormones influence virtually all bodily activities. The glands we are most concerned with in this section are the pituitary gland and the adrenal glands, although all the glands are involved to some extent in the stress response.

The amygdala, hippocampus, and frontal lobes of the brain are extensively connected with the endocrine system. When a stressful event occurs, cortisol is released. People who recover quickly from stress have lower baseline levels of cortisol. When cortisol is present at high levels over a long period of time, it may kill cells in the hippocampus. This is documented in posttraumatic stress disorder and severe depression (Goleman 2003).

The Pituitary: The Master Gland

The intimate relationship between the hypothalamus and the pituitary gland can be seen in Figure 2.1 . As various areas of the hypothalamus are stimulated, it in turn stimulates corresponding areas in the pituitary. Thus, thoughts, anticipations, and nervous-system responses can and do become hormonal actions. Some portions of the hypothalamus stimulate the parasympathetic nervous system and inhibit the stress response. Other areas of the hypothalamus activate the sympathetic nervous system and increase the stress response.

Hormone-releasing factors are produced in the hypothalamus and released into a local bloodstream to the anterior pituitary, which releases pituitary hormones into the bloodstream and to their target organs. This is an example of hormonal stimulation of the pituitary gland. The hypothalamus also executes nerve control over the pituitary through neurological connections between select nuclei in the hypothalamus and the posterior portion of the pituitary gland. The hypothalamic cells that produce hormone-releasing factors and the ones that stimulate neurological release of pituitary hormones are neurologically linked with the limbic system and the cortex. These links constitute a basic connection between our thoughts and emotions and the onset of psychosomatic disease (Rossi 1993).

The Adrenal Glands

Although all the endocrine glands may eventually become involved in the stress response, the adrenal glands are responsible for most of the physical manifestations of stress arousal, such as increased heart and respiration rates. There are two adrenal glands, one sitting over each kidney. The adrenal consists of two parts: an inner section called the medulla and an outer layer called the cortex (see **Figure 2.5** and **Table 2.2**).

The medulla responds to the hypothalamic messages that travel along sympathetic nerves extending into the medulla. When the hypothalamus is alerted, an impulse is sent to the adrenal medulla, and this area immediately releases the hormone epinephrine (commonly called adrenaline), which primarily affects the cardiovascular system. With the effects of this hormone, along with its close kin, norepinephrine (noradrenaline), and a third hormone, dopamine, the stress response is fully manifested throughout the body. As long as the control centers of the brain perceive the need for arousal, stimulation of the adrenal medulla continues. Prolonged stress can eventually fatigue the medulla.

The hypothalamus acts on the adrenal cortex not through nerve impulses but by means of a hormone secreted by the pituitary gland in response to a hypothalamic hormone-releasing factor. This hormone, adrenocorticotropic hormone (ACTH), circulates through the bloodstream to the adrenal cortex. Once the adrenal cortex is stimulated, it in turn secretes hormones into the blood that manifest the stress response in a number of ways. The two primary secretions of the adrenal cortex are **glucocorticoids** (primarily cortisol) and **mineralocorticoids** (primarily aldosterone). Cortisol affects metabolism (that is, the total body processes) by increasing the availability of energy (in the form of glucose, fatty acids, and amino acids), either for the stress response or for recovery from an extreme period of overactivity. It increases, as much as tenfold, a metabolic process of the liver called **gluconeogenesis**, through which the body forms glucose out of available glycogen and amino acids. This assures the body, especially the central nervous system, of an adequate supply of the most efficient energy source (blood glucose) for use during this period of heightened need. Furthermore, during gluconeogenesis, cortisol decreases the use of glucose by muscles and fatty tissue, probably by making the system insulin resistant, thus producing a mild diabetic effect.

During the stress response, cortisol mobilizes both fatty acids and proteins in the blood. The mobilization of protein reduces the stores of protein in all body cells (except

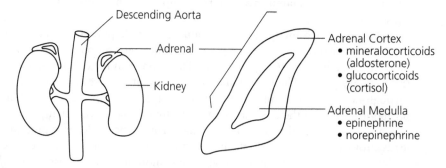

Figure 2.5 Adrenal Glands and Hormones

Table 2.2 The Endocrinology of the Stress Response

Endocrine Gland	Location	Hormones Released	Effects
Adrenal Medulla	The core of the adrenal glands, which lie atop the kidneys	Adrenaline (epinephrine)	Increased heart rate, increased force of heart contraction, increased muscle tension
		Noradrenaline (norepinephrine)	Increased vasoconstriction causing increased blood pressure
Adrenal Cortex	The covering of the adrenal glands	Cortisol	Increased fat mobilization, increased muscle wasting, immune suppression, increased serum cholesterol, increased blood glucose
		Aldosterone	Increased sodium retention, increased water retention causing increased blood pressure and potential irritability and moodiness
Thyroid	Neck	Thyroxin	Increased metabolism

in the liver and the gastrointestinal tract, which is where the mobilization takes place). Hence, if the stress response is maintained for a long period, the supply of protein available for the formation of mature white blood cells and antibodies diminishes to the point of disease susceptibility. In this way, prolonged stress can promote muscular wasting and impair the immune system.

When fatty acids are mobilized from adipose stores, they circulate through the bloodstream in order to be available as an energy source for muscle tissue. When fatty acids are actually used for physical resolution of the stress response, they present little health threat. However, high levels of fatty tissue in the blood appear to promote atherosclerosis (fatty plaquing of the arteries), especially when they are present over time. In this day of "pseudostressors" such as caffeine, nicotine, sedentary lifestyles, and nonassertive response to stress, the fatty acids called out during the stress response may circulate in the bloodstream for hours until they are taken up by the tissues and stored away for future use. There is some evidence that the body prefers to store fat near the liver, which processes it, and fat cells near the abdomen appear to be particularly sensitive to glococorticoids. Thus, people under chronic stress may tend to deposit more fat around their abdomen even when they are not particularly overweight. As we have mentioned many times, the body is an extremely efficient organism and will change its form and function to realize efficiency. In this case, it is to keep fat near where it is needed, and in general, it is to maintain arousal if that appears needed to solve ongoing threats, whether real or imagined.

Aldosterone is the other major adrenal cortex hormone secreted in increased amounts during the stress response. The body reacts to aldosterone by preparing itself for increased muscular activity and better dissipation of heat and waste products. It does this by retaining extra sodium (salt), which results in increased water retention. This leads to increases in blood volume, blood pressure, and the amount of blood the heart pumps out with each beat. As with other body systems, prolonged manifestation of the stress response can endanger the cardiovascular system.

SUMMARY

Stimuli (stressors) trigger a response by the body (stress). Understanding how the response occurs and which systems control arousal completes the picture and brings into focus the right choice of stress management activities. Consider the following points:

- The central nervous system and the endocrine system are both involved in controlling stress arousal.
- The central nervous system is divided into the autonomic and voluntary control system.
- The autonomic nervous system is more involved with stress than the voluntary system. It has two divisions: the sympathetic, which sets off the stress response; and the parasympathetic, which is more associated with normal and more relaxed functions.
- The stress response, often referred to as the fight-or-flight response, is a sympathetic nervous system function.
- All areas of the brain and nervous system are involved in the stress response; however, the limbic-hypothalamic complex, which controls emotions, is key.
- The reticular activating system (RAS) is also stimulated during the stress response and is responsible for heightened awareness, which provides the increased background arousal needed for the fight-or-flight response.
- The endocrine system, which is a series of glands secreting hormones, is essential, especially for the prolongation of the stress response.
- The adrenal glands are the primary endocrine glands involved in the stress response.
- The adrenal cortex, located on the outside of the adrenal gland, secretes cortisol, which controls stress metabolism, and aldosterone, which controls electrolyte balance (sodium and water retention).
- The inside of the adrenal gland, the medulla, secretes the neurohormones epinephrine (a.k.a. adrenaline) and norepinephrine (a.k.a. noradrenaline), which act primarily to stimulate the cardiovascular system.

SOURCES CITED

Benson, H. (1992). *The relaxation response.* New York: Avon.

Bloom, F., Lazerson, A., and Hofstadter, L. (1995). *Brain, mind, and behavior.* New York: W. H. Freeman.

Chan, O., Inouye, K., Vranic, M., and Matthews, S. G. (2002). Hyperactivation of the hypothalamic-pituitary-adrenocortical axis in streptozotocin-diabetes in associated with reduced stress responsiveness and decreased pituitary and adrenal sensitivity. *Endocrinology, 143,* no. 5, 1761–68.

Davidson, R. J., Jackson, D. C., and Kalin, N. H. (2000). Emotion, plasticity, context, and regulation: Perspectives from affective neuroscience. *Psychological Bulletin, 126,* no. 6, 890–906.

Ekman, P. (2003). *Gripped by emotion*. New York: Times Books/Henry Holt.

Eriksson, P. S., Perfilieva, E., Bjork-Eriksson, T., Alborn, A. M., Nordborg, C., Peterson, D. A., and Gage, F. H. (1998). Neurogenesis in the adult human hippocampus. *Nature Medicine, 4,* no. 11, 1313–17.

Ganong, W. (1995). *Review of medical physiology,* 14th ed. Los Altos, CA: Lange.

Gellhorn, E. (1970). The emotions and the ergotropic and trophotropic systems. *Psychologische Forschung, 34,* 48–94.

Gellhorn, E., and Keily, W. F. (1972). Mystical states of consciousness: Neurophysiological and clinical aspects. *Journal of Nervous and Mental Diseases, 154,* 399–405.

Glaser, R., and Kiecolt-Glaser, J. K., eds. (1994). *Handbook of human stress and immunity.* New York: Academic Press.

Goleman, D. (2003). *Destructive emotions.* New York: Bantam Books.

MacLean, P. D. (1949). Psychosomatic disease and the "visceral brain": Recent developments bearing on the Papez theory of emotion. *Psychosomatic Medicine, 11,* 338–53.

McEwen, B. S. 2000. Effects of adverse experiences for brain structure and function. *Biological Psychiatry,* 48, 721-31

Metcalfe, C., Davey Smith, G., Sterne, J. A., Heslop, P., Madeod, J., and Hart, C. L. (2005). Cause-specific hospital admission and mortality among working men: association with socioeconomic circumstances in childhood and adult life, and the mediating role of daily stress. *Europeans Journal of Public Health,* 15, 238–44.

Moruzzi, I., and Magoun, H. (1949). Brain stem reticular formation. *Electroencephalography and Clinical Neurophysiology,* 1, 455–73.

Pert, C. (1999). *Molecules of emotion: Why you feel the way you feel.* New York: Simon and Schuster.

Robinson, D. L. (1996). *Brain, mind, and behavior: A new perspective on human nature.* Westport, CT: Praeger.

Rossi, E. L. (1993). *The psychobiology of mind-body healing.* New York: W. W. Norton.

Weil, J. L. (1974). *A neurophysiological model of emotional and intentional behavior.* Springfield, IL: Charles C. Thomas.

Wolf, S., and Wolff, H. G. (1947). *Human gastric function,* 2nd ed. New York: Oxford University Press.

Stressed Person/Relaxed Person

PART 1

First, think about what it's like to be stressed or what someone else looks like when they're stressed. Then describe a stressed person in the categories below.

Next, think about what it's like to be relaxed or what someone else looks like when they're relaxed. Then describe a relaxed person in the categories below.

When Stressed	**When Relaxed**
Physical	Physical
Mental	Mental
Emotional	Emotional
Social	Social
Spiritual	Spiritual

PART 2 Optimal You

On the left-hand side of the page, describe the attributes you want for yourself from Part 1. In the other column, write what you would take as proof that you have these attributes.

Examples

Attributes	Proofs
Physical: I'd just like to generally slow down my pace instead of running from one place to the next.	I'd look and feel more "put together" when I get to class, lunch, or wherever I'm going.
Mental: I'd like to quit worrying all the time.	I'd wake up some morning and discover that I haven't spent all night worrying.
Emotional: I'd like to quit being so angry.	I'd have better friendships. People would probably like me better.
Spiritual: I'd like to be at one with myself.	I'd meditate every day.

Attributes	Proofs
Physical	
Mental	
Emotional	
Social	
Spiritual	

What do the attributes you have written down tell you about your life as you are living it now? Are you basically a stressed person, or are you basically a relaxed person?

Write a positive word or short phrase about using your recognition of the stressed state and the relaxed state that will be useful to you in future situations.

CHAPTER 3

The Body's Response to Stress

The Stress-Response Pathway

Stress follows a predictable route. A leads to B, and B leads to C. If A is stress, B is system dysfunction, and C is disease and premature death. This was known to the Greek philosopher Epictetus, who wrote that death was a "common consequence of chronic perturbation" and that anxiety was a disorder of the "will to get." He believed that it was better to die of hunger exempt from grief and fear than to live in affluence with perturbation. The exact path and mechanisms of this relationship between stress and premature death have been identified. This chapter discusses how the body's major systems respond to stress.

Although the central mechanisms for short-term arousal, as outlined in Chapter 2, are basically the same for everyone, each person reacts to prolonged stress arousal in different ways. Why some individuals respond to their stressors by developing back pain, others by becoming hypertensive, and others by exhibiting behavioral effects such as depression, withdrawal, or abuse of alcohol, drugs, or other people has been questioned since the inception of the study of stress. How a person "assigns" the stress response to a particular organ is called organ specificity. Franz Alexander (1965), one of the early pioneers in mind-body medicine, proposed that just as pathological microorganisms have a specific affinity for certain organs, so also do certain emotional conflicts afflict certain internal organs and behaviors. Bernie Siegel (1994) concluded that individuals suffering from stress-related disease sensitize specific organs of the body. Ernest Rossi and Milton Erickson (Rossi 1993) propose that the person who experiences stress reacts in an appropriate way to alleviate that original stressful situation. However, the individual then becomes conditioned to that mind-body response, so that even when the original stress is over, the body tends to continue to react in this newly learned way. Eventually the organ or system that is responding to prolonged stress arousal breaks down due to exhaustion, or, as we explain in Chapter 5, emotional patterns become conditioned and individuals tend to continue to react inappropriately long after the initial arousal.

Regardless of whose theory of organ specificity is "right," the points that are important to the discussion of stress-related disease include the following:

- Stressful events, situations, or experiences elicit the generalized stress arousal discussed in Chapter 2 and summarized in Table 2.1.

- The stressor is appraised immediately at the hypothalamic level, and the arousal response begins.

- Simultaneously, the hypothalamus alerts the limbic system and the higher cortical levels.

- Feeling tone is added by the limbic system and fed back to the lower centers of the brain, and in this manner the stress response may be prolonged. The cortex adds perception and conscious thought, further stimulating arousal.

- Depending on the emotional value (positive or negative) along with the conscious appraisal of the stressor, the appropriate systems of the body are asked to help solve the stressful problem.

- Upon solution of the problem or disappearance of the stressor, the trophotropic system attempts to return the system(s) to normal.

- RAS arousal may continue, increasing the reactivity tone of the central nervous system.

- If a person is often confronted with stressors causing central-nervous-system arousal, the system develops a higher resting nervous reactivity.

- Upon responding to the initial stressor, the body learns a response that, although appropriate at the time, may become inappropriate with prolonged arousal.

Prolonged duration of the stress response is the factor that causes the most harm. It is not so much the one-shot, generalized alarm reaction that brings about illness; it is the prolonged state of arousal, in response to which we somehow "choose" one or more systems to defend the body against stress. These systems become susceptible to all kinds of stressors and keep fighting until exhaustion. The resulting diseases and conditions might be called diseases of prolonged arousal. **Figure 3.1** illustrates the flow of stress arousal from the brain to the stress response.

Harold G. Wolff (1968), an early proponent of stress management, considered stress to be an internal or resisting force that is usually stirred to action by external situations or pressures that appear as threats—especially symbolic threats (i.e., threats involving values and goals). However, mobilizing our physical defenses (which were originally designed for battling physical threats) in response to symbolic (social or psychological) sources of threat produces an inappropriate response. To determine whether a response is appropriate, we must consider the outcome. Physical arousal to physical threat is appropriate: It usually is short lived and dissipates with action. Physical arousal to symbolic threat is problematic in at least two ways:

1. In our modern society, we can seldom resolve psychological threats to the ego with physical activity in order to resolve stress.

2. Symbolic threat tends to last longer because of emotional input and internal dialogue, and therefore is not as easily dissipated.

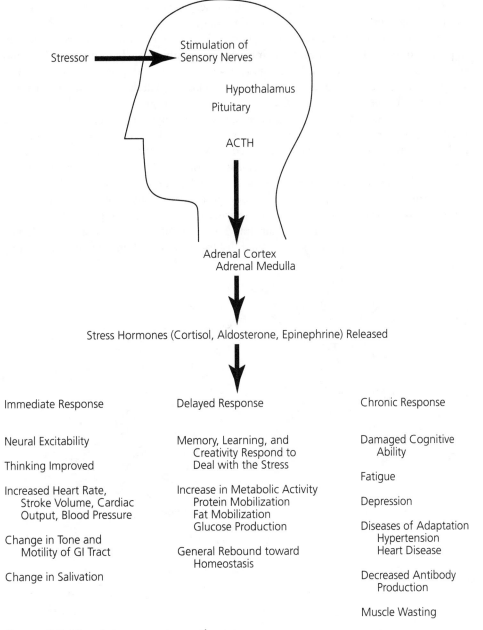

Figure 3.1 The stress-response pathway

When physical action is not warranted, it is not performed, but the stress reaction persists and becomes detrimental to the body.

Hans Selye, perhaps the most noted stress researcher of the twentieth century, contributed a concept that is fundamental to the understanding of stress-related disease. In 1926, as a second-year medical student, he first noted that patients suffering from a number of diverse diseases displayed a common set of symptoms. At the time, he called this the "syndrome of just being sick" (Selye 1974).

Selye took his interest in the "sick syndrome" into the laboratory, where he injected impure and toxic gland preparations into laboratory animals. Regardless of the gland tissue and hormones injected, the animals developed a stereotyped syndrome (a set of symptoms that occur at the same time). These symptoms included increased activity and enlargement of the adrenal cortex, atrophy of the thymus gland and lymph nodes, and development of ulcers in the gastrointestinal system. Selye soon found that this same syndrome occurred in response to other kinds of stress: heat, cold, trauma, infection, and many others. This syndrome identified by Selye became known as the biological stress syndrome or the general adaptation syndrome (GAS). The three stages of the GAS, (see **Figure 3.2**), are alarm, resistance, and exhaustion (Selye 1956).

Alarm is the initial response to a stressor. In the **alarm stage,** the body shows generalized stress arousal. This stage is characterized by widespread sympathetic discharge, increased ACTH secretion by the pituitary, and stimulation of the adrenal glands. Adrenal stimulation in turn assists in the full-blown fight-or-flight response. The body

1. Alarm Phase
Complex physiological response
Initiated by presence of stressors
Triggers release of adrenaline,
muscle tension, increased heart
rate and blood pressure

2. Resistance Phase
Body mobilizes to
combat stressor

3. Exhaustion Phase
Resources become depleted
Resistance breaks down
Disease or death may result

Figure 3.2 General adaptation syndrome

shows generalized stress arousal, but no specific organ system is affected, although most, and in some cases all, of the body systems show measurable changes.

The **resistance stage** is marked by the channeling of the arousal into one or several organ systems. This is the body's unique intelligence of directing the stress response into the specific organ system most capable of coping with the stressor. Dealing with the stressor is a complex phenomenon encompassing physical, mental, emotional, behavioral, and philosophical coping mechanisms. In addition to mustering the forces to deal with the stressor, the body begins to adapt to the stress arousal. This process may be thought of as bending a little so as not to remain rigid and break. However, this adaptation process contributes to stress-related illness. The specific organ system becomes aroused, and with prolonged arousal and chronic resistance it may fatigue and begin to malfunction. As the system deteriorates, problems specific to the system begin. For example, stress arousal in some parts of the nervous or cardiovascular systems can produce life-threatening debilitation in a short time.

The resistance stage becomes particularly troublesome when resistance goes beyond responding to the initial stressor. It is as though the body has learned a new mode of defensive adaptation and continues it until it becomes a disease or condition in itself.

Exhaustion occurs after prolonged stress because the organs and systems of resistance have been depleted of their energy to perform. During this final stage, the organ system or process involved in the repeated stress response breaks down. ACTH secretion increases, and the response takes on the generalized character of the alarm stage.

In the **exhaustion stage**, disease or malfunction of the organ system or even death may occur. Sometimes exhaustion of one weakened system will shift the resistance to a stronger system, forcing that system into the adaptation process. To illustrate the damage that can be caused by adaptation, let's consider hypertension as a response to stress. The body must react to the stressor, so it needs to pump more blood to the muscles. This is accomplished by increased blood pressure. The increased blood pressure sets off another set of alarms so the body can eventually normalize the pressure. If the stress is prolonged and increased blood pressure is part of the response, the body will adapt and shut off the alarm, thus decreasing its internal struggle of lowering the pressure. It learns to live with the elevated pressure—it adapts. The body can adapt to high blood pressure without constantly eliciting an alarm reaction, but the increased pressure promotes kidney and heart damage, which can eventually kill the individual if the situation is allowed to continue. Adaptation may be a lifesaving process, but it must also be recognized as a type of disease process. In fact, Selye often referred to stress-related symptoms as "diseases of adaptation."

What has intrigued researchers for years is that the stress symptoms can provide information about the nature of the stress. There are noticeable differences between anger and fear responses, for example. As outlined by Selye, there are two arousal paths that lead to physical symptoms. One pathway is that of abnormal physiological processes provoked by the failure of general coping abilities. The other is triggered by appraisals of specific threats, which may be channeled to specific organ systems for resolution. If resolution does not occur and the threat continues, a symptom of continued arousal of the specific organ will eventually become noticeable. A specific symptom is merely the specific locality in the body that has taken up the stress response. The brain is responsible for thinking and for emotional storage and retrieval, but it cannot move or act. Action belongs to the organs, especially the muscles. In a stressful situation, all emotional and thought processes occur in a directed attempt to resolve conflict. Organ systems are activated in an attempt to resolve stress arousal; however, coping strategies can misfire. Even when behavior or action is inhibited, the physiological aspect is expressed as getting ready (background action). Inhibited behavior can still leave a person excited. The physiological aspects of a blocked action can be continued or repeated because no appropriate cutoff signal is received. Throughout the day, each new stressful situation leaves a residual amount of tension in the body, the accumulation of which results in an inability to dissipate all the residual tension.

Individuals can remain in a phase of active coping or resistance almost indefinitely. Patients with stress-related symptoms show many signs of being in an active coping phase too long. In the muscle system, there is excessive muscular contraction as the individual prepares for a specific intentional response. Emotions, defined as "directed energy," are often the cause of prolonged muscle contraction. Emotional energy is intentional, meaning it is directed at resolution of the problem. Sometimes general arousal is used for resolution, and other times very specific mechanisms are targeted for coping with the emotional problem. For example, anger can result in generalized muscle contractions needed for a total body response to run away from danger, or anger may result in contraction of the hand muscles to make a fist to strike back.

As one might expect, understanding of stress symptoms varies with an individual's experience and beliefs. Some individuals make an instant connection between a particular symptom and their lifestyle and stressors. They intuitively understand the symptom and are ready to do something about it. They understand that they are responsible for their health, just as they are responsible for their economic well-being, their relationships, and their happiness. They are willing to be responsible for the positive and the negative behaviors and events in their lives.

The body is so hardy and programmed for survival that it takes months or years of stress arousal, incompetent coping, and unhealthy lifestyles to break down organ systems. If we choose to listen to these symptoms—the messages from the body—we may be able to prevent more serious conditions from developing. If we listen to the symptoms and make changes in our lifestyle, we can create good health. These conditions present an important learning component and they appear to be closely related to the stress, struggles, and coping endeavors of everyday life.

To Selye, stress was more than a response; it was a process that enabled the body to resist the stressor in the best possible way by enhancing the functioning of the organ system best able to respond to the stressor (Rosch 1997). Understanding the body's response can be the first step in mapping out a competent coping strategy.

The following sections describe how the body's major systems respond to stress.

The Muscles' Response

The muscles are our only means of expression. We cannot move toward pleasure or away from danger without muscle movements. Speech, facial expression, eye movements, and indeed every mode of expression, feeling, and resolution of an emotion are achieved through muscle movement. Yet the muscles are under the command of the will, awaiting orders and obligingly obeying them. Oddly enough, many of the orders are given subconsciously, are counterproductive, and contribute significantly to stress and tension. This is because chronically tense muscles complete a feedback loop and further stimulate the mind, resulting in increased stress, which appears as irritability and hostility. Chronically tense muscles also result in numerous stress-related disorders, including headache, backache, spasms of the esophagus and colon (the latter resulting in either diarrhea or constipation), posture problems, asthma, tightness in the throat and chest cavity, some eye problems, lockjaw, muscle tears and pulls, and perhaps rheumatoid arthritis.

It is important here to reemphasize the word **chronic**. Stress disorders are caused by chronic, long-term overactivity. Acute, even violent, muscle contractions are not as harmful to the body as are slight or moderate contractions sustained over a long period.

Muscles have only two states, contraction and relaxation—although varying degrees of contraction, called tension, occur. Relaxation occurs when there is an absence of muscle contraction or tension. In this sense, activities that we commonly call relaxation (as in the sentence "I am going to the movies to relax") are better termed recreation. Movies may be recreational, but seldom do they produce muscle relaxation.

A muscle is a mass of millions of cells that can shorten when stimulated by nerve impulses. This shortening moves bones, causes traction, and creates tension, but no work is done. This situation is referred to as muscle tension and is linked with the stress-related disorders previously mentioned. Pain develops when a partially contracted muscle closes a blood vessel, causing an inadequate amount of blood to be delivered to the tissues. Pain can also develop when a chronically shortened muscle exerts an abnormal pulling pressure on a joint, when a chronically shortened muscle is overexerted and its fibers thereby torn, or when the proper function of an organ is disrupted, which is the case in smooth-muscle disorders such as diarrhea, constipation, and esophageal spasms.

Even though muscles maintain their own resting level of contraction, purposeful movement is under the control of the central voluntary parts of the brain, primarily the cerebellum and motor cortex. The most specific and exacting control comes from the motor cortex, which contains specific areas corresponding to particular areas of the body, such as the finger area, leg area, and neck area. Stimulation of any of these areas of the brain results in the movement of muscles in the corresponding body area. When the brain finally decides on an action, impulses are directed from the motor cortex, and the muscle contracts.

Remember that muscle cells receive only two commands—contract or relax; this is the limit of their capabilities. A finely coordinated action involves an unbelievable number of contract and relax commands, the sequence of which must be learned, practiced, and stored in the memory. Even then, a coordinated movement is impossible without constant feedback about the result of the contraction. This feedback allows a person to instantly approve and refine the muscle action until the brain can accomplish the act without conscious control. A person has only to think, "Pick up the pencil," not figure out how to accomplish the act.

Let's now consider this in relation to stressful muscle tension. Imagine a potentially threatening situation in which you are contemplating some defensive action. You think defensively, you prepare to move, and you automatically assume a defensive posture. Whether you are correct in interpreting the situation as a threat is not important. What is important is that you have engrams (learned patterns) for this type of reaction, and they can be assumed without your consciously thinking about it. The muscle action for bracing, defensive posturing, or preparing for action can be completed even though your mind is not consciously considering such action. Thus you can see how hidden fears or anger can result in chronic stressful muscle tension. Stress in general and the especially the psychological factors have been extensively studied and show a significant relationship to muscle-related back pain (Hellsing and Bryngelsson 2000, Lee et al. 2005). Emotional distress and catasrophizing or imagining the worst case scenario was shown to be most related to the risk of back pain (Linton 2005).

Although anticipation is necessary for preparation, it has been found that muscle tension develops and remains until a task is completed or until the mind is diverted to a new thought process. Interestingly enough, successful completion of a task results in more rapid resolution of muscle tension than does failure to complete the task. Also, if you imagine a muscle movement or an action (for example, a defensive posture), you will experience the same preparatory muscle tension that occurs when you are actually engaging in the activity. This may explain why highly anxious people who are often in a high state of expectation frequently prove to have a great amount of muscle tension.

The muscle tension and movements described in the last few paragraphs are controlled by the motor cortex of the brain. Impulses from the motor cortex are normally carried to the muscles by the spinal cord and a cable of neurons called the **pyramid tract.** In addition, a pathway called the **extrapyramidal motor system** sends signals from the hypothalamus and upper limbic area to the muscles. Stimulation through this pathway causes a variety of unconscious postures and rhythmic movements. Like the reticular formation, discussed in Chapter 2, this system seems to be both specific and nonspecific. Nonspecific activation may result in **nonspecific tonus,** or increased general tension throughout the system. This hidden state of tension may last over time and can augment a "voluntary" bracing action or cause a muscular overreaction. Either stimulation results in chronic muscle tension, which can lead to illness. Of course, relaxation can replace tension if the inherent rhythm is dominated by a low-arousal, tranquil rhythm. Such is the purpose of the relaxation exercises and techniques given in later chapters.

The Gastrointestinal Response

When Hans Selye conducted his classic experiments on stressed laboratory animals, he found ulcerations of the stomach lining to be one of the responses. But why would the gastrointestinal (GI) system be involved? It serves no function in the fight-or-flight response and logically should not be controlled by the parts of the brain that anticipate or interpret possible threats. Nevertheless, GI disorders are responsible for filling more hospital beds in the country than any other disorders, and science has clearly established that many GI disorders have stress-response roots.

The gastrointestinal system (see **Figure 3.3**) is responsible for accepting food, mechanically breaking it down by churning it in the stomach, moving it through the intestines, and supplying enzymes that will finally convert small food particles into the blood sugar, simple fatty acids, or amino acids the body uses for energy or for building tissue. The GI system has an inherent rhythm and is governed by numerous automatic

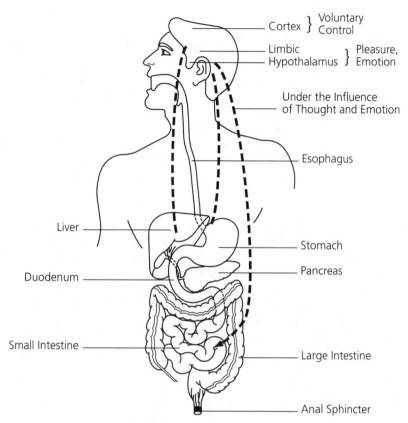

Figure 3.3 The gastrointestinal system

reflexes that control its movements, its emptying, and its secretion of enzymes. The GI system is also associated with the motivation system, in that hunger must lead to food-gathering behavior. The centers that control hunger and appetite are located in the hypothalamus and are closely related to pleasure and displeasure (see the discussion of the limbic system in Chapter 2). Hunger and satiety are definitely emotional states and, as such, affect the functioning of the GI system.

The GI system responds to emotional situations in a more complex manner than the typical sympathetic versus parasympathetic process described in the preceding chapter. Research over the last several decades has added greatly to our knowledge of the relationship between the gastrointestinal system and excess stress arousal. This greater understanding of the GI system dispels the stereotype that the sympathetic system arouses and the parasympathetic relaxes, for overstimulation of either of those two divisions of the autonomic nervous system can result in disease (Bhatia and Tandon 2005)

Response to stress arousal can be measured in every structure along the alimentary canal, starting with the mouth. Since Pavlov's classic studies, it has been clearly demonstrated that emotional states influence the flow of saliva. You may have had the experience of getting up before an audience to deliver a speech and finding your mouth dry.

This occurrence has long been used as a measure of fear: In ancient China, suspected criminals were made to chew rice, and the lack of a mucous wad was taken as an indication of guilt. On the other hand, seeing the dentist preparing to drill a tooth often turns on saliva to the point that the dentist must continuously vacuum it away.

The emotions can also induce spastic contraction of the muscles in the esophagus, which leads to the stomach. These contractions disrupt peristalsis (the rhythmic movement that carries food through the digestive system) and make swallowing difficult and in some situations impossible. The stomach, too, has been recognized as part of the emotional response system. Most anxiety tests take into consideration the state of the stomach. Statements such as "I have no appetite," "I have a gnawing feeling in the pit of my stomach," and "I feel nauseated" are the most often described physical symptoms of anxiety and emotional arousal.

Researchers have been able to observe the activity in the stomach lining. They have noted that in situations producing anger, resentment, or aggression, the lining increases its secretions of hydrochloric acid and various enzymes and becomes engorged with blood. The membrane eventually becomes so frail that eruptions occur spontaneously and ulcerations develop. Situations producing fright, depression, listlessness, and withdrawal produce the opposite reaction—the stomach lining functions below its normal level. But even that situation is not without problems: Decreasing the blood flow to the secreting glands reduces the natural protection of the area against certain harsh substances such as hydrochloric acid, which helps break down food in the stomach. Stress arousal has long been associated with the onset and exacerbation of stomach ulcers.

In the intestines, similar patterns have been observed. Stress arousal has been shown to alter peristaltic rhythm. This alteration in normal peristalsis in both the small and large intestines is responsible for two of the most classic stress responses: diarrhea, if movements are too fast and normal drying through water absorption does not take place; and constipation, if movement through the intestines is very slow and excessive drying occurs. Chronic constipation can lead to more severe intestinal blockage. Blockage of the bile and pancreatic ducts as well as inflammation of the pancreas (pancreatitis) has been linked with stress arousal, although little research has been conducted in this area. There is a long but inconsistent relationship between inflammatory bowel diseases and stress. Excess stress arousal is more implicated in exacerbating the conditions than in causing them. The exact mechanisms are not fully known, but there appears to be a relationship between the nervous, endocrine, and immune systems and stress-related dysfunction (Maunder 2005; Levenstein 2000; Hart and Kamm 2002). Pert's study of neuropeptides indicates that from top to bottom, the gut has receptors that respond to the various molecules of emotion (1999).

The Brain's Response

The brain was discussed as part of the control system in Chapter 2. Although the brain is the primary control organ, it is also part of the response to stress arousal, which illustrates the circular nature of the stress control-response mechanism. Brain arousal stimulates brain response, which is ultimately responsible for changes in behavior. Brain neurons constantly exchange ions (atoms that carry tiny electrical charges) across their cell membranes. This activity forms wave patterns, which can be followed through the use of an electroencephalograph (EEG). This instrument measures the frequency or rate of the wave pattern in cycles per second, or hertz (Hz). Unlike the muscles, which remain electrically inactive until they are stimulated into action, the cells of the brain emit a constant electrical rhythm.

The dominant, quiet rhythm of the brain has been designated the *alpha wave pattern*. It is characterized by a wave pattern that fluctuates at the rate of 8 to 13 cycles per second, and it emits energy that typically varies from 25 to 100 microvolts. An increase in the brain's activity changes this basic alpha rhythm, producing a wave pattern that is higher in frequency (13 to 50 cycles per second) but emits less energy. This faster wave pattern of lower voltage has been designated *beta*. Another common wave pattern, called *theta*, fluctuates at the rate of 4 to 7 cycles per second, and an even slower wave pattern, *delta*, fluctuates at fewer than 4 cycles per second and usually occurs only during sleep.

Analysis of complex brain-wave patterns has been used to diagnose abnormal brain states. More recently, the practice of referring to wave patterns to describe various activation states has become popular. The alpha wave has been associated with the absence of meaningful cause-and-effect thinking; this is a quiet state of mind in which stress arousal is at a minimum. The beta pattern is characterized by focusing attention, problem solving, and relating the self to the external world. Although this is not necessarily a stressful state, stress arousal is more possible in the beta state. Less is known about the mental state associated with the theta pattern, although researchers report that the thought patterns are directed internally and are less related to specific external events. Daydreams, fantasies, and what some researchers call "creative images" are more likely to occur during the theta state. More information on the brain wave and its associated mental states is presented in Chapters 13 and 16 on relaxation and meditation.

Apart from the more measurable physical responses of the brain to stress, psychological or mood responses occur as well. Besides the "hardwiring" of the brain (such as we see in axons, dendrites, and the synaptic activities between them) is the constant chemical exchange in the brain cells, especially in the nerve complexes, or nuclei. Receptors for endogenous mood changers (from endorphins and myriad other neuropeptides) are found in abundance in the pleasure–pain pathway from the hindbrain to the forebrain, in areas where the five senses bring their information to be shared, throughout the forebrain where ethical decisions must be made, even the supportive glial cells. Emotional states and moods are produced by the various neuropeptide ligands (Pert 1999).

During rest and relaxation, the brain is said to be in **homeostasis,** which means that the subjective moods of the individual are in harmony, promoting a healthful relationship between mind and body. During stress, the psychological mechanisms of the mind are thrown into turmoil. A "mood disturbance" is one common characteristic of the stress reaction. Stress commonly elicits confusion, fear, extreme emotional sensitivity, and feeling of ego threat.

The Cardiovascular Response

Not all diseases are stress related. However, in the case of cardiovascular disease, stress is highly implicated. The question is exactly how much of a contributor stress is in relation to the other risk factors. The indirect nature of stress and the long-term development of this chronic disease obscure the answer.

Diseases of the cardiovascular system (see **Figure 3.4**) include problems related to the heart itself (its basic structure and rhythm), to systemic blood flow and blood pressure, to the structure of the blood vessels, and to the makeup of the blood. It is obvious that each aspect cannot be considered separately from the others; they are all intricately related, and malfunction of one affects the others.

The heart's job is to pump blood to the body's cells. The blood contains oxygen and energy-producing substances that are the basic necessities for the life of the cell. To pump blood, the heart, a cavity surrounded by muscle, must contract. As the muscle contracts, the cavity becomes smaller. This increases the pressure of the blood within the chamber.

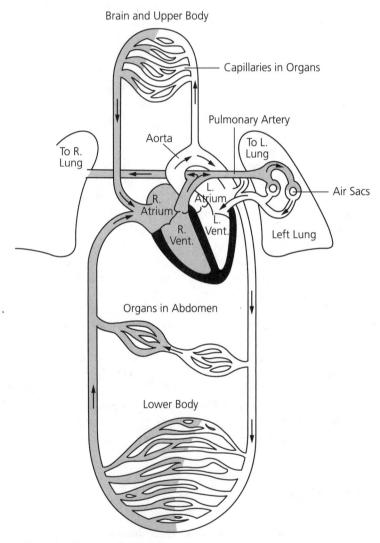

Figure 3.4 The Cardiovascular System

When the pressure in the cavity is greater than that outside it, the blood is ejected into the miles of blood vessels, arteries, and veins that travel to every part of the body. Each blood vessel contracts in a similar manner, thus helping to maintain the pressure and aid the movement of the blood traveling through the system. Once ejected, the blood is pushed along under pressure, which in the average adult male is about 120 millimeters of mercury (slightly less for females). When the heart completes its contraction phase, it relaxes, and the pressure in the system drops to about 80 mmHg in the average male (again, slightly less for females). These pressure indications (120/80) are used to express blood pressure, which is easily measured by a cufflike instrument called a *sphygmomanometer.*

It should be obvious that the fewer times a heart must contract or beat to accomplish the necessary supply functions, the more rest it will get. The heart has an inherent rhythm that is determined by the membrane potential of a special area in the right atrium called the *pacemaker.* Even when the heart is denied nervous stimulation, it is capable of independent action; however, the heart is constantly receiving impulses from the brain, and its inherent rhythm is continually influenced by the central nervous system. The heart receives impulses from both the sympathetic and parasympathetic nervous systems (see Chapter 2). Thus, it is under moment-to-moment control by various centers of the brain that are in touch with the body's metabolic and physiological demands. In addition to neural regulation, the heart can also be influenced by the hormone epinephrine, which can increase the contractibility of the heart muscle (the *myocardium*), increasing the speed and strength of the contraction.

Research evidence suggests that chronic stress is implicated in enhanced cardiovascular reactivity, elevations in stress-related hormones, and depressed immune function. Uchino and colleagues (1992) studied older subjects who were long-term caregivers for Alzheimer's disease patients and found that the chronic stress of caregiving increased cardiovascular reactivity. (See also Baum, Cohen, and Hall 1993.) Caregivers had a substantially greater incidence of depressive disorders than matched control subjects, and the caregivers were also found to have poorer immune function than controls. Chronic stressors seemed to produce longer-term autonomic, immune, and endocrine alterations. It has been known for some time that prolonged stress increases glucocorticoids, especially cortisol as discussed in Chapter 2, and one effect is to suppress testosterone levels in males (Filaire et al. 2001). More recent study has linked what is termed the cortisol-testosterone ratio to increases in ischemic heart disease (Davey-Smith et al. 2005)

A significant survival mechanism of the cardiovascular system is that the heart is capable of anticipating physiological and metabolic demands by increasing its action before it actually has to. As we have seen, however, the anticipation of such demands very often increases the activity of the system, but then the final action is thwarted by the conscious cortex. In this case, the cardiovascular response is to no avail. Similarly, many psychological states increase cardiovascular activity when no action is actually required. A new or unusual experience frequently elevates the heart rate, as do fear, anger, anxiety, and most situations that threaten the ego. You may recall Harold Wolff's definition of stress as a physical response to a psychological or symbolic threat that is inappropriate in kind and intensity in our complex society. These stressors are usually symbolic, requiring no physical action. The response, nevertheless, is physical. Thus, a chronically stressed person often has a chronically overworked heart.

Another cardiovascular problem related to stress is chronically elevated blood pressure, or **hypertension.** It has been estimated that perhaps 15 to 20 percent of the adult population suffers from hypertension, usually considered to be a pressure above 160/95. Approximately 90 percent of the cases are called *essential hypertension,* meaning the origin is unknown. Because the primary work of the heart is to overcome the pressure in the arteries through which the blood must flow, high blood pressure greatly increases the work of the heart and contributes to cardiovascular problems.

Like the heart, the blood vessels have an inherent tone that can be altered moment to moment by both parts of the autonomic nervous system and by hormones (epinephrine and norepinephrine) to reflect the physiological demands placed on the system. Anticipation and psychological states such as fear, anger, and anxiety will alter the diameter of blood vessels, producing a physical response to symbolic or imagined threats.

A third problem concerning the cardiovascular system is **atherosclerosis,** the destruction of the vessels by the infusion of fatty plaques, which contain cholesterol, triglycerides, and other fatty elements. The relationship between stress and vascular problems appears to be that during stress arousal, the hormones epinephrine and cortisol mobilize fats and cholesterol for use by the muscles, and the fats and cholesterol circulate in the bloodstream until they are used or reabsorbed. (The process was described in Chapter 2). Although there are many factors in the development of atherosclerosis, constantly saturating the system with unneeded fats through the stress mechanism can only exacerbate the problem. Research has shown that a complex interplay between the neuroendocrine, the inflammatory system, and hemostatic mechanisms including blood platelets and blood cell fragments may be the link between stress and coronary risk (Nijm et al. 2005). An artery infused with such plaques will eventually lose elasticity and harden, producing **arteriosclerosis** (an advanced form of atherosclerosis). This disease is directly responsible for more than half a million deaths annually in the United States.

When an artery in an advanced state of disease loses its elasticity, it elevates the blood pressure, thus contributing to hypertension and disease of the heart itself. In addition, atherosclerotic plaques, by narrowing the diameter of the blood vessels, diminish oxygen delivery and may bring on a *myocardial infarction,* or heart attack, if the coronary arteries are affected. Many factors contribute to the development of atherosclerosis and hypertension, including a diet high in cholesterol and saturated fats, which add to the amount of potential fatty deposits in the blood vessels; lack of exercise; smoking, which mimics sympathetic nervous system stimulation, narrowing the blood vessels and increasing the heartbeat; obesity; sex (males are more at risk); age; heredity; and, of course, stress, which underlies many of the others. That being said it should also be said that historically most research has been done on males. Most recent research indicates that females have the same adverse effects to stress as males and the same cardiovascular risks (Buchner et al. 2005).

Another vascular problem associated with stress is the vascular headache, also known as the migraine headache. Migraines are thought to be caused by an exaggerated constriction of blood vessels in and around the brain. This constriction is followed by a reflex dilation or enlarging of those vessels, which causes the release of toxic chemicals that irritates local nerve endings and adds to the pain. The root of this type of attack is complex and appears to involve, in a headache-prone individual, a psychogenic trigger of the sympathetic nervous system, which then causes the initial constriction of the blood vessels. This phase, known as the prodromal phase, is characterized by nausea, increased irritability, and an unusual sensitivity to noise and light. Physiologically, this phase seems to deplete the level of the hormone serotonin in the system. It may be the loss of this hormone that causes the reflex dilation of the vessels and the accompanying intense pain. Little is known of the underlying cause of migraine. The migraine-prone individual may have abnormal metabolism of serotonin or may be deficient in an enzyme that oxidizes this hormone. Recent clinical investigations have shown that certain types of migraine headaches can be alleviated by controlling the central nervous system through elaborate relaxation training. This points not to the alleviation of any chemical imbalance but to control over the initial psychogenic trigger.

The Skin's Response

It is sometimes difficult to think of the skin as a separate system capable of responding to stress arousal, but its complex function and intricate nervous control make it a sensitive response system, and its accessibility makes it a convenient window into the body. When you observe the stress response of any body system, you are looking through that system into the mental activity responsible for the response.

The skin has two basic response patterns that show the world what is going on in the body and in the mind. One is often referred to as electrical language because it seems to speak if you have the proper listening device. Each of the millions of cells that constitute the skin system contains chemicals that have an electrical nature. As the body expresses itself, the chemical activity of the skin cells changes, producing different patterns of electrical activity. This electrical activity can be measured on the skin surface. The constant but ever-changing activity of the skin appears as "chatter," and although complex and sometimes difficult to interpret, it is used by police authorities in most lie-detector systems and by health professionals to help understand an individual's emotions, motivations, and problem-solving techniques.

The second basic response system of the skin is its temperature. Under the skin are small blood vessels that change in response to emotion. During tense, anxious periods they shut down and allow less blood to pass, causing the skin to appear pale and the skin temperature to decrease. At other times, the blood vessels open and allow the skin to flush with blood, thus increasing the skin temperature. Determiners of blood flow in the skin include the neuropeptides.

With this type of response pattern, it is not hard to visualize how prolonged emotional responses could change the activity of the skin long enough to result in malfunction and disease. Certain skin conditions or illnesses have been found to have roots in our psychological response patterns. For example, eczema, a skin lesion characterized by redness, swelling, itching, and fluid discharge, has been associated with emotional stimulation. The reddening and itching are indicative of abnormal blood flow to the area, while the fluid discharge is indicative of an increased rate of fluid production by the skin cells. Laboratory studies have established that in eczema-prone individuals, emotional arousal increases the amount of fluid exuded by the skin cells, whereas relaxation diminishes it. Eczema patients have been classified as being restless, impatient, and unduly irritable, but the relationship of these characteristics to the skin condition has not been clearly established. Similar preliminary work has been done with patients suffering from urticaria (hives), psoriasis, and acne, but these investigations are still in their infancy.

Structure and Function of the Immune System

The frontal lobes, the amygdala, and the hippocampus are all extensively connected with the body, in particular with the immune system. People who recover more rapidly from stress have better immune system function. They have higher levels of natural killer cells, a defense that the immune system uses to fight off foreign antigens from cancer to the common cold (Goleman 2003).

The immune system (see **Figure 3.5**) provides natural and acquired defense against foreign elements that enter the body through the air we breathe, the food we eat, or in other ways. The immunity we are born with, **innate immunity,** is provided by the skin, the acidic secretions of the stomach, mobile white blood cells, and other natural body structures and biochemicals that defend against all invaders in a nonspecific manner. Also, we develop what is called **acquired immunity.** This is a process whereby the body recognizes foreign agents called **antigens** (bacteria, toxins, and viruses) and responds to each by producing antibodies specific to it. Two lines of acquired immunity defense, *humoral* and *cellular,* are very important to our discussion of stress and psychosomatic disease. Both originate in the bone marrow, where undifferentiated stem cells are produced (see **Figure 3.6**).

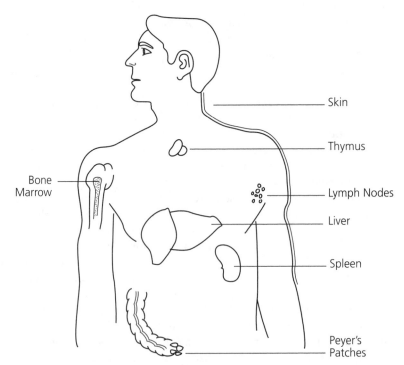

Figure 3.5 Major centers of immune system tissue

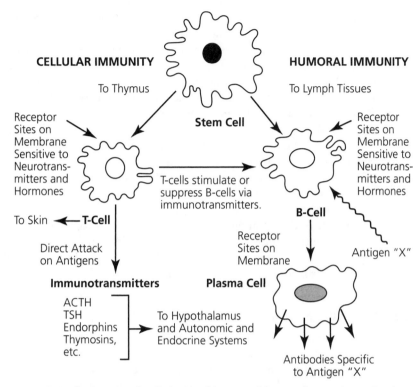

Figure 3.6 Development of cellular and humoral immunity and production of immunotransmitters

In humoral immunity, the stem cells migrate from the bone marrow to the various lymphatic tissues throughout the body, where they mature into white blood cells called *beta-cell lymphocytes* (B-cells). When an antigen enters the body and is taken up by the bloodstream, it is detected by the B-cells as the blood is filtered through the lymph nodes, spleen, and so on. The antigen stimulates the B-cells to evolve into plasma cells that then synthesize specific antibodies that attack the invading antigen. Figure 3.6 depicts this process.

The development of cellular immunity is similar to that of humoral immunity, except that the stem cells of the bone marrow travel to the thymus gland, where they mature into *T-cell lymphocytes* (T-cells) that attack invading antigens directly. Some of these T-cells travel to the skin to make the entire surface of the body part of the immune system (Glaser and Kiecolt-Glaser 1994). It is important to the discussion of stress and disease to note that T-cells and B-cells have receptor sites that respond to neurotransmitter substances of the autonomic nervous system, to hormones of the endocrine system, and to other informational substances that keep the whole body's communication network up to speed. This means that the immune system can influence and be influenced by the control systems discussed in Chapter 2.

In the 1960s, immunology came of age as a science, and it is now one of the most exciting branches of research into illness and disease, especially pertaining to AIDS,

SARS, and other developing diseases. For years, immunologists were so busy discovering the complexity of the immune system itself that they paid little attention to its communication with the other systems of the body. More recently, however, research in psychoneuroimmunology (PNI) has begun uncovering the physiological mechanisms that control the intimate communication among the nervous, endocrine, and immune systems. It is this research that gives us the missing link between how our thoughts and emotions influence our health and disease states.

Immunological research has found that neurotransmitters (such as epinephrine and norepinephrine) can attach to immune cells and change their ability to multiply and destroy invading agents. Furthermore, research has identified the "hard-wiring" system of nerve fibers that transmit messages between the brain and lymphocytes that fight infection and cancer in the body (Pert 1999).

In addition to immune-cell response to neurotransmitters and hormones of the endocrine system, the immune system apparently talks to the other control systems through immunotransmitters such as ACTH, thyroid-stimulating hormones, and other polypeptides such as the endorphins and thymosins. T-cells also have the ability to stimulate or suppress B-cells.

Stress and the Immune System

Our current knowledge of the coherent mechanisms of communication among the nervous, immune, and endocrine systems is altering the old medical belief that thoughts and emotions had nothing to do with disease. The medical findings of world-renowned physicians and researchers such as O. Carl Simonton, Stephanie Matthews-Simonton, Bernie S. Siegel, Joan Borysenko, and Norman Shealy, to name a few, have led to widespread recognition that thoughts, emotions, attitudes, and beliefs have a great bearing on health, disease, and the ability to rebound from illness (Borysenko 1999; Borysenko and Dveirin 2005; Davidson et al. 2003; Matthews-Simonton et al. 1992; Myss and Shealy 2002; Siegel 1994; Simonton 1994). Candace Pert might be called the "mother of emotional research" with her groundbreaking study of the neuropeptides published in her book, *The Molecules of Emotion* (Pert 1999). Her continued work gives us insight into what's going on at the subconscious level to harm or heal us (Pert 2004, 2006).

The immune system may become dysfunctional and lead to stress-related illnesses in basically three ways: (1) underactivity, (2) hyperactivity, and (3) misguided activity (Rossi and Cheek 1994). Characteristic diseases caused by these three types of dysfunction are, respectively, cancer, asthma, and rheumatoid arthritis. Underactivity or depression of the immune system occurs in response to stress-induced release of adrenal cortex hormones. Various researchers (Cohen et al. 2003; Gomez-Merino et al. 2005; Smith and Nicholson 2001) have found that even slight depression of the immune system greatly increases susceptibility to pathogens. The hyperactive immune response seen in asthma involves a highly irritable mucosal lining of the lungs. When the lining is irritated, the resulting hyperimmune response can cause symptoms ranging from mild discomfort to respiratory failure. Autoimmune diseases are examples of a misguided immune system that attacks its own tissues as well as those of invading antigens. Autoimmune disorders are often associated with immune-deficiency syndromes, injuries, aging, and malignancies

(Rossi 1993). It appears that breakdown in communication within the nervous, endocrine, and immune systems through neurotransmitters, endocrine hormones, and immunotransmitters is basic to all immune dysfunctions (Padgett 2003).

Studies in which volunteers were exposed to pathogens such as cold viruses provide direct evidence that stress modulates the speed and potency of immunological defenses. For example, to study the effects of academic stress on immune response, Glaser and colleagues (1992) gave a series of hepatitis B inoculations to forty-eight second-year medical students on the last day of a three-day exam series. Students who were less stressed, less anxious, and who reported greater social support demonstrated a stronger immune response. Conversely, Liu and colleagues (2002) found that school examinations enhance airway inflammation to antigen challenge. In both cases, the stress of school exams can diminish the immune response, and stress management techniques can help to strengthen the immune system.

If stress arousal is prolonged, any or all of the biochemicals, organs, and systems involved will be affected until fatigue occurs. At that point, infections, common colds, and slight skin conditions appear. As the fatigue continues, the conditions worsen and more serious illnesses develop. When the immune response to disease elements is diminished by 50–60 percent, the body may respond with persistent and repeated infections requiring antibiotics, with summer colds, with serious skin-disease inflammation, and with chronic respiratory conditions such as bronchitis, asthma, or tuberculosis. Immune-system fatigue diminishes the body's ability to resist all invading viruses, bacteria, and toxins.

The Prevention and Treatment of Diseases of Arousal

The first section of this chapter outlined the stress response pathway or how stress generally manifests itself in the body. The second section briefly further looked into how each system of the body is affected and how disease may result. Stress management is not intended to treat disease, but to reduce the stress that research continues to show is a significant factor in the development and exacerbation of certain diseases. That being said, if stress does exacerbate the disease it stands to reason reducing the stress may in fact help the treatment regime. In addition, some of the standard stress management techniques used in the prevention of stress are likewise used in various treatments. This section takes a look at some of those techniques and the philosophy behind the use and concludes with a look at the power of the mind in making "stress wise" choices and the wisdom of listening to our bodies for messages of health and illness.

Hans Selye formulated the concept of mind-body diseases of adaptation many years ago (Selye 1974). He suggested that medication could be given to counteract stress hormones that ravage the system or that the adrenal glands could be removed surgically. Seyle also noted that if a nonspecific shock could cause these conditions (which he characterized as "getting stuck in a groove"), perhaps various forms of nonspecific shock therapy could counteract the conditions. Nevertheless the traditional medical system continues to be perplexed by the potential for the concept in the prevention and treatment of disease. However, as more evidence is discovered about the mind-body connection in the genesis of disease, there is growing acceptance in the medical community of the addition of more holistic practices in the fight against mind-body disease.

One of the most highly researched diseases is cancer. The etiology of cancer is complex and the theories of causation and success in treatment are varied. Psychological aspects of stress are thought by some to be involved and to others there appears to be little relationship. Cancer may serve as an example of how holistic modalities based on mind-body theory may facilitate healing. A major line of evidence both classic and more recent shows a mind-body connection with various cancers and the stress of life change (Dohrenwend and Dohrenwend 1974; Golden-Kreutz et al. 2005; Meador 1992; Kroneke et al. 2004; Nielsen et al. 2005, Ollonen et al. 2005). It appears that any form of trauma involving a significant life change can activate the cortical-hypothalamic-pituitary-adrenal response, producing the adrenal cortical hormones that suppress the immune cells that continually search out and destroy cancer cells in the system. In addition, a negative self-concept, depression, and anxiety are all associated with immune-system suppression or under activity. Coping ability is also a significant factor in whether stress will have an immunodepressant effect (Poikolainen, Kinerva, and Lonnquist 1995).

A research study to show the influence of behavioral intervention on cancer development or progression involved health education, enhancement of problem-solving skills regarding diagnosis, stress management techniques, and psychological support for stage I or II malignant melanoma patients (Fawzy et al. 1993). Intervention patients who were seen in groups of seven to ten for ninety minutes every week for six weeks exhibited reduced psychological distress and more significant immunological changes than the control group. The intervention group showed significant increases in the percentage of natural killer cells, as well as increased natural killer cell activity. A six-year follow-up of these patients showed a trend toward greater recurrence and a statistically significant higher mortality rate in control patients than in the intervention group patients. Similar results were found in the progression and regression of cervical cancer (Tiresma et al. 2005)

Data suggest that psychological and behavioral outcomes for women with gynecologic, breast, and colorectal cancers and men with digestive tumors, prostate, and bladder cancers can be improved with psychological interventions, and it is likely that even greater gains could be achieved if more health behavior components were added (Anderson 1994). To address the stress component of this disease directly, prevention of prolonged stress arousal is the first line of defense. Prevention can take the form of learning to avoid stressful situations, restructuring or reframing events previously thought of as stressful (through assertiveness training, realistic setting and attaining of interpersonal and professional goals, and so on), and learning to reduce the arousal tone of the central nervous system through meditation or other quieting activities.

If disease has become apparent, these preventive measures are also used in treatment (Siegel 1994). In addition, active intervention in the form of imagery has been found helpful in some cases of cancer. The reasoning behind the use of imagery in fighting disease is that mind modulation of body processes is considered to be a psychoneurophysiological fact; if the mind can contribute to the sickness, it can also contribute to getting well. Matthews-Simonton and colleagues (1992) and Simonton (1994) have successfully used imagery and the technique of cognitive reframing to treat cancer and found that their methods seem to enhance cellular immunity. Whereas such therapists and researchers as Matthews-Simonton, Simonton, and Creighton have found the use of active imagery to be successful, others such as Siegel (1994) and Benson (1999) have approached prevention and treatment through quieting the mind. Herbert Benson's "relaxation response" was designed to bring about an inner stillness of central origin (Benson 1992). The combination of imagery and some form of meditation is used by most current practitioners of psychosomatic medicine (Rossi and Cheek 1994).

Mind-Body Unity

Whether the psychosomatic approach to treating diseases like cancer has potential will be determined sometime in the future. For now it remains a very minor part of the treatment regimen. Potential progress has been slowed by our view of medicine that sees the body and the mind as separate entities. Perhaps ultimate success will accompany changes in our approach to mind-body unity or disunity that we know profoundly affects our health.

Physically, there are only minute differences between modern man and the caveman. We have the same central nervous and endocrine systems—that is, the brain, nerves, and hormones—that allowed our ancestors to meet physical emergencies. What has changed is the extent to which the conscious mind has taken control of the body and the extent to which our total being has been transformed into ego consciousness, that is, into logical, rational thinking that protects and preserves the psychological/emotional self. In other words, there has been an emphasis of personality or ego and a deemphasis of our physical aspects.

The ancient Greek and Far Eastern philosophies did not separate mind from body, and did not even recognize differences between physical matter and spirit, or between the inanimate and the animate. Gradually there was a change from the mind-body unity philosophy (known as holism or monism) to a separation of mind and body (dualism). With the dualistic philosophy of Descartes in the seventeenth century, the world further identified with the mind rather than with a complete mind-body organism. Man was considered an ego being carried around inside a machinelike body, which was ruled and used by the mind. "Lower" animals were seen not as being similar to humans though functioning on a different plane, but rather as inferior life. Indeed, nature itself was treated as inferior as the natural environment became a resource or commodity to be used by humans.

The philosophy of Descartes compartmentalized life into specialties—science, religion, philosophy, politics, and medicine—with each segment of society being governed by specialists. Man was either philosopher or scientist or politician or physician. No one could be all, even though those activities related to each individual's expertise. Even the care of one's personal health was left to others.

As the balance between the mind and body gradually shifted in favor of mind dominance, the products of the mind (technology) advanced, often unchecked. We have now become so dependent on machines, external expertise, and a gigantic bureaucracy to run our complex society that most of our activities seem to be various forms of endless technological education whereby we attempt to learn to use our resources most efficiently.

The increased birthrate and the growth of urban areas have resulted in overpopulation, noise, air and water pollution, job dislocation, and decreased individual privacy and self-reliance. As a result of improved methods of communication and transportation, we have been driven to accomplish more in less time. Trying to keep pace with our technological advancements has drastically affected our value systems: basic values that once took generations, even centuries, to change are now in a constant state of flux. For example, family structure, religion, education, work, communication, and sexual identity are now constantly changing, some for the good of human growth, some not so good. Most important to the basic concept of this book is change itself, because it epitomizes psychological pressure.

Coping with change has become a preoccupation in our society. The coping styles in turn have become mind games. Thus we have developed a vicious cycle: Increased thoughts lead to stress arousal, and the conceiving of ways to reduce stress just adds to the arousal. The harder we try to reduce stress, the more stress we subject ourselves to, so we try even harder. In our efforts to think our way out of this dilemma, we have created a condition in which our most important channel to the basic natural truths (our bodies) has been demoted to a second-class status. We do not act as we feel; we act as we think we ought to feel, or as we would like to feel, or as others expect us to feel. We do not listen to the subtle messages of our bodies; we can now only hear the cacophony of major illness. Stress management tries to teach us that we cannot totally subdue the innate stress response that we share with the caveman. That vestige of our physical past is ever present to remind us that we cannot totally "civilize" this natural creation. It reminds us we cannot conquer nature; we are nature. The denial of this naturalness pits mind against body, a needless battle that has no winner.

One does not have to "go back to nature" to be more natural. All one must do is stop gratifying the mind at the expense of the body. We have tuned our ear to the message of the mind; now we must do the same and listen to the message of the body. However, it is difficult to hear over the din of the engine; and even in quiet, it is impossible to hear over the constant chatter of the mind. The inner life of the body cannot be controlled, only encouraged. That was the opinion of the ancient scholars and it still is the opinion of current scholars (Sands 2002).

Distress and tranquility are opposites. When distressed, the mind is bombarded with stimulation of thoughts, plans, schemes, worries, constant reenactment of an event, or mental preparation for it. Tranquility is quiet, it's peace, and it's somewhat of a void that can be filled with a sense of feeling the self. You cannot act or create if you are reacting. You cannot "feel" your body when your body is feeling the pain of stress. Your spirit cannot be free as long as it is burdened with worry.

The fantastic proliferation of knowledge in recent centuries has not led to new enlightenment. Humans have not become wiser, we are not significantly happier, and in many respects we are less healthy. But happiness is relative and can to a degree be conditioned; health, on the other hand, is more absolute and thus becomes a concrete focus of our attempts to regain our balance.

We will further explore mind-body unity throughout this book, as it becomes the central tenet in understanding of the nature of health and disease and is the primary building block in developing a stress management program.

SUMMARY

The stress response begins the moment you are exposed to a stressor, whether it be physical (such as an attack), psychosocial (such as an insult), or a sympathomimetric stressor (such as caffeine or nicotine). The stress response begins immediately, often before the threat is realized. If the stressor is appraised as threatening, an increased response is evoked. This response is a hypermetabolic response set off by stress hormones released from the brain and endocrine system. These cause an increase in heart and respiratory rates; an increase in blood pressure; the mobilization of fat, blood glucose, and cholesterol; immune suppression; and sodium and water retention. Consider the following points:

- The stressor is appraised immediately at the hypothalamic level and the arousal response begins. Simultaneously, the hypothalamus alerts the limbic system and the higher cortical levels.
- Feeling tone is added by the limbic system and fed back to the lower centers of the brain, and in this manner the stress response may be prolonged. The cortex adds perception and conscious thought, further stimulating arousal.
- Depending on the emotional value (positive or negative) along with the conscious appraisal of the stressor, the appropriate systems of the body are asked to help solve the stressful problem.
- Symbolic threat tends to last longer because of emotional input and internal dialogue, and therefore is not as easily dissipated.
- When physical action is not warranted, it is not performed, but the stress reaction persists and becomes detrimental to the body.
- Upon solution of the problem or disappearance of the stressor, the trophotropic system attempts to get the system(s) back to normal.
- Alarm is the initial response to a stressor. In the alarm stage, the body shows generalized stress arousal. This stage is characterized by widespread sympathetic discharge, increased ACTH secretion by the pituitary, and stimulation of the adrenal glands.
- The resistance stage of the GAS is marked by the channeling of arousal into one or several organ systems.
- Exhaustion occurs after prolonged stress because the organs and systems of resistance have been depleted of their energy to perform.
- A prolonged high level of stress will cause chronic muscle tension, leading to numerous musculoskeletal disorders.
- Stress arousal affects the gastrointestinal system by situationally causing greater saliva flow or dry mouth, increased or decreased stomach secretions, and changes in gastric motility.

- Effects of stress on the cardiovascular system are hypertension, placquing of the vessels, and changes in heart rhythm.

- Psychoneuroimmunology (PNI) has begun uncovering the physiological mechanisms that control the intimate communication among the nervous, endocrine, and immune systems. It is this research that gives us the missing link between how our thoughts and emotions influence our health and disease states.

- When overstimulated by stress, the immune system becomes depleted and fatigued, which compromises the ability to resist disease.

SOURCES CITED

Alexander, F. (1965). *Psychosomatic medicine.* New York: W. W. Norton.

Anderson, B. L. (1994). Surviving cancer. *Cancer,* 74, 1484–96.

Bhatia, V., and Tandon, R. K. (2005). Stress and the gastrointestinal tract. *Journal of Gastroenterology and Hepatology,* 20, 332–39.

Baum, A., Cohen, L., and Hall, M. (1993). Control and intrusive memories as possible determinants of chronic stress. *Psychosomatic Medicine,* 57, 274–86.

Benson, H. (1992). *The relaxation response.* New York: Avon.

Benson, H. (1999). *Timeless healing: The power and biology of belief.* Audiocassette. New York: Simon and Schuster.

Borysenko, J. (1999). *Fire in the soul: A new psychology of spiritual optimism.* Elizabeth, NJ: Replica Books.

Borysenko, J., Borysenko, M., and Kramer, J. eds. (1994). *The power of the mind to heal.* Los Angeles: Hay House.

Borysenko, J., and Dveirin, J. (2005). *Saying yes to change.* Los Angeles: Hay House.

Buchner, B., Kleiber, C., Stanske, B. and Herrmann-Lingen, C. (2005). Stress and heart disease in women. *Herz,* 30, 416–28.

Cohen, S., et.al. (2003). Emotional style and susceptibility to the common cold. *Psychosomatic Medicine,* 65(4), 652–57.

Davey Smith, G., Ben-Shlomo, Y., Beswick, A., Yarnell, J., Lightman, S., and Elwood, P. (2005). Cortisol, testosterone and coronary heart disease. *Circulation,* 112, 332–40.

Davidson, R. J., et al. (2003). Alternations in brain and immune function produced by mindfulness meditation. *Psychosomatic Medicine,* 65(4), 564–70.

Dohrenwend, B., and Dohrenwend, B., eds. (1974). *Stressful life events: Their nature and effects.* New York: Wiley.

Fawzy, F. I., Fawzy, N., Hyur, C., Elashoff, R., Guthrie, D., Ashey, J., and Morton, D. (1993). Malignant melanoma: Effects of an early structured psychiatric intervention, coping and affective state on recurrence and survival 6 years later. *Archives of General Psychiatry,* 50, 681–89.

Filaire, E., Bernain, X., Sagnol, M., and Lac, G. 2001. Preliminary results on mood state, salivary testosterone: cortisol ratio and team performance in a professional soccer team. *European Journal of Applied Physiology and Occupational Physiology,* 86, 179–84.

Glaser, R., and Kiecolt-Glaser, J. K., eds. (1994). *Handbook of human stress and immunity.* New York: Academic Press.

Glaser, R., Kiecolt-Glaser, J. K., and Esterling, B. A. (1992). Stress-induced modulation of the immune response to recombinant hepatitis B vaccine. *Psychosomatic Medicine,* 54, 22–29.

Goleman, D. (2003). *Destructive emotions.* New York: Bantam.

Golden-Kreutz, D. M., Thornton, L. M., Wells-Di, G. S., Frierson, G. M., Jim, H. S., Carpenter, K. M., Shelby, R. A., and Andersen, B. L. (2005). Traumatic stress perceived global stress and life events: Prospectively predicting quality of life in breast cancer patients. *Health Psychology,* 24, 288–300.

Gomez-Merino, D., et al. (2005). Effects of combined stress during intense training on cellular immunity, hormones and respiratory infections. *Neuroimmunomodulation,* 12, 164–72.

Hart, A., and Kamm, M. A. (2002). Review Article: Mechanisms of initiation and perpetuation of gut inflammation by stress. *Alimentary Pharmacology and Therapeutics,* 16, 2017–28.

Hellsing, A. L., and Bryngelsson, I. L. (2000). Predictors of musculoskeletal pain in men: A twenty-year follow-up from examination at enlistment. *Spine,* 25, 3080–86.

Kroneke, C. H., Hankinson, S. E., Schernhammer, E. S., Colditz, G. A., Kawachi, I., and Holmes, M. D. (2004). Caregiving stress, endogenous sex steroid hormone levels, and breast cancer incidence. *American Journal of Epidemiology,* 159, 1019–27.

Lee, C. Y., Kratter, R., Duvoisin, N., Taskin, A., and Schilling, J. (2005). Cross-sectional view of factors associated with back pain. *International Archives of Occupational Environmental Health,* 78, 319–24.

Levenstein, S., Prantera, V., Varvo, M. L., Scribano, A., Andreoli, A., and Luzi, C. (2000). Stress and exacerbation in ulcerative colitis: A prospective study of patients enrolled in remission. *American Journal of Gastroenterology,* 95, 1213–20.

Linton, S. J. (2005). Do psychological factors increase the risk for back pain in the general population in both a cross-sectional and prospective analysis? *European Journal of Pain,* 9, 355–61.

Liu, L. Y., et al. (2002). School examinations enhance airway inflammation to antigen challenge. *American Journal of Respiratory Care Medicine,* 165, 1062–67.

Matthews-Simonton, S., Simonton, C. O., and Creighton, J. L. (1992). *Getting well again.* New York: Bantam Books.

Maunder, R. G. (2005). Evidence that stress contributes to inflammatory bowel disease: Evaluation, synthesis and future directions. *Inflammatory Bowel Disease,* 6, 600–8.

Meador, C. K. (1992). The person with the disease. *Journal of the American Medical Association,* 268, 1, 35.

Myss, C., and Norman Shealy, C. (1998). *The creation of health.* New York: Three Rivers Press.

Nielsen, N. R., Zhang, Z. F., Kristensen, T. S., Netterstrom, B., Schnohr, P., and Gronbaek, M. (2005). Self reported stress and risk of breast cancer: Prospective cohort study. *British Medical Journal,* 331, 548.

Nijm, J., Wikby, A., Tompa, A., Olsson, A. G., and Jonasson, L. (2005). Circulating levels of proinflammatory cytokines and neutrophil-latelet aggregates in patients with coronary artery disease. *American Journal of Cardiology,* 95, 452–56.

Ollonen, P., Lehtonen, J., and Eskelinen, M. (2005). Stressful and adverse life experiences in patients with breast symptoms; a prospective case-control study in Kuopio, Finland. *Anticancer Research,* 25, 531–36.

Padgett, D. A., and Glaser, R. (2003). How stress influences the immune system. *Trends in Immunology,* 24, 444–48.

Pert, C. (2006). *Everything you need to know to feel go(o)d.* Carlsbad, CA: Hay House.

Pert, C. (2004). *Your body is your subconscious mind.* Audio CD. Boulder: Sounds True.

Pert, C. (1999). *Molecules of emotion.* New York: Simon and Schuster.

Poikolainen, K., Kanerva, R., and Lonnquist, J. (1995). Life events and other risk factors for somatic symptoms in adolescence. *Journal of Psychosomatic Research,* 39, 1, 53–62.

Rosch, P. J. (1997). Reminiscences of Hans Selye, and the birth of "stress." *Health and Stress: The Newsletter of the American Institute of Stress,* no. 9, 1–4.

Rossi, E. (1993). *The psychobiology of mind-body healing.* New York: W. W. Norton.

Rossi, E. L., and Cheek, D. B. (1994). *Mind-body therapy: Methods of ideodynamic healing in hypnosis.* New York: W. W. Norton.

Sands, R. (2002). The power of the parasympathetic nervous system. *Stress News,* 14, no. 4, 4–8.

Selye, H. (1956). *The stress of life.* New York: McGraw-Hill.

Selye, H. (1974). *Stress without distress.* New York: Signet.

Siegel, B. S. (1994). *Love, medicine and miracles: Lessons learned about self-healing from a surgeon's experience with exceptional patients.* New York: Harper and Row.

Simonton, O. C. (1994). *Healing journey: The Simonton Center program for achieving physical, mental, and spiritual health.* New York: Bantam.

Smith, A., and Nicholson, K. (2001). Psychosocial factors, respiratory viruses and exacerbation of asthma. *Psychoneuroendocrinology,* 26(4), 411–20.

Tiersma, E. S. M., van der Lee, M. L., Garseen, B., Peters, A. A. W., Visser, A. P., Fleuren, G. J., van Leeuwen, K. M., le Cessie, S., and Goodkin, K. (2005). Psychosocial factors and the course of cervical intra-epithelial neoplasia: A prospective study. *Gyneologic Oncology,* 97, 879–86.

Uchino, B. N., Kiecolt-Glaser, J. K., and Cacioppo, J. T. (1992). Age and social support: Effects on cardiovascular functioning in caregivers of relatives with Alzheimer's disease. *Journal of Personal and Social Psychology,* 63, 839–46.

Wolff, H. G. (1968). *Stress and disease.* Springfield, IL: Charles C. Thomas.

Journal Entry 3

Your Body's Response to Stress

To further your insights about how stress affects you and to begin developing that awareness, complete the following exercise.

Your responses to this exercise may indicate which systems in your body are likely to be subjected to stress arousal and become weakened. This exercise lists some of the potential arousal signs in three major categories. Check the symptoms you usually experience, then describe any additional symptoms you may also experience.

Signs and Symptoms. Check the items that you often experience.

_____ stiffness in neck

_____ fingers and hands tremble or shake

_____ twitch in muscles (specific muscle:_____)

_____ difficulty standing still or sitting quietly

_____ stuttering or stammering speech

_____ frequent headaches (location on head:_____)

_____ muscle tension (specific muscles:_____)

_____ voice quivers

_____ nervous mannerisms; for example, biting nails, twisting hair, tapping feet, and so on

_____ heart pounding

_____ feeling lightheaded or faint

_____ cold chills

_____ cold hands

_____ cold feet

_____ dry mouth

_____ profuse sweating (location:_____)

_____ upset stomach

_____ sinking feeling in stomach

_____ frequent digestive disturbance

_____ moist or sweaty palms

_____ flushed or hot face

_____ preoccupied

_____ frequent insomnia

_____ uneasy or uncomfortable

_____ nervous or shaky

_____ confused

_____ forgetful

_____ insecure

_____ overexcited

_____ angry

_____ irritated

_____ worried

_____ anxious

_____ exhausted

_____ heart beats faster and harder

_____ backache

_____ shaky hands

_____ shallow, rapid breathing

_____ increased blood pressure

_____ stomachaches

_____ frequent diarrhea

_____ frequent constipation

_____ frequent indigestion

_____ hyperventilation

_____ skin rashes

_____ teeth grinding

_____ tension in the jaw (TMJ)

_____ chronic exhaustion

_____ inability to concentrate

_____ forgetfulness

_____ inability to concentrate

Can you identify which system(s) of your body is/are most likely to respond to stress? Tally your responses above to fit into the main headings in this chapter given below.

Musculoskeletal _____   Skin _____

Cardiovascular _____   Brain/Mind _____

Gastrointestinal _____   Immune System _____

1. What does this tell you about your stress response in general?

2. Have you been able to identify your major stress response system(s)? Do you think knowing this will be instrumental in your stress management program? How?

3. Write a positive word or short phrase about reading the messages from your body that will be useful to you in future situations.

CHAPTER 4

The Human Spirit

The stress that each person encounters throughout life may be seen as a battle with three basic elements:

1. What we need to survive physically

2. What we need for ego, emotional, and mental survival

3. What we are willing to do to live by a deep philosophical or spiritual construct.

The physical stress and pain we encounter and endure has its roots in beliefs and behaviors that we learn early in life that make it possible for us to survive both physically and emotionally. As we grow older, many of these beliefs and behaviors may no longer be beneficial to us. Emotional behaviors (pouting, throwing a fit, or crying to get your way) may have worked in childhood, but are no longer appropriate in an adult world. These then become sources of personal and interpersonal stress. As we mature, we continue to try to resolve our stress problems in a more rational way, hoping that peace and serenity, happiness and joy, love and compassion, healing and abundance will be the final outcome. Somewhere, we picked up that expectation. When these hopes become real expectations, they become the core of our belief system, and when we finally learn to live by the spiritual laws that will provide these dividends, stress diminishes and often disappears from our lives. Stress management methods such as meditation, visualization, Eastern movement arts (such as Tai Chi), and other introspective techniques are invaluable during this process.

A decade ago it may have been strange to see a chapter devoted to philosophy and the human spirit in a book about stress and stress management. Within that time frame, though, acceptance of matters regarding the human spirit have become more commonplace, even highly sought by men and women of all ages and religions. Government and private research continually illustrates the relationship between spirituality and health, prayer and healing, meditation and relaxation (Barnes et al. 2004; McCaffrey et al. 2004; Walker 2005).

Spirituality is one of the four basic areas of health (physical, emotional, mental, and spiritual), and it can be described in either secular or religious terms. The common thread to all religions is the desire to help people live a more spiritual life and to learn about spiritual leaders and their living examples of a spiritual life. Isn't it interesting that between 600 and 500 BCE (Before the Common Era) five highly important spiritual leaders were born? Buddha, Lao Tzu, Confucius, Zoroaster, and Mohammed entered this earth plane during that short span of time (and Christ, just 500 years later). They all sought deep personal change, greater inwardness in their spiritual lives, sought to become one with a spiritual reality that transcended their mundane conditions—and in so doing, became examples for millions who followed. This period of time (circa 600 BCE) has been called the *Axial Age* (Armstrong 2001), the beginning of humanity as we know it. During this time men and women endeavored to become conscious of their existence in an unprecedented way. Therein are the roots of spiritual possibility that each person feels at some time in life.

These early spiritual leaders professed a philosophy not unlike that of the ancient Taoists or the Native Americans: Live simply with loving kindness and equality toward all. As the people of the world parted into various religions and their particular dogmas, separation of one sect from another became the norm, and we often still see religious rivalry, persecution, and death as a consequence. As we have seen throughout history, strict or fanatical adherence to religious dogma tends to separate, whereas our true spiritual nature is to connect, to join, and to love unconditionally without judgment.

Spirituality is our relationship with some higher power or source of energy and also our relationship with others and the environment. Spirituality develops over time, and that development goes through a number of stages, beginning with an egocentric and unprincipled life. This is characterized by young children and self-serving adults. The next stage is characterized by strong belief in religion and churchgoing. The individuals here are strongly tied to their religious dogma and are not very tolerant of spiritual practices that differ from theirs. The next stage is the questioning stage, when the individual begins to examine set religious practices and keeps only those that seem right and truthful to him or her. The last stage is one of universal loving and acceptance, and it can occur within one's religion or outside of a set religion. People at this stage accept all others, regardless of their religion, race, age, economic class, sexual preference, status, or any other divisive classification. In this stage, people see the spirit that connects all living things.

Deepak Chopra, in discussions with noted physicists, persists in asking whether there is not a universal intelligence that governs all of life. Either there is a plan or there is no plan. Even molecules in seeming chaos, when gently nudged, fall into order. In this order can come peace, and the peace and quiet can hopefully reduce the stress in our lives.

Living the Spiritual Life

Simple words of wisdom that contain the essence of the spiritual life come from the ancients. Their descriptions of the serene and happy life appear more as philosophical reminders of how one should live than as a specific dogma of what one must think and do in order to receive the rewards of a possible later life. Somehow we know that spirituality has something to do with truth, caring, trust, and loving kindness.

Consider the spiritual direction given by Lao Tsu on Taoism and by a Cheyenne medicine man regarding the medicine wheel.

The Tao

Famous quotes from the *Tao Te Ching* by Lao Tsu include, "The Tao that can be told is not the eternal Tao" and "The nameless is the beginning of heaven and earth." Such is the difficulty of defining spirituality. The *Tao Te Ching* is thought to have been written in the sixth century BCE and has been translated more than any work other than the Bible. It is the epitome of a spiritual treatise, a philosophy of how to live a life of health and happiness. The philosophy of Lao Tsu was simple: Accept what is in front of you without wanting the situation to be other than it is. Study the natural order of things, and work with it rather than against it because to try to change what is only sets up resistance. Nature provides for all without discrimination—therefore let us present the same face to everyone and treat all as equals, however they behave. If we watch carefully, we will see that work proceeds more quickly and easily if we stop trying, if we stop putting in so much extra effort, and if we stop looking for results. In the clarity of a still and open mind, truth will be reflected.

The Medicine Wheel

The Native American philosophy of life, with its own colorful images and symbols, brings the nature of spirit closer to our times and place. Hyemeyohsts Storm, in his book *Seven Arrows,* offers insight into the spiritual life of the Plains Indians. The Medicine Wheel is a sacred symbol of the Plains Indians that shows how each person must make a conscious journey for spiritual fulfillment.

As the very Way of Life of the People, the Medicine Wheel gives an understanding of the universe. It is the Great Shield of Truth, the Heart, and the Mind. The Medicine Wheel Way begins with the touching of the brothers and sisters, then of touching the world around (all living things), and finally of teaching to Sing the Song of the World in order to become Whole (Storm 1972).

The Medicine Wheel is to be thought of as a mirror in which everything is reflected: nature, ideas, and other people. **Figure 4.1** depicts a simple Medicine Wheel. Usually constructed of small stones, each stone of the Wheel represents one of the many things in the universe and differs from person to person, depending on who is constructing it. Stones might represent family members, animals, religions, philosophies, or even nations. All things within the Medicine Wheel are equal, as it is in the universe. In order to become whole, everyone must learn harmony with all the spirits of the Universe. To do this, they must learn to seek to find their place or purpose. They must learn to Give-Away (give the gift of themselves as the buffalo or deer gave of itself so that people might eat).

The basic starting place for the journey is the direction of birth on the Medicine Wheel. Each of the four directions, or the Four Great Powers, has a symbolic color, animal totem, and philosophic meaning. As described by Storm, the top of the Medicine Wheel is North. Its color is white, the buffalo is its medicine animal, and its meaning is Wisdom. The South is represented by the color green, the mouse is its

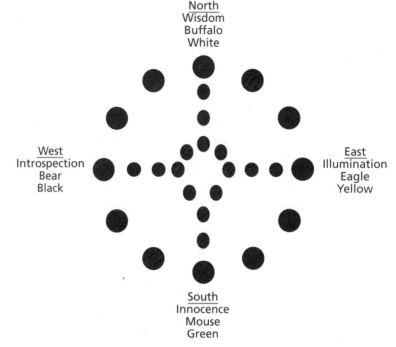

Figure 4.1 The medicine wheel of seven arrows

medicine animal, and it is the place of Innocence and Trust and for being close to what has heart and meaning. The West is the place of Looks-Within or introspection. Its color is black and the bear is its sign. The East is the Place of Illumination, where we see clear and far. Its color is yellow and the symbol of place is the Eagle. We are each born to a starting place that gives a way of seeing and experiencing the world. Our starting place will be the easiest way for us to interact with others all our lives, but in order to be whole, we must visit all four directions and learn how to live each. For instance, if a person is "born of the North," they show the inherent ability to ponder and make wise decisions. However, to become spiritually integrated, they must also learn innocence and trust, learn the ability to see (perceive) clearly, and look deep within their own soul.

Stress in Seeking Spirit

This brings us then to the connection between stress management and spirituality. Perhaps the deepest roots of human stress—buried, invisible, and unconscious to many—are the four basic spiritual questions of humankind:

1. What is the basic energy that moves the universe?

2. What is life, where did it come from, and where is it going?

3. What is the human role on this earth, and where are we going as a species?

4. Who am I? What is my purpose, my function, and my destiny?

Spiritual philosophy (as in, "We are spirits that happen to be living inside human bodies") teaches us that the answers to these questions are inherent in every human being. Spirit and individual souls are indivisible partners in the power that moves the universe, and all material things are produced by that power. This knowledge is buried in the "mind" of everyone, and this knowledge is real and true for all time. It urges us toward fulfilling our spiritual goal. It is almost as though we just have to know the part of us that is forever unchanging. Aldous Huxley called it the "Perennial Philosophy": that there is something beyond the world of change, and philosophers from every age seek to know what that is.

We concentrate most of our lives on survival of the psyche and the physical body, and so the spiritual questions often go unanswered. As egocentric beings, we spend most of our time on Question 4: "Who am I?" and, as a subset, "Why are all these other people making it so difficult for me?" In reality, the four questions are upside-down. We start with the known, physical, material self and then proceed to relationships with others and the environment. Then, perhaps, we begin to question things larger than ourselves and our physical space. Then (again perhaps) we get to the "God" question. What is the energy that's putting this all together, and how am I a part of that? *Am* I a part of that?

In birth as we move from soul energy to human energy, we are set apart from others, we are divided against one another by our selfishness and competition, yet we yearn for harmony and togetherness. We have a need to love and be loved, yet few among us obtain the harmonious loving state of unified separateness until we have paid our dues. Individualization, self-discovery, feelings, risk taking, and confiding are part of the process of relating to others who act as mirrors for us so that we can learn to do it better next time. Our emotional relationships become a win/loss column, a see-saw process that ebbs and flows between sublime comfort and intense stress.

After birth, the human infant is in servitude for months upon months, learning how to get its needs met. It learns that behaving in certain ways can be bartered for being fed, held, loved, and cared for. In order to survive in this world of other people, many of whom hold the reins of acceptance or denial, we learn to judge and compete. We orient ourselves, what we know, what we feel, and what we value by banking it off the outside world. From the earliest of times and the very depths of our knowing come comparison and judgment (also called reflection, relativity, or relationship).

To become human means to be separate from all other material things. Our goal is to use the other material things as teachers to remind us how to get back to a perfect soul state. It is trial-and-error learning, and it takes as long as it takes. Until the process is a gift and a friend, anxiety and stress fill the mind.

Mindfulness, or consciousness, becomes the path to peace.

In our search for love, we want to grasp, to hold, to cling, and to possess. We know that we are part of something larger and want to belong. But does peace come from the conditional type of loving that we see in most human relationships? More likely, such relationships are fraught with unmet expectations and unspoken barter and become the breeding ground of stress.

Most of us think of relationship as in "significant other," family, and friends. Yet, relationship occurs between us and all other aspects of our lives, such as money, time, religion, and, yes, even ourselves. Some believe that love relationships are primarily and simply to ensure the propagation of the species. In fact, we must seek relationships in order to learn to think and behave skillfully. Doing so brings the rewards we require on a soul level.

Seriously searching for "who we really are" slowly turns our head toward the more philosophical questions. When we begin to consider the meaning of life, the power that moves the universe, and the collective human role, our human relationships come into perspective, and we become more skilled, more mindful in our behavior.

Managing stressful behavior begins at a survival level. We do what we have to do to save our skin! We become more skillful as we learn about human psychology and apply it to ourselves and others. The continuum of skillful behavior continues as we move toward worldly understandings and on to universal philosophical understandings.

We learn the fear of rejection, the anger of being thwarted, and the guilt of unacceptable behavior, and we experience the anxiety of struggle between needs and what we have to do to get our needs met. Until each person releases the tension between what they are and what they think they should be, anxiety and the discomfort of stress will be their companions.

Stress will change our minds and mold our bodies. It will influence the length and quality of life. It will determine the amount of peace we enjoy or struggle we endure. Interactions with other people will be largely responsible for the amount of stress we experience. Stressful events and relationships could be considered the basic classroom in which we either learn to do better or not.

Purposefully seeking the answers to life's basic questions and constructing a conscious philosophy to live by will concomitantly enhance the quality of human relationships.

Two Insights from Science

For those of a scientific bent, two scientific paradigms offer insight into the mystery, definition, and interpretation of spirit and spirituality. The earlier of the two is that of quantum physics. Einstein presented to the world an equation that allowed the interchangeability of mass and energy ($E = MC^2$). At the quantum level, where energy can become mass and mass can become energy, all material things begin. The human body is energy that has been materialized. The macro human body and all its cells are surrounded by and infused with energy that is not as visible as the material self. Each level of manifestation is characterized by its own degree of consciousness, which is one octave removed from the other. This is discussed at greater length later in the chapter under the topic of personality and individuality. The basic message is that *everything* is interwoven as energy—whether it is physical, emotional, mental, or spiritual.

The second paradigm is that of psychoneuroimmunology or mind-body medicine. Although this laboratory research has identified the amino-acid structure of many ligands or neuropeptide messengers that influence cells all over the body via receptors on cell membranes, it brings up questions that pique the minds of spiritual philosophers. If all cells of the body are "in on" everything that happens (or has ever happened) to it, is the physical body, in fact, the mind? Candace Pert (2004) insists that "your body is your subconscious mind." We know that the body remembers traumas and that bodywork of various kinds may trigger memory of those traumas.

Then comes the big question: What is the intelligence or wisdom that directs the physical body toward balance, health, or homeostasis? When Walter B. Cannon coined the term homeostasis, was he talking merely about the physical feedback mechanisms that keep the body in balance, or was he philosophically asking the question, "Do we have consciousness, or does consciousness have us?" Is there invisible life energy that originally programs the body toward health and happiness?

Personality and Individuality

To use quantum physics to describe our world, we would note that the molecular masses that vibrate the most slowly are those that we can see and touch, that is, that we can use our physical senses to explore. There is little doubt that there are human energy fields that we cannot so easily explore with the physical senses. Emotions and thoughts are energy fields, and although we may interpret them through overt behavior, their very essence is extrasensory. The most elusive of the human energy fields is the spirit.

Ouspensky (1949), Gurdjieff (see Speeth 1976), James (1890), Jung (1933), and countless other philosophers/psychologists since their time speak of two coexisting entities within humans: One is *personality,* consisting of the physical body, its emotional makeup, and its mental makeup (see **Figure 4.2**). The *physical* or material layer of our existence is the most basic. It includes not only simple mass but also the vegetative state wherein the mass searches for food, takes it in, and digests it. As we've noted before, the physical body is often our main focus because we can see it, touch it, and understand its physiology down to the microscopic functioning of RNA and DNA (and beyond).

Figure 4.2 Personality and individuality

For most people it is difficult, if not impossible, to comprehend the idea of the other "invisible" supportive energy layers around the physical body. The early Greek philosophers Socrates, Plato, and Aristotle (as with modern physicists) sought to define what was "real" by being able to physically measure it. Only through deductive reasoning could they examine spirit (Wolf 2002).

The next layer of energy outward from the physical is the *emotional* (sometimes called the "animal") layer that adds emotion, drives, antipathy, and desires to the physical. Chapter 5 delves deeper into the emotions and how they function as basic stressors throughout our lives. Next, the *mental* layer adds intellect and consciousness, that is, doing things on a "conscious" level. In some teachings, these three layers are simply called "man," characterized by the human intellect. Others, including the great psychiatrist Carl Jung, called it the personality.

The second of the two coexisting entities is *individuality*, which consists of free will, the soul, and divine energy (see Figure 4.2). Jung felt that the purpose of life was far greater than just learning how to cope with maladjustment in one's psychosexual makeup: There was also a challenge to cooperate with a profound impetus from deep within one's own being, an impetus toward wholeness. He proposed that there was a level of mind that contained "archetypal" or universal themes, a collective unconscious to which we all have access. One of those archetypes is the Self, that part of humans that seeks to find its spiritual purpose and connection. In our dichotomy here, that would be the search for individuality.

The behaviors that issue from one's personality and one's individuality are quite different. The response from personality is more of a childhood-learned behavior. On our most basic physical level, the personality makes choices that satisfy our most immediate physical needs. The hungry choose food and the cold choose warmth. At the next level, personality choices are further influenced by emotions. The lonely choose company or often self-nurturing with food, drugs, and alcohol. The fearful choose to withdraw or to hide in the emotional world of depression. Add to this physical-emotional mix a human's unique intellect, and the choices become even more complex. Knowledge can be spun by the personality into elaborate webs of revengeful deception or it can be translated by one's individuality into loving activities.

Individuality is a higher order of being, of eternal dimension, richer in meaning and relationships. It is the awakening of one's "right use of will," connecting us with a higher order of behavior. Behaviors that issue from individuality stem from wisdom, compassion, and a higher consciousness. Individuality is ever present and available to guide the personality. It is one's individuality that more closely defines the real self, who we really are. Its nature is to be innovative and creative, happy and peaceful, loving and generous.

Free will is foundational to spiritual advancement because it demands that conscious decisions be made; conscious decisions about which thoughts to have, which feelings to nurture, and which behaviors to perform. It is not just knowing what your mission is but also how to live it. Will allows us to give attention to specific ideas beyond mere physical survival. We are constantly given the opportunity to shape experiences with the will.

Hidden from our immediate senses are myriad decisions about which thoughts to have, which feelings to nurture, and which words to say to elicit a desired reaction. Choices that are mindful do not follow the logic of the personality. Not seeking revenge when hurt or not insulting those who disagree with us are examples of mindfulness. Purposefully going against lifelong conditioning of personality by not choosing greed or prolonged grief are acts of mindfulness. The first step in moving toward a mindful response is controlling destructive emotions. Separating emotion from the event produces detachment. Mindfulness is the freedom to be aware of the moment without reacting with old automatic responses from childhood, the unskillful past.

Philosophy and religion tell us that free will is inherent in each soul; that it is inborn. It is a key element to becoming more spiritually enlightened, because it demands that we make conscious decisions about which thoughts to think, which feelings to nurture, which words to speak, and which behaviors to perform. We are constantly given the opportunity to shape experiences with the will and the very depths of our soul. Little free will can be exercised when we let others make our decisions for us. Early survival depends on learning and doing what others want us to do, so a large part of become a conscious adult is discovering that we have the ability to make free-will choices that affirm our real selves and then begin to think, speak, and act from our inner spirit nature. The force of old habit is stronger than the force of ideal action unless the soul is awakened. The space between is called "stress."

Compassion and Mindfulness

Lucky for us, connecting the personality and one's individuality is a compassionate/intuition energy, which is also called the genius level, characterized by intuition. Compassion, or listening to our inner voice, puts us in touch with our higher spiritual nature, which is ever present and available to guide the personality layers. If the personality does not allow feelings and thoughts that nurture spiritual search, the process may be delayed for a lifetime. Living one's life at a higher level requires that one get past the knee-jerk reactions of the personality and learn more skillful responses to painful experiences. Compassion guides this process, especially compassion for oneself.

Compassion is the key to mindfulness, and the ultimate expression of compassion is forgiveness. To forgive is to no longer blame, and without blame, all that is left is the acceptance of responsibility. This means being responsible for your thoughts and feelings as well as your actions. It means shedding the psychological myth of conditioned responses, scripts, and roles that most of us have been taught and have virtually constructed in our cells. It means taking responsibility for the stress we cause ourselves and being gentle with the love and support of those who accompany us. It means choosing to act out of compassion and understanding. It means making mindful choices. The goal in decision making, especially when it involves others around us, is harmonious coexistence in which there are no thoughts, feelings, and actions that cause separation. Rather than using the personality to create separation, in mindfulness we use compassion to create union.

In illustration, **Figure 4.3** shows the difference between making a decision from a conditioned personality response and from a mindful response. The personality-based response likely involves anger or fear, is less skillful, *even stressful*. If motivated by wisdom, love, and compassion, the decision becomes mindful, and a peaceful resolution is accomplished. Mindfulness of the highest order requires compassion and intention.

Just what is this "mindfulness?" Aren't we mindful when we intentionally get even with someone, or when we purposefully withhold from someone? Mindfulness as we

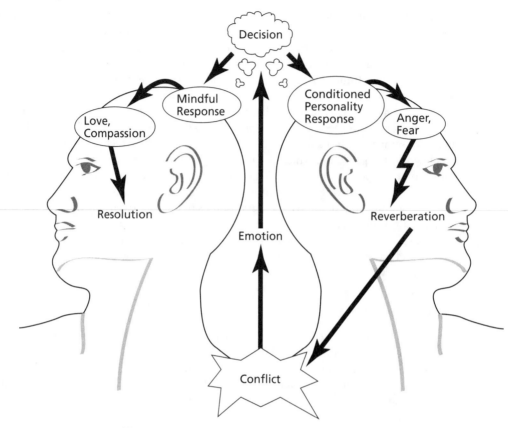

Figure 4.3 Difference between making a decision from conditioned personality response and mindful response

use it here in conjunction with spiritual development is less what to think and more how to think—more a description than a prescription. It is demonstrated in subtle differences—not so much in technique but in motivation. Abraham Maslow (1968), generally credited with founding the humanistic psychology movement, explains this fundamental difference as acting (1) from intellectual self-serving objectivism (usually fear based and competitive) or (2) from the intuitive belief in truths beyond ourselves, cooperation, and belief that humans can fulfill their highest potential. The point on which this skill turns is the "right use" of free will—being free enough from immediate gratification and debilitating emotions to make choices based on universal truths. This is not to say that one cannot consciously check decisions against the "yardstick" of options drawn from wisdom. One can understand the concepts involved and believe in both the possibilities and their own potential abilities and practice.

Connecting with divine spirit, the very essence of being, is our spiritual goal. It motivates us, guides us, and coaxes us toward consciousness. Stress-producing behaviors we engage in and observe in others are all the proof we need that we spend much of our time in the unconscious state. To become spiritually conscious (or mindful) is a choice (series of choices) we must make, and then we must practice it as a skill to eventually own it as a living philosophical art. Much of this book gives direction for solving stress issues in accepted cognitive-behavioral ways, yet the human spirit draws us to the ultimate stress management techniques—compassion, love, kindness, faith, honesty, and trust.

The Forces

Within us are several basic forces or voices. First is the voice of our social environment—family, friends, church, and other institutions. As we become enculturated or socialized by these people, we adopt their belief system or pay the consequences. We are taught what we must do in order to survive in this social environment. This is "tribal power" that is instilled early in life and seeks to control the group's behavior. The mind of the tribe changes slowly, over decades or even centuries (Myss 2007).

A second voice, the individual voice that recognizes that all is not well, begins to speak within us when we accumulate the knowledge, experience, and self-esteem to question the tribe's power and decisions. Many times it is awakened by a stressful situation. This is the individual voice of the human spirit, and it begins to speak to us when we are no longer content to be controlled by the "tribe," money, acceptance, or other external rewards. The individual mind can change much more quickly than the tribal mind. Reading a book, taking a seminar, or talking with a mentor may change one's outlook. An epiphany may come overnight.

The third voice is a voice of divine guidance. We are so thoroughly trained to obey the laws of the tribe and then urged by inner desires to take command of our own lives that it is difficult to switch to a release of the self to the divine. From the third voice we learn that we are not the ocean; we are a droplet of water in and of the ocean, and there are universal laws that bring happiness and peace.

These forces might also be called the outer, inner, and innate voices.

Steps Toward Enlightenment

How many experts does it take to change a lightbulb? Many or few, depending on whether it wants to change. How do we get to conscious behavior? We do not just trip over it and then pick it up when we turn twenty-one or forty or some magical age. The motivation to become conscious comes first. Consider the man who could not dance:

> There once was a man who couldn't dance, yet he imagined he could. He invited a woman to go dancing with him, and although they enjoyed each other's company as they dined and chatted, the dance floor experience was a disaster. He stepped on her toes, bumped into other dancers, and twirled her into walls, and the beat of the music completely evaded his feet. On the dance floor he realized he had made a terrible mistake: He had chosen a woman who could not dance! It took him dozens of women before he realized that it was he who could not dance. He went to a dance studio and learned all the steps and became quite a dancer and lived happily ever after.

How long does it take to recognize that what we are doing is not working? How long do we curse and blame others when things continue to turn out poorly? It takes the willingness to look at our life and admit that something is not working here. Perhaps it is a habitual anger response or jealousy or how we shrink back in fear. Whatever stresses a person gives him or her a clue that change is due. If the stressor can be perceived as a gift and a piece of information, it can propel a person forward.

As physical beings, we all inevitably experience pain. How long we suffer from it depends on our perception. Much of suffering is caused by trying to avoid situations that we expect will be painful. Suffering is like an untreated disease that festers and gets worse, yet it is the suffering that finally gets our attention. The cataclysmic events in life act as lightning rods that draw insight to those who are willing to understand the message that comes with the event.

What causes suffering? A two-and-a-half-century-old response given by Eastern spiritual masters would be ignorance, craving, and hatred—the three poisons of the mind. Ignorance was defined as not having the perception of the true nature of the self or soul; craving (or greed) was defined as an insatiable overwanting; and hatred encompassed fear, anger, jealousy, and envy. All of these poisons stem from attachment—attachment to material things, relationships, and mental states to which the person has become accustomed. Change becomes the enemy, yet change is so constant that if befriended, it becomes the expected rather than that which renders surprise.

Ignorance may be the first hurdle—ignorance of the true nature of the self. The true nature of the human spirit cannot be explained in personality terms. The spirit does not necessarily follow the physical laws that humans have established while trying to ensure "civilized" societies. The spirit follows divine law that truly makes all people equal, sharing universal intelligence and benevolence. Divine law puts us all in the same pool; no one soul is better or worse than another because the true self is a part of this divine pool. Each person has ideas and beliefs about this pool. Many call it God/Goddess, the Great Spirit, Allah, or universal benevolence or goodness.

The first step toward enlightenment is the step from outer control to self-control. At some time, each person makes the decision to listen to an inner voice rather than to external voices. The tribe has a great deal of power, and the individual must go beyond that power. Each person must make his or her own decisions, even though these decisions may cause trouble. The "mistakes," however, are the individual's own mistakes, and they are lessons to be learned.

It is as though the individual knows we all have the birthright of happiness, yet the person keeps putting up roadblocks with fear, anger, greed, procrastinations, and prevarications. The individual does this because his or her personality (our conditioned physical, emotional, and mental aspects) has learned to protect and to ensure the survival of the psyche and physical body. Human spiritual nature pushes us toward refining our thoughts and actions to uncover the soul. It does this by helping us find ways to unlearn old, no-longer-useful personality behaviors that separate us from others and from our own souls and to begin to become mindful of every choice we make.

This step may take the person out of his or her job, marriage, or family. Depression may occur. The fear of aloneness is often strong during this time, yet it is a time when learning to live happily with oneself is a high priority. It does not mean a life of celibacy or living alone in a cave; it is a time of getting to know and enjoy the self. Remember that this is the step from outer to inner guidance.

When self-concept is strong enough and the choice is made to continue toward finding spirit, the next step evolves. This is the step of losing the self and entering the symbolic, looking at things from a transcendent, universal, or spiritual view rather than a material view. Rather than depending on the received, or heard, wisdom learned from others—or the intellectual wisdom that occurs after one has learned from others and then examines for its rationality, benefit, and practicality for oneself—the individual finally depends on personal experiences and has his or her own realization of truth. This is the step from inner voice to innate voice. It is governed by one's individuality, the spirit nature that has always been there even though it had been buried by material worries. This is where the true self resides. The last stage of this last step is living a life of appreciation or gratitude.

On a personal level, being off your spiritual course feels negative, and you may experience remorse for your actions, thoughts, or words. Remorse, like all negative feelings, is a signal that you have strayed off course. Joy, on the other hand, is a signal that you are keeping to the course you have charted. Thomas Jefferson had it right when he said, "You feel good when you do good, and you feel bad when you do bad."

"Right action" is choosing the action that results in joy rather than in remorse, yet feeling remorse can motivate you to seek a different way to do it in the future. Remorse is often not apparent on a conscious level. However, it must be brought up to a conscious level in order to stimulate behavior change. When you are off your spiritual course, you create situations that become opportunities to bring remorse to your consciousness. Although remorse can be beneficial, lasting guilt is useless and paralyzing because it keeps one focused on the past. Even though glancing back may be useful, you cannot steer ahead while looking backward.

We all ultimately search for one thing: happiness. The key elements that contribute to happiness are health, wealth, and friendship, yet the master key is perception—how we think about what we have. True happiness is of the heart.

Exercises

The following exercises are presented here to help you recognize where you may be creating stress in your life by following or not following your philosophical/spiritual path.

Honor Code

What is your honor code with the universe? First, write in your journal or notebook the items that make up your personal honor code. Likely items would be truth, acceptance, loving kindness, and so on. List as many things that you can think of that govern your behavior.

Second, take each item and write about a recent scenario in your life in which you used that item. An example might be the item of "truth." You were asked why you did not like someone's response, and you told them the truth in a kind, assertive manner.

Third, after you have completed the first parts of the exercise, think about what you have written. Was it difficult to come up with examples that prove your honor code? Did it seem easier to come up with examples that disproved your honor code? Is your professed honor code different from the code you actually live by? Remember that you are as you act.

Lies I Have Told

In this exercise, keep a notebook handy for a full week to write down all the lies you tell during that time. Big lies, little lies, mean lies, and white lies. Leave some room between your lies. The second part of the exercise is to write an explanation of why you told the lie. Were you tired, scared, ignorant, or what? Also write down how you felt after you did the deed.

Then think again of your honor code (as in the first exercise). Was truth part of your code? What is happening in your life that keeps you from telling others the truth? Is there one particular aspect of your life where truthfulness is especially lacking? Is it easier to tell some people the truth than others? Who? Why?

Mysteries and Miracles

Keep an ongoing journal of the mysteries and miracles in your life. Write about how your spiritual questions are answered, how unexpected good things happen to you, the "spooky" things that have happened to you and others you know well, when you feel out of spiritual alignment, and what you plan to do to realign yourself.

SUMMARY

Spirituality is one's personal relationship with a comforting higher power or source of energy. Consider the following points:

- Spiritual health is one of the four basic components of personal health (also emotional, mental, and physical).

- Although religions are built on spirituality, spirituality and religiosity are not necessarily synonymous. A person may be one and not the other.

- Fanatical adherence to religious dogma tends to separate, whereas true spiritual nature is to connect.

- Our physical nature separates us from others; spirituality joins us.

- The personality is ingrained in our physical nature and manifests as learned behavior that takes care of physical, psychological, and emotional survival.

- Individuality, through wisdom and compassion, leads toward soul discovery and divine guidance.

- The spiritually bound person is first shaped by the social environment, then by his or her own philosophy, and ultimately by divine guidance.

- The first step toward enlightenment is from outer control to inner control.

- When inner control (self-concept) is strong enough, one may choose to enter the symbolic world of spirit and view the world in a transcendent or spiritual way rather than materially.

- The spiritual journey can be made less stressful by focusing on the process of personal integrity.

SOURCES CITED

Armstrong, K. (2001). *Buddha.* New York: Penguin.

Barnes, P. M., et al. (2004). Complementary and alternative medicine use among adults: United States, 2002. *CDC Advance Data Report #343.*

James, W. (1890). *Principles of psychology.* Mineola, NY: Dover.

Jung, C. G. (1933). *Modern man in search of a soul.* New York: Harcourt Brace Jovanovich.

McCaffrey, A. M., et al. (2004). Prayer for health concerns: Results of a national survey on prevalence and patterns of use. *Archives of Internal Medicine, 164*(8), 858–62.

Myss, C. (2007). *Entering the castle.* New York: Free Press.

Ouspensky, P. D. (1949). *In search of the miraculous.* New York: Harcourt Brace Jovanovich.

Pert, C. (2004). *Your body is your subconscious mind.* Audio CD. Boulder, CO: Sounds True.

Rinpoche, Y. M. (2007). *The joy of living.* New York: Random House.

Speeth, K. (1976). *The Gurdjieff work.* New York: Harper & Row.

Storm, H. (1972). *Seven arrows.* New York: Ballantine.

Walker, D. (2005). Prayer and spirituality in health: Ancient practices, modern science. *CAM at the NIH, Focus on Complimentary and Alternative Medicine, 12*(1), 1–6.

Wolf, F. A. (2002). *Matter into feeling.* Needham, MA: Moment Point Press.

Journal Entry 4

What Is the Basis of My Beliefs?

You have been asked in this chapter to think about whether you have consciousness or if, perhaps, consciousness has you. Are you a separate entity with mere social ties to the rest of humanity, or are we all "cut from the same cloth"? A very deep sense of anxiety comes from not having a guiding belief about life itself or, perhaps worse yet, from professing a guiding belief and not acting accordingly.

To help you identify your beliefs, your tenets regarding life and all living things, we present four major universal questions and space for you to journal your answers.

The Four Major Questions

1. What is the basic energy that moves the universe?

2. What is life, where did it come from, and where is it going?

3. What is the human role on this earth? Where are we going as a species?

4. Who am I? What is my purpose, my function, and my destiny?

Journal your answers, keying in on how you go about living them in your daily life.

1. If you believe that a spiritual power exists, describe it. Is it an entity, an energy, nature, and so on? What are the characteristics of this power? Is it benevolent and all goodness? Describe the goodness. Is it a mixture of goodness and something else? Describe that. How does this energy affect you?

2. How did life originate? What is life? Was there a beginning? What came before the beginning? Is there such a thing as death? What about life everlasting? Where do you go when you die? What do you think of reincarnation? Karma?

3. How did humans come to take on material life? Why do we have to come and take on the miseries of being human? Just what is it that we are supposed to do here as a human race?

 4. Do you know what your purpose in life is? Is it merely a way to make a living, or is there a bigger reason why you are here? Did you choose your parents, or did they choose you? Do you choose your opportunities, friends, where you live, and other experiences in life, or do they choose you?

 5. Did your philosophy of life change as you went through this introspection? How?

 6. How are spiritual questions and answers related to your stress? To your calmness or serenity?

 7. Can we learn to live at peace with ourselves and others?

 8. Write a positive word or short phrase that reflects your life philosophy and that you can use when you lose sight of what is important.

5

Stressful Emotions, Thoughts, and Beliefs

Negative emotion is the tinder that feeds the fire of stress. Emotion is expressed in the contraction of fear and the explosion of anger; it is the slow cooker of revenge, the cancer of depression, the stealth of guilt, the blanch of terror. Everyone experiences negative emotion, and some cultivate it until it kills them. At some point in life, most people decide that negative emotions are luxuries that they cannot afford and begin to give them up.

What is emotion? In its broadest definition, emotion includes the commonly used terms such as anger, fear, joy, guilt, jealousy, love, courage, and sadness; the drive states such as hunger and thirst; and basic sensations of pleasure and pain. Early scientific arguments between Walter Cannon and William James questioned whether emotions originated in the brain and then messages were sent out to the body so that it would respond appropriately, or whether emotions originated in the body on a feeling level and then were worked on by the brain. As in all great arguments, each side probably offers something to ponder. From Pert's research (1999, 2004) on what she terms the "molecules of emotion," we find what Oriental healers and philosophers have proclaimed for centuries: The body and mind are one. Although various parts of the body have their own specificity of action (the heart pumps blood, the lungs aerate the blood, etc.), an interconnecting network of neuropeptides allows all cells of the body to have their own mobile phone, so to speak, to talk with everyone else—the human Internet.

There is a growing body of literature linking immune function to emotions. For instance, Insel and Fernald (2004) found that involvement in distressing relationships was associated with increases in stress hormone levels that damage genes identified to control virus-fighting cells. McClain, Rosenfeld, and Breitbart (2003) noted that Interleukin-6, the immune marker most highly correlated with mood states, is one of several markers of inflammation, an important process in a variety of diseases like heart disease, diabetes, and stroke, and is associated with increased stress and depression. Research done at NIH's Complementary and Alternative Medicine branch continues to study the links between emotion, mood, stress, disease, and health (Barnes, Powell-Griner, and Nahin 2005).

We do learn (become accustomed to using specific neural and chemical pathways) to expect emotions to feel a certain way and lead to certain outcomes, yet it is a total mind-body learning rather than memories laid down in certain parts of the brain. Once an emotional response is formed and stored away in the limbic part of the brain, it colors later actions and decisions. We know the amygdala (an almond-shaped structure deep in the limbic system) has emotional "hot spots" or nuclei. When something scares or otherwise upsets us, the amygdala is at the center of the brain's circuits for stamping that moment in memory, and communicates with other brain sites to determine the valence of the emotional input. Thereafter, when something seems to resemble that original moment of distress, the amygdala recognizes that similarity and dictates our response in a few hundredths of a second, even before the forebrain has had time to fully mull over what is going on—or what the consequences of our reaction will be (Goleman 2006a, 2006b). Recent research in the field of drug addiction and treatment notes that the cingulate cortex (illustrated in Figure 2.2) has important function in detecting and controlling emotions—feelings, pain, and associated bodily arousal (Kosten et al. 2006; Whitten 2007).

An interesting part of this neurophysiology of emotion (and important to the study of emotional stress) is that although the amygdala is the emotional message–receiving center, its wiring provides *no* direct access to the centers for speech! When we receive emotion-stimulating input from the various parts of our brain, instead of sending a message to the verbal areas where we could verbalize what we're feeling, the body has no choice but to mimic that emotion in its structure; that is, instead of being able to talk about it we literally "put it in our body" (Goleman 2006b). What an important insight to interpersonal relationships! Everyone knows at least one person who can't seem to "talk about his/her feelings." It is not impossible to talk about your emotions; you just have to consciously *want* to, as we will see later in this discussion.

Emotion is an energy complex involving nerves, muscles, gut, bone marrow, glandular activity, and other diverse cells of the body. Over time it may be learned as a physical pattern that readies the body for confrontation, retreat, expression, or no expression. Emotions are instantaneous forms of experience and reaction. When people are being emotional, their body expresses immediate physical reality, and this expression takes place before they can even be consciously aware of it. Emotions are forms of immediate experience. When individuals experience emotion, they are in direct contact with physical reality and even if they are excellent poker players, to some degree, it will show on their face (Goleman 2006; Manstead et al. 2003).

Emotional responses learned in early life are reactions to basic needs and external stimuli, and as people grow older they also learn to create emotional patterns from their thoughts (Goleman 2006). Even before emotional patterns are learned by any kind of cognitive conditioning, however, there is an innate feedback system that is designed to keep the mind and body in balance. We call this the "wisdom of the body," or perhaps **homeostasis.** In early life, babies practice emotional patterns until they are fairly habitual reactions. Because children are taught directly or indirectly to not show their emotions, especially unpleasant ones, they develop negative self-talk (an inner dialogue with one's self) that also becomes part of their emotional patterns (Bradshaw 2005). If children do not like the way an emotion feels, or cannot (or are not allowed to) express it, they may "block" it out of their consciousness altogether and it lives at a somatic level. Emotional reactions become part of the basic personality.

The Development of Human Emotion

MacLean explains that, anthropologically, the brain developed as three distinct parts (see **Figure 5.1**):

1. a brain that relates to the physical world,

2. a brain that relates to the inner world, and

3. a brain that relates to abstraction and creativity (1990).

We might think of these parts as physical, emotional, and mental (just as we saw these three aspects defined in the last chapter as "personality"). The evolution of the brain began as brain 1, the physical brain. It helped life survive for hundreds of millions of years by registering and responding to physical input. It was merely instinctual and reflexive.

Following the adage "ontogeny recapitulates phylogeny" (meaning that, as an organism develops, it passes through, or repeats, each phase of the evolution of its species), the physical brain was complemented with brain 2, the emotional brain. The emotional brain wrapped around the physical brain, and these two areas developed an intimate communication network. Now, explains MacLean, in addition to responding to physical stimuli, humans began to place an emotional value on their relationship to the physical world and to each other. The emotional brain handles not only emotions but also all internal images. It receives concrete, physical images from the lower brain and abstract images from the cortex, and its job is to make some kind of cohesive relationship out of those images. Pearce (1994) calls the midbrain the "heart" of the central nervous system, for it handles love, hate, fear, attraction, aversion, bonding, and all other relationships.

Finally, with further evolution, the third brain (the thinking brain, or cortex) enveloped the other two parts. It enabled us to work with abstract imagery, think on an intellectual plane, and create thoughts and forms not necessarily based on physical input. The thinking brain, or cortex, makes it possible for us to analyze, synthesize, create, compute, and otherwise play with the information furnished by the two lower brains. Especially important to our study of stress is the development and functions of

The Thinking Brain (Cortex)
• Intellectual
• Abstract Imagery

The Emotional Brain (Limbic System)
• Emotional
• Dream Imagery
• Metaphoric Imagery

The Physical Brain
• Physical Input/Output
• Concrete Imagery

Figure 5.1 The triune brain and its intercommunication links (adapted from Pearce 1985)

the forebrain or frontal cortex. This area of the brain is responsible for our being able to be consciously responsible. It gives us the ability to plan for the future, to delay gratification, to formulate intent and make changes toward intent, and to make conscious decisions. It is the seat of our moment-to-moment emotional reactivity. Pert (1999) explains that this part of the brain does not fully develop until the early twenties in humans, which might explain unsocial behaviors of youth.

The two hemispheres of the cortex are not connected at birth and therefore undergo concurrent development. At about age one, the corpus callosum begins to provide a communication link between the two hemispheres, and specialization begins to occur in each (see **Figure 5.2**). Before the development of the corpus callosum is completed (somewhere around age four), the two hemispheres communicate only with their respective parts of the lower brains. Once the corpus callosum is developed, the hemispheres can communicate freely without any input from the physical and emotional brain functions, making it possible for us to think and plan without emotional and physical interference. This ability has created the double-edged sword of being able to think and create on a very high plane but without compassion for the physical body, for our emotions, or for human relationships and ethics.

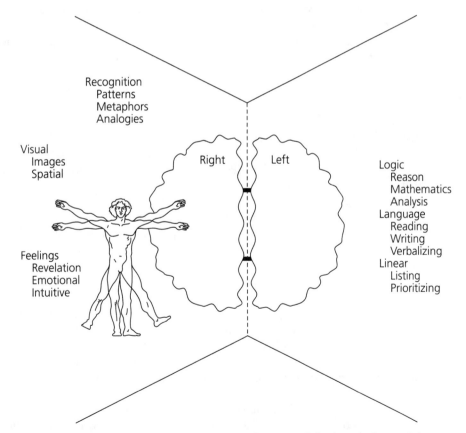

Figure 5.2 Right- and Left-Brain Functions (in most right-handed people)

A very important aspect of emotional health rides on the lines of communication among the three parts of the brain. The physical and emotional brains communicate in both directions, showing the constant synchrony of these two areas. There is also strong bidirectional communication, although not as complete a synchrony, between the emotional brain and the right hemisphere of the cortex. However, that same bidirectionality is not seen between the emotional brain and the left hemisphere of the cortex; in fact, it appears that the two are only casually connected. Therefore, the lower-brain nerve signals that *do* reach the left hemisphere must travel through the right hemisphere and across the corpus callosum (Pearce 1985).

In other words, the emotional brain is in close neural communication with the functions of the right hemisphere but not with the functions of the left hemisphere. In a culture that rewards left-brain functions very highly, it is likely that emotional messages are not necessarily received, recognized, nor communicated by the rational left hemisphere. The right hemisphere of the brain cannot write or speak, so it must send emotional messages via the body (i.e., physical signs and symptoms) or consciously try to figure out what a particular emotional situation means.

By understanding the original nature and development of these three parts of the brain, which in current terminology are the **thalamus, hypothalamus,** and **brain stem** (the physical brain); the **limbic system** (the emotional brain); and the **cortex** (the thinking brain), we are afforded insight into the neural connections of mind-body disease (Wallenstein 2003). With the acceptance of neural plasticity (that the brain changes through experience), we know that chronic emotional states actually change the structure of the brain (Siegel 1999).

Beyond the neural connections, the neuropeptide system is also at work. These peptides are important keys to the understanding of emotion in that their receptors are found in extremely high concentration not only in the hippocampus, amygdala, and hypothalamus but also throughout the autonomic nervous system, in nerve ganglia on either side of the spine, in internal organs, on the surface of the skin, in the dorsal horn of the spinal cord (which is the first synapse where all somatic-sensory information is processed), and in other locations (Pert 1999). With this information, it no longer holds that the emotional brain is housed only in the limbic system and hypothalamus.

According to Pearce (1985), during the first year of life, babies develop and use primarily the physical brain to sense and respond to their world. At about age two, the emotional brain centers begin to develop. The physical brain still receives all the outside messages, but the emotional linkage now begins coloring the information with "like" and "dislike" immediately upon receipt of the information from the physical brain. With the development of emotional learning, the child becomes not only a physical self but also an emotional self, relating outside events with feelings of joy and laughter, fear and crying, love and happiness. These actions take on a stimulus-response form as memory patterns develop. For example, a child may form a negative emotional memory pattern from being left with a sitter when the parents go out. After the first traumatic time, the child may begin to cry whenever either parent merely prepares to leave. In fact, the child's reaction to early separations from the parents becomes the basis for his or her reaction to all separations and losses later on in life.

As growth and development continue, the functions of the neocortex are added to the functions of the midbrain and old brain. This makes it possible for the child to just think about the parents leaving him or her alone, which elicits the emotional habit form of fear, anger, and even rage. In this instance nothing external or physical has actually happened, such as the parents preparing to leave, calling a sitter, or telling the child that they plan to go out. Because the child can now think in "what if" terms, any emotional pattern with an experiential base can be voluntarily brought back. Accompanying this pattern may be subconscious beliefs such as "They must not love me, or they wouldn't go away without me," and an even more basic belief, "I must be an unlovable person" or "I must be a bad person." Unless these beliefs and thought forms are changed, they are carried into adulthood and used as a belief in other negative emotional experiences. It is not difficult to imagine how traumatic real abandonment or abuse can be and what long-term risk factors can develop. Individuals tend to block emotional memories of childhood traumatic experiences, and when emotional energy is blocked, the mind loses its full capacity to analyze, evaluate, and synthesize situations and experiences (Viscott 1997). When negative emotions are blocked, the mind cannot integrate the experience, and what is more, the blocked emotional energy continues to build with new experiences that resemble the original traumatic experience. This further diminishes the mind's ability to function clearly, and behavior in response to the new stimulus becomes less logical because it is based on an old experience that probably happened when the child was not old enough, powerful enough, or skilled enough to do anything about the situation.

Because emotional patterns learned in response to actual physical stimuli are stored in the mind and body, they can later be stimulated by merely thinking about them or by having a certain part of the body stimulated. Neurolinguistic Programming, a system of communication that professes a neurological response with every word we know, would explain this as an "anchor." Through the ability to relive stressful situations, people learn how to scare themselves to death, worry themselves into an anxiety attack, and catastrophize even the most harmless situation. By the same token, however, people can retrieve pleasure, joy, love, and happiness by thinking about times when they felt those emotions. More important to the study of stress management, we know that changing one's permanent outlook to one of joy, pleasure, and happiness actually changes the structure of the brain in health-enhancing ways.

Richard Lazarus (1998), a leader in research concerning emotional stress, noted several decades ago that we should speak less of stress and more of emotion because stress primarily concerns destructive personal-environmental relationships that stimulate and perpetuate negative states such as fear, anger, jealousy, and shame that fall under the heading of emotion. Slaski and Cartwright (2002) add that we usually define stress in terms of emotional experiences—when asked to tell about their stress, most people relate their "feelings" of stress as fear, anger, guilt, shame, and so on.

Current researchers of emotional stress think that the emotional aspects of life play a more important, and perhaps the most important, role in the study of stress (Ekman 2003). One of the more recent developments of research in this area has been the concept of emotional intelligence and emotional quotient.

Pain and Pleasure

Broken down to basic physiology, initial emotions arouse only two feelings: pain and pleasure. Psychiatrist David Viscott (1992, 1997) reduces the emotional complexity of young and old alike to a single process that is repeated time and time again in everyone's life. The process begins in the present where only pain or pleasure are felt. These are the immediate unconscious emotional responses at the amygdala level. As we live with and process these basic emotions, we turn them into feelings such as guilt, anger, and depression, all of which are centered in the past. The following is a progression that is important to recognize and then combat if you do not wish to live with emotional stress:

Pain in the present is experienced as hurt. If released here, it goes no further.

If held, the pain of the past is remembered as anger.

Pain created by thoughts of the future is perceived as anxiety.

Unexpressed anger redirected against one's self and held inside is called guilt.

Anger directed inwardly toward one's self creates depression.

The main insight from Viscott's work is that much of our stress and distress comes from stored hurt, which disguises itself as anger, anxiety, guilt, and depression and manifests itself as behavioral patterns. Look under depression and you will find anger. Look under guilt and you will find anger. Look under anger and you will find hurt and sadness. Look under hurt and sadness and you will find fear—what you have been hiding all along.

Self-Assessment   EXERCISE 1

Place your answer to each of the following questions in the space provided before each number.

_____ **1.** I know when something is emotionally upsetting me.
 a. almost always   c. seldom
 b. often   d. almost never

_____ **2.** My choices are strongly colored by my emotions.
 a. almost always   c. seldom
 b. often   d. almost never

_____ **3.** When anger or depression strikes, it overwhelms me.
 a. almost always   c. seldom
 b. often   d. almost never

_____ **4.** When I'm angry, everyone around me pays for it.
 a. almost always   c. seldom
 b. often   d. almost never

_____ **5.** I have the ability to wait long periods of time to get what I want.
 a. almost always   c. seldom
 b. often   d. almost never

_____ **6.** I experience test anxiety.
 a. almost always   c. seldom
 b. often   d. almost never

_____ **7.** Setbacks don't keep me down for long or keep me from doing my job.
 a. almost always   c. seldom
 b. often   d. almost never

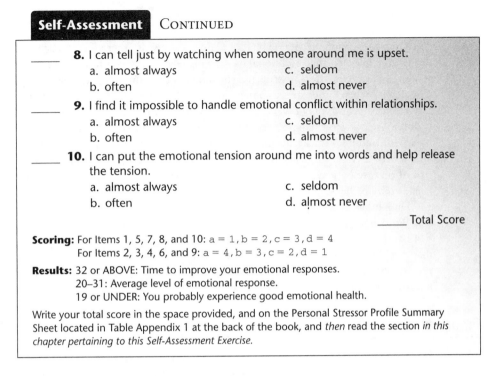

_____   **8.** I can tell just by watching when someone around me is upset.
    a. almost always   c. seldom
    b. often   d. almost never

_____   **9.** I find it impossible to handle emotional conflict within relationships.
    a. almost always   c. seldom
    b. often   d. almost never

_____   **10.** I can put the emotional tension around me into words and help release the tension.
    a. almost always   c. seldom
    b. often   d. almost never

_____ Total Score

Scoring: For Items 1, 5, 7, 8, and 10: a = 1, b = 2, c = 3, d = 4
For Items 2, 3, 4, 6, and 9: a = 4, b = 3, c = 2, d = 1

Results: 32 or ABOVE: Time to improve your emotional responses.
20–31: Average level of emotional response.
19 or UNDER: You probably experience good emotional health.

Write your total score in the space provided, and on the Personal Stressor Profile Summary Sheet located in Table Appendix 1 at the back of the book, and *then* read the section *in this chapter pertaining to this Self-Assessment Exercise.*

Yale psychologist Peter Salovey (Salovey and Mayer 1990) proposed the concept of "emotional quotient" in the early 1990s, and Dan Goleman (2006a, 2006b) subsequently popularized the topic in an effort to help people understand the role that emotion plays in successful interactions with others. He pointed out that an individual may have a high intelligence quotient, yet be emotionally inept. The emotionally inept suffer poor interpersonal relationships, whether at home, work, or school.

Goleman found five basics that are involved in emotional intelligence: (1) self-awareness: being aware of what you feel and using inner knowing to make skillful decisions; (2) self-management: being able to control anxiety and impulses and to use anger appropriately; (3) self-motivation: using inner zeal and optimism when setbacks occur; (4) empathy: being able to recognize unspoken emotional states in others and being able to respond in a compassionate way; and (5) interpersonal skills: skillfully interacting with and handling emotional reactions of others.

Women and Men React Differently

In the stress management world, it has now become apparent that men and women react to stress differently, not just through learned behavior but also through basic physiological nature. A landmark UCLA study (Taylor et al. 2000) identified that women respond to stress with certain brain chemicals that cause women to "tend and befriend" other women. Until this study was published, it was generally believed that when people experience stress, they react with the fight-or-flight syndrome. Period. Now it seems that women have another choice, the lifesaving option of banding together for mutual support.

When the hormone oxytocin (a hormone instrumental to birth and lactation processes) is released as part of the stress response in a woman, it affects the fight-or-flight response, encouraging the woman to tend children and gather with other women instead of running or fighting. In doing this, additional oxytocin is released, which further counters stress and produces a calming effect. Estrogen also enhances the calming. Men release high levels of testosterone when under stress, so they don't get the calming response of oxytocin.

Future research may reveal more ways that oxytocin encourages women to care for children and develop female friendships, but the "tend and befriend" notion developed by Taylor and her colleagues may explain why women consistently outlive men. Study after study cited by Taylor and her colleagues has found that social ties reduce women's risk of disease by lowering blood pressure, heart rate, and cholesterol. Having female friends may be helping women live longer.

Dr. Ruthellen Josselson, coauthor of *Best Friends: The Pleasures and Perils of Girls' and Women's Friendships* (1999), laments that it seems that when women get busy with work and family, the first thing they do is let go of friendships with other women. She feels that this is a grievous mistake because women are such a source of emotional strength to each other. They need to have unpressured space in which they can have the special kind of talk that women experience with each other, thus relieving emotional stress.

Emotional Energy

Deepak Chopra (1998) explains emotional energy with the most dynamic of new sciences—quantum physics—and also through ancient Indian spiritual philosophy. Chopra makes a convincing case that we all exist in a common field of intelligence in which solid material structure, time, and space are merely concepts. Further, the body is a field of intelligence, or mind, that has produced a physical body through thought. When a thought occurs, the message is known to all parts of the body—every cell—simultaneously. All parts of the body then produce the hormone(s) responsive to the particular thought. When an individual thinks of an experience as exhilarating, all cells respond with the physical (neuropeptide) correlate of exhilaration. When the thought response to a situation is depression, the entire body hormonally expresses depression. Thoughts produce emotion; emotion produces thoughts.

Emotional energy carries messages that each individual names fear, anger, and so forth on the basis of experience. Lazarus (1998) observes that regardless of whether there is a label or a universally correct word for an emotion, all of us have had the following emotional experiences:

1. anger
2. anxiety
3. sadness
4. guilt
5. shame
6. envy
7. jealousy
8. disgust
9. hope
10. pride
11. gratitude
12. happiness
13. love
14. compassion

These experiences are stored in the mind-body in the form of memory patterns, and when the body is triggered, it responds with a pattern. To illustrate, take a moment to gasp as though surprised or frightened. The body instantaneously braces itself. Muscles contract, the lungs and heart modify their action, and if taken to great extent, this "as if" situation can cause all the systems involved in this emotion to alter their functions. Through nerve stimulation, the muscles tense, the heart beats faster and/or harder, respiration quickens and/or deepens, the pupils dilate, and glands are stimulated to either reduce or increase their secretions, depending on the function of the gland. The adrenals are stimulated and begin dumping out hormones to help answer the emergency signals that have been given at the brain level. The emergency signal is the perception of a situation that demands attention. It may be a situation wherein joy or humor is perceived, or the signal may be perceived as danger. Also, it may have its roots in the external world or within a thought pattern that has little external base. The response to the emergency signal is the emotional reaction pattern, or—as we first identified it in this book— the stress response.

Emotions such as anger, fear, happiness, and jealousy are expressed more actively than guilt, background anxiety, or contentment; yet all of them have a total-body response pattern. Pert (1999, 2006) explains that all emotions have a neurological-hormonal profile and that we can categorize emotional response patterns as either healthy or unhealthy by their impact on the immune system. Furthermore, each person's learning experience and cognitive control may help to place all of his or her emotions in the healthy category through recognition, restructuring the meaning of the emotion, and letting go of an "unhealthy" emotion once the associated emotional experience is over (Bradshaw 2005).

If the emotion you experience is positive, tension builds and then is released as perhaps a shout or laughter. Pleasure is felt with the release of emotional tension. When the emotion is negative, tension builds up and tends to be stored. Usually, during this time, negative self-talk increases the tension. Pain is caused by extreme and unrelieved tension.

Emotional messages do not dissipate until they are delivered, and delivery means that the message is recognized and allowed to play itself out. When blocked-up emotional energy is released, certain body aches and pains may also go away.

Stressful Emotional Patterns

At a very early age, little girls and boys learn that very few emotions are acceptable (Ekman 2003). At first, laughter and giggling are usually highly prized by adults, but as children grow into adolescence, they quickly learn that loud laughter and silly giggling are not acceptable in public. Children are rewarded for not crying, reprimanded harshly for displaying anger, and chided for being fearful. They are asked to not show that they have been emotionally hurt, to be selective about whom they should love, and to contain their exuberance. Thus, it is no wonder that most adults engage in negative mind-talk when they get angry, are hurt or fearful, or even want to shriek in happiness and joy.

Because of the years of negative mind-talk that accompany emotions, everyone denies negative emotions to some degree or another. When a person gets angry and says, "This is really silly to get mad," the emotion is not honored. But it happens anyway.

And it is stored in a favorite place (or places) in the body, with all the other anger that has been denied and not released. Release of an emotion is necessary before the body can go back to a relaxed state, or back into balance. Most people know the effectiveness of a good laugh or cry as a release to make them feel better.

Bradshaw (2005) points out that dysfunctional families deny their children the right to feel or to talk about feelings. This keeps the children from being in touch with what they are feeling because, first of all, they are shamed out of expressing any feelings and, second, they aren't allowed to talk about their feelings. In some families, children are allowed to express only certain emotions, such as guilt. This early learning forms the child's emotional quotient.

Mind and Life Conference on Destructive Emotions

Recently Western science and Eastern philosophy met when the Mind and Life Institute sponsored a retreat that studied the topic of destructive emotions. A number of important new neuroscientific findings about human emotions and how they relate to stress and the alleviation of it were uncovered (Goleman 2004). Several findings pertinent to the management of stressful emotions, thoughts, and beliefs follow:

1. In their study of emotions, Davidson and his colleagues at the University of Wisconsin (2000) have found dramatic increases in key electrical activity in the left middle frontal gyrus, a zone of the brain previous research had pinpointed as a locus for positive emotions. When people have high levels of this brain activity in that specific site of the left prefrontal cortex, they report feelings such as happiness, enthusiasm, high energy, and alertness.

   They also found that high levels of activity in a parallel site on the other side of the brain—in the right prefrontal area—correlate with reports of distressing emotion. People with a higher activity in the right prefrontal site and a lower level in the left are more prone to feelings such as sadness, anxiety, and worry. An extreme ratio of right-to-left activity in these prefrontal areas predicts a high likelihood of clinical depression or an anxiety disorder.

   The balance between right and left activity might be termed one's "emotional set point," what we have referred to earlier in this text as emotional reactivity.

2. The phenomenon of neuroplasticity has been confirmed. The brain, through fresh connections between neurons or through the generation of new neurons, changes through experience. This is meaningful to the discussion of stress management because we now know that practicing constructive emotions enhances the positive emotion portion of the brain. This points to the use of meditation, positive imagery, and other stress management techniques to actually modify the brain to create a greater peace and happiness in life. However, Goleman (2004) cautiously points out that the possibility of freeing the mind completely from the hold of destructive emotions surpasses any assumptions of modern psychology.

3. The destructive states of mind, according to Wallace (1998), include low self-esteem, overconfidence, harboring negative emotions, jealousy and envy, lack of compassion, and inability to have close interpersonal relations. Wallace points out that these can be boiled down to hatred, desire, confusion, pride, and jealousy or to the "three poisons"

of Buddhism: anger, craving, and delusions. These are the destructive emotions that bring stress into our lives. Their antidotes are the constructive states of mind:

Self-respect	Compassion
Self-esteem (to the extent deserved)	Benevolence
Feelings of integrity	Generosity
Seeing the true, the good, and	Love
the right	Friendship

4. Recognizing triggers of destructive emotions and then applying appropriate antidotes (e.g., compassion applied to anger) become a universal stress management technique. The ultimate step for individuals is to see if they can find one antidote for all their negative emotions. Many find that antidote to be compassion. When practiced diligently, it changes the brain, the mind, and the body.

Breaking Unhealthy Emotional Cycles

Because most negative emotional responses are old, habitual responses to perceived dangers, people can learn to break those patterns in various ways. One is by relaxing. Movement of energy occurs in the body as it carries out an emotion. The instantaneous constriction of muscles becomes such a part of the emotional response that the physical reaction to stress cannot occur if the muscles will not respond. Therefore, one way to break the emotional stress response is to RELAX. A time-honored, efficient, and effective way to relax in any situation is to do deep, diaphragmatic breathing. Chapter 12 describes the use of breathing exercises as a method of general relaxation.

Another way to break old negative emotional-response patterns is to act on them as soon as you notice that you are thinking negative thoughts or saying negative things to yourself. At that time, tell yourself, "Stop it!" Then, after noting your negative thinking pattern, replace it with relaxation and/or positive thoughts, or just focus on and enjoy what you are doing and experiencing at the present time (Dusek and Girdano 1995).

As you are learning how to break negative emotional-response patterns, those patterns will still occur. However, it is healthy to experience the patterns, honor them, and learn to release the tension that could otherwise lead to poor health. If the emotional energy is not released, disease or behavioral symptoms will occur. The following exercise gives explicit directions for turning unhealthy emotional responses into healthy ones:

1. Allow yourself to focus on the emotion; really focus on how it feels.

2. Ride out the unpleasant feeling, allowing it to vibrate throughout the body, even if it appears as physical symptoms.

3. Assist the process by finding the thought form that is blocking you. Test thoughts and phrases that come to you to determine whether they are the cause. Sample phrases might be: "I am scared," "I am lonely," "Quit picking on me!" "I give up," "No, No, No!" Scan your body for the feelings that come up with each one of the statements.

4. When you discover the restricting thought, change it into a new, productive one, such as "I can work through this," "I am happy to spend some time with myself," "There is nothing to fear."

5. Continue to work on using the old thought form less and less as the new thought form is patterned by use. Imagine making a new path through the grass and letting the old one you used to take grow over. If you do not change the causal situation (the old, negative thought form), any symptom relief is temporary.

6. Write your experience as a journal entry.

Thoughts and Beliefs

Once we have recognized an emotional pattern, we can learn from it something about our basic attitudes and opinions in life. An emotional response to a situation is always produced by a belief, attitude, or opinion. Most of the time we are not aware of the thought pattern because the reaction is a habit, not a well-thought-out response.

Thoughts

Our states of health, physical development, coping behaviors, moods, feelings, emotional response, and level of stress are all expressions of our thoughts. They are also subject to alteration by a change in thoughts (Goleman 2004, 2006a, 2006b). Our thinking or belief system can be the ultimate control system in our lives. The conscious mind attempts to control our stress by controlling our actions and behaviors. Control is the way we function to get our needs met. When the mind focuses on some goal, our thoughts can control and manipulate our world (including our unconscious mind) until the goal is achieved.

If we do not wish to display our emotions, we can suppress them with the mind. The left hemisphere of the brain has the ability to bypass feeling input, and we learn to do that well when there are negative consequences of emotional feelings. If the body cannot be controlled by covering up symptoms (such as by wearing deodorants or taking drugs), the conscious mind can choose to ignore the symptoms up to a point of endangering health. On the positive side, the thought system can change stressful situations into controlled ones. When people are depressed or unhappy, they can choose to do activities they did when they felt good, and this activity is likely to make them feel better (Glasser 1994, 1999).

Thoughts allow us to anticipate a situation, assume a defensive posture, and increase background arousal if necessary. In a situation of prolonged stress arousal, thinking efficiency may be decreased due to overload. What you believe dictates how you will react to a stressor and what you will experience from the situation. Control is maintained by taking small steps that do not exceed your ability to cope.

Small steps may mean engaging in new behaviors that you can manage. Large steps, in the form of behaviors that challenge deep beliefs, usually force individuals beyond their normal ability to cope. At this point, recruitment occurs. Recruitment is the use of negative maladaptive behaviors—for example, ego defense, rationalization, withdrawal, and illness—as helpers in the attempt to cope. Attempts at controlling stress in these times of overload usually result in what is known as incompetent coping. When one feels out of control, it is usually the result of too much input demanding too many responses (Colbert 2003).

Thus far, we have noted that the physical body is aroused by emotions. Emotions may be thought of as the "middle man" between the body cells and the mind. In the final analysis, most causes of stress stem from the thought process, how we perceive our world. Patent (1998) points out that we have 50,000 or more thoughts a day (most of them being the same ones we had the day before) and that the majority of our thoughts are in the form of beliefs, which are necessary to interpret the world around us.

Mind- or thought-control approaches to stress management range from the more spiritual/religious system of Scientology to the more current and popular "Secret" system (Byrne 2007). They provide step-by-step guides to identifying the current uncomfortable situation, what it is that the individual is aiming at both short- and long-term, and then methodologies to change thoughts, beliefs, and behaviors to get to their desired goal(s). Between these two mentioned systems are myriad proscribed procedures for using the mind to identify irrational thoughts and beliefs. For example, Albert Ellis's (2006) Rational Emotive Therapy is based on his belief that: (1) both rational and irrational beliefs determine how people respond to events, (2) thoughts cause us to feel, (3) thoughts can be old and go unchallenged, (4) thoughts and beliefs are accessible to conscious reflection, and (5) people have the ability to choose to work at achieving happiness. His ABC Model of Emotional Reaction contends that when a person has a self-defeating negative feeling (C) about an activating event (A) that blocks a goal, a person usually holds a dysfunctional or irrational belief (B). His system then proceeds to help his clients find the thoughts that are harassing them and set them up as hypotheses to be tested. When clients strenuously question the validity of their irrational hypotheses, they find that the thoughts behind their inappropriate emotions do not conform to reality, are self-defeating, and merit change of mind, change of belief, change in behavior.

Beliefs

Beliefs are enduring patterns of thought. Most beliefs are learned early in life from parents, relatives, peers, and authority figures. The beliefs that are accepted from others and formed on our own become the programs that determine behavior on emotional, mental, physical, and spiritual levels. A true belief is a nonconflicted, solid idea that governs our day-to-day thoughts and actions. The beliefs that people hold about themselves and about life in general are the foundations on which they base all their behavior. Beliefs provide a framework through which experience is measured, analyzed, and evaluated, and that determines the response to experience. As such, they provide a sense of security even when an experience is negative.

If information about reality is not consciously rejected by the mind or if it does not directly conflict with existing beliefs, then an individual accepts it as true. Virtually all humans, no matter how they are raised, have an innate tendency to take their strong desires and preferences and construct them into "musts"; and therefore have an inborn propensity to needlessly upset themselves.

Once incorporated as a belief, it is generally forgotten even though it continues to operate. This does not mean that beliefs are lost to conscious awareness, only that the mind no longer pays attention to them most of the time. It is something like having money in the bank. Even though you may not be using it right now, it influences how you live and affects many of your decisions. In the case of beliefs, they become such a familiar way of interpreting the world that they are completely taken for granted.

The self-image is an example of a belief, a base, or a foundation upon which an individual's entire personality and behavior (and eventually their reaction to stressors) are built. (Chapter 6 explains self-concept in depth). For example, if the self-image is strong and positive, day-to-day experiences will seem to verify, and thereby strengthen, the self-image. If the self-image is weak or negative, day-to-day experiences will seem to verify that and thereby weaken the self-image. People with a strong belief in self have what some call an "internal locus of control" and are likely to meet life in an unconflicted manner. Conversely, people who are lacking in belief of self will have a more external locus of control, which sets them up for conflict and stress.

Beliefs act as guidance systems for the flow of life. Where there is conflict, the flow is distorted, and this distortion may lead to acute or chronic tension, often expressed on the muscular, organ, or cellular level. Such tension can lead to pain and illness, and this is the basis for the mind-body philosophy. Some experts in the field believe that the source of all illness is in conflicting personal beliefs, ideas, and actions.

Milton Erickson, the famous hypnotherapist and behavior-change artist, believed that every person has his or her own unique map of the world, an inner belief system that is unconscious and constitutes a kind of hypnotic trance (Erickson and Rossi 1980). It is as though we go through life with a posthypnotic suggestion that we act in a certain way to certain stimuli. It is the "inner child" who forms this core belief system. Core material, according to Kurtz (1997), is the way our internal experience is organized. It is composed of our earliest feelings, beliefs, and memories that are made in response to the stresses of our childhood environment. This core material is nonlogical and primitive; it was the only way a child knew how to survive. Once these core beliefs, feelings, and memories are formed, they become the basis of future responses.

Deepak Chopra (1998) explains this concept in another way, using the term "premature cognitive commitment." He notes that the brain and body form an early response to an object/situation and that response is embedded there. It becomes an actual neurophysiological pattern. All future experiences in any specific area are based on this premature cognitive commitment.

Two examples given by Chopra in his book, *Ageless Body, Timeless Mind* (1998), are the following:

1. When newly hatched fish are placed in an aquarium that has been separated down the middle by a Plexiglas divider, the fish learn to stay on their own side of the divider. When the divider is removed, the fish still stay on their side of the aquarium.

2. One litter of newborn kittens was reared in a "vertical" environment—all the objects and lines in their space were vertical. Another litter was reared in a "horizontal" world—all the objects and lines in their space were horizontal. When the kittens grew to adulthood and were placed in the opposite environment, they actually could not see physical barriers that were different from those where they were reared. That is to say, kittens from the "horizontal" world ran into the vertical legs of chairs and tables. Even though there was nothing wrong with their sight, these animals had given premature cognitive commitment to their early environment.

Abraham Maslow (1999) is probably best known for developing a hierarchy of motivation and the developmental progression of human needs, growth, and potential. The lower-level human needs, starting with the most basic and moving upward, include:

1. physical: fulfillment of basic physical needs

2. safety: need to feel secure and protected

3. love: the ability to love and be loved, and to belong and be accepted

4. self-reliance, dignity, and respect

5. self-actualization and fulfillment of personal growth and development.

What motivates the child in early infancy are the first rungs on Maslow's motivational hierarchy: getting physical needs (such as hunger) met and feeling safe and secure. In order to do that, the baby is at the mercy of the older people in its environment. It must meet the demands and adapt to the reality of significant others. In computer language, this becomes the hardwiring of the individual (Maslow 1968). Since these needs are hierarchically arranged, the individual must satisfy lower needs in order to achieve satisfaction of higher needs.

At the core of our being is the basic belief structure that has guided our thoughts and actions throughout our lives. Positive changes must be made at this level so that they reflect a change in our perceptions and, in turn, the way our bodies react to the mental and emotional input. In order to use beliefs and thoughts to change an emotional reaction, we must perform five basic operations:

1. Recognize and honor the emotion rather than deny, repress, rationalize, or otherwise not honor it.

2. Identify the negative thought complex that is behind the negative emotion. Every stressful situation in life has an old, outdated, negative belief behind it. That belief was formed when it was useful. In adulthood, it is no longer so.

3. Break the habitual loop that the emotion triggers.

4. Replace the negative thought complex with a new, positive thought complex.

5. Respond to situations from the new belief complex.

SUMMARY

It is impossible to separate emotion from thought from belief. Every interaction has an immediate, subconscious emotional subtext. Emotion drives everything else: hence the word, "e-motion," put energy into motion. If you were to outline the procedure, it might look like this:

1. An interaction (novel input) occurs.

2. The amygdala, in nanoseconds, scans for danger (fear arouses it the most).

3. The amygdala commandeers key parts of the brain to respond immediately.

4. The amygdala then connects with other points in the brain that direct thoughts, attention, and perception toward the novel input.

What this iterates from earlier chapters is that before thoughts, speech, or behaviors occur, the subconscious mind has registered emotion. Emotional feelings have no voice, so the body just incorporates the feeling. Conscious effort is necessary to get to the meaning of the feelings.

Since people usually describe stress in terms of emotional experiences (such as burnout, jealousy, anger, or fear), the study of emotion is an important part of stress management. Consider the following points:

- Emotions are reactions to internal needs and external stimuli, which in turn prompt action.
- Emotion can be consciously denied, leaving the unconscious mind to resolve the stress—oftentimes resulting in disease or debilitation.
- Emotional response patterns are stored in the brain and other cells throughout the body, all of which communicate with each other.
- Although humans share common emotional experiences (such as anger, fear, and love), individual emotional responses are learned and unique to each person.
- Emotions are categorized as healthy or unhealthy by their impact on the immune system.
- Stressful emotional patterns can be broken.
- Thoughts can change stressful emotional situations into controlled ones.
- Beliefs are the foundations of thoughts, emotions, and behavior.
- Destructive emotions such as anger and fear can be alleviated with meditation and other relaxation techniques.
- Emotions don't just happen. They are the direct result of the way we choose to look at ourselves and the world around us.

SOURCES CITED

Barnes P. M., Powell-Griner, E., McFann, K., and Nahin, R. L. (2005). Complementary and alternative medicine use among adults: United States, *CDC Advance Data Report #343*.

Bradshaw, J. (2005). *Healing the shame that binds you.* Deerfield Beach, FL: HCI.

Chopra, D. (1998). *Ageless body, timeless mind: The quantum alternative to growing old.* New York: Three Rivers Press.

Colbert, D. (2003). *Deadly emotions.* New York: Thomas Nelson.

Davidson, R. J., Jackson, D. C., and Kalin, N. H. (2000). Emotion, plasticity, context, and regulation: Perspectives from affective neuroscience. *Psychological Bulletin, 126,* no. 6, 890–906.

Dusek, D., and Girdano, D. (1995). *Emotional risk factors.* Winter Park, CO: Paradox.

Ekman, P. (2003). *Emotions revealed.* New York: Times Books/Henry Holt.

Ellis, A. (2006). *How to stubbornly refuse to make yourself miserable about anything.* Capetown, South Africa: Citadel Press.

Erickson, M. H., and Rossi, E. (1980). *Hypnotic investigation on psychodynamic processes.* New York: Irvington.

Glasser, W. (1994). *Control theory manager.* New York: Harper & Row.

Glasser, W. (1999). *Choice theory: A new psychology of personal freedom.* San Francisco: HarperCollins.

Goleman, D. (2004). *Destructive emotions.* New York: Bantam.

Goleman, D. (2006a). *Emotional intelligence.* New York: Bantam.

Goleman, D. (2006b). *Social intelligence.* New York: Bantam.

Josselson, R., and Apter, T. (1999). *Best friends: The pleasures and perils of girls' and women's friendships.* New York: Crown.

Kosten, T. R., et al. (2006). Cue-induced brain activity changes and relapse in cocaine-dependent patients. *Neuropsychopharmacology,* 31, no. 3, 644–650.

Kurtz, R. (1997). *Body-centered psychotherapy: The Haikomi method.* Mendocino, CA: LifeRhythms.

Lazarus, R. (1998). *50 years of the research and history of R. S. Lazarus.* Mahwah, NJ: Lawrence Erlbaum.

MacLean, P. D. (1990). *The triune brain in evolution: Role in paleocerebral functions.* New York: Plenum.

Manstead, A., Frijda, N., and Fischer, A. (eds.) (2003). *Feelings and emotions: The Amsterdam Symposium.* Cambridge: Cambridge University Press.

Maslow, A. (1968). *Toward a psychology of being.* New York: Van Nostrand Reinhold.

Maslow, A. (1999). *Toward a psychology of being,* 3rd ed. New York: Wiley and Sons, Inc.

McClain, C. S., Rosenfeld, B., and Breitbart, W. (2003). Effect of spiritual well-being on end-of-life despair in terminally-ill cancer patients. *Lancet,* 361, no. 9369, 1603–1607.

Patent, A. (1998). *Bridges to reality.* New York: Celebration Publishers.

Pearce, J. B. (1985). *The magical child matures.* New York: Bantam.

Pearce, J. B. (1994). *Magical child, magical adult.* New York: Sound Horizons.

Pert, C. (2004). *Your body is your subconscious mind.* Audio CD. Boulder, CO: Sounds True.

Pert, C. (1999). *Molecules of emotion: Why you feel the way you feel.* New York: Simon & Schuster.

Salovey, P., and Mayer, J. D. (1990). Emotional intelligence. *Imagination, Cognition, and Personality,* 9, 185–211.

Siegel, D. (1999). *The developing mind: How relationships and the brain interact to shape who we are.* New York: Guilford Press.

Slaski, M., and Cartwright, S. (2002). Health, performance, and emotional intelligence. *Stress and Health,* 18, 63–68.

Taylor, S. E., et al. (2000). Female responses to stress: Tend and befriend, not fight or flight. *Psychological Review,* 107, no. 3, 410–29.

Viscott, D. (1992). *Emotionally free.* Chicago: Contemporary Books.

Viscott, D. (1997). *Emotional resilience: Simple truths for dealing with the unfinished business of your past.* New York: Crown.

Viscott, D. (2003). *Finding your strength in difficult times.* New York: McGraw-Hill.

Wallace, A. (1998). *The bridge of quiescence: Experiencing Tibetan Buddhist meditation.* Chicago: Open Court.

Wallenstein, G. (2003). *Mind, stress, and emotions.* New York: Commonwealth Press.

Whitten, L. (2007). Cocaine abusers' pretreatment cue responses predict recovery success. *NIDA Notes,* 21, no. 2, 7–8.

Journal Entry 4

Expressing Emotion

We noted in this chapter that pain in the present is experienced as hurt (Viscott 1997). If hurt is released here, it goes no further; but if allowed to fester, it can turn by degree into anger, anxiety, guilt, and depression. Realize that hurt is a basic negative feeling. You cannot be in the present without the willingness to feel hurt. Be with your sensations. Resist the impulse either to deny what you feel or to turn it into anger.

Work through this journal exercise to find where hurt has been positive and/or negative in your life.

 1. Write down an instance when you think that hurt can be positive:

 2. Give an example of an experience in your life where you let hurt become anger.

 3. Write down here what could you have said in this situation (#2) that would have allowed you to resolve your emotion and move on? Remember, "I feel hurt" doesn't mean that someone was meant to hurt you. There's always another side to the story, despite the hurt you felt.

 4a. Write down an instance when you were on the other side of a "hurt" situation; that is, when you felt that someone's feelings were hurt by what you did or said. Did you feel caught up in your own motives without thinking about the other person? Did you give any more importance to the other person's hurt than you felt was given to yours (as in #2)? Explain.

4b. This incident can help you if you want to find out the kinds of things that create threat in you. See this as an opportunity to take responsibility for your feelings. That makes it easier to forgive, since anyone who teaches you something about yourself deserves your thanks. Write a brief paragraph about forgiveness.

5. Write a positive word or short phrase about recognizing anger or fear that will be useful to you in future situations.

6

Patterns of Behavior

"A man's fate is his character," said the famous philosopher Heraclitus. The study of character styles, that is, the study of personal behavior choices, offers some order and congruence to all the different kinds of stressful behavior in which the individual engages.

One's response to stress is clearly affected by one's behavioral habits. Character styles and behavioral habits, both stable and transient, are often referred to as personality and point to dispositions within a person that affect their ability to process and respond to stress (Contrata and Guyll 2001). The famous physician Sir William Osler once suggested that where malignant disease is concerned, it may be more important to understand what kind of patient has the disease rather than what kind of disease the patient has.

In this chapter, we examine how selected features of personal behavior, habits, skills, and choices interact with stress. The first part will consider the more stable character trait of self-concept and the effect on behavior and health. The second part will consider the behavioral habits and response patterns of anger/hostility, fear, and anxiety and how these relate to the need for control, and interact with stressors, stress, and symptoms of disease. Each section is preceded by a self-assessment exercise; complete each one before reading about the topic relating to it, and learn about yourself as you learn about behavior in general. Each section concludes with some effective stress management tools that have been reported in the literature.

Self-Concept

For many years, psychologists have been pointing to **self-concept**, or the way we perceive ourselves, as perhaps the single most influential factor in behavior. It would follow that self-perception plays an important role in stress and stress management, also. Simply put, the stronger the self-concept, the more resources a person can bring to bear to avoid stressful situations and respond to stress arousal.

Self-concept (how we think of ourselves) is constructed from beliefs of how we actually are, what we want to be, and what we think we ought to be. These beliefs evolve through personal observation and comparisons, and by accepting and believing what others tell us about ourselves. How we are treated by the significant people in our lives, especially in childhood, determines to a great extent how we feel about ourselves. The childhood environment that produces guilt, feelings of inferiority, learned helplessness, and self-consciousness diminishes the likelihood of developing a healthy self-concept.

Erik Erikson (1986), noted developmental psychologist, outlined eight stages of development (and subsequently expanded it to nine; see Erikson and Erikson 1997) that one must successfully complete in order to have a healthy self-concept. In looking at the positive learning and the lack of learning at each stage (as in Table 6.1), we can see the characteristics of the healthy and the unhealthy self-concept. Table 6.1 shows Erikson and Erikson's (1997) developmental stages, each building on the stage previous to it. Erikson has given each of the stages a name that describes the accomplishments or nonaccomplishment that a person may make at a given stage. Each stage is also assigned the age or ages at which this stage normally develops. Table 6.1 lists the expected results of positive learning and what the lack of learning results in at each stage.

Many adults are stuck in Stages 5, 6, or 7 (possibly from ages twelve to forty) and never reach Stage 9. Being stuck in Stages 5, 6, or 7 may derive from lack of completion of the very early stages. John Bradshaw's term "adult children" applies to those individuals who are stuck in an early stage of development (Bradshaw 1992). Adult children behave from childhood scripts rather than from more highly developed states of being.

People of any age can enhance their self-concept. An imperative thing about self-concept is that the individual is the only one who can increase the positive feelings that he or she has for self. Each of us can encourage, support, love, and help create a positive environment in which others may learn to love themselves, internalize their self-worth, know that they have impact in the world, and develop self-confidence and self-esteem. The final work of self-concept enhancement, however, has to be done by ourselves. Nobody can do it for us.

What is your image of yourself? Self-Assessment Exercise 2 was designed to provide some insight into your self-concept. If you scored from 10 to 19 points, you have a high self-concept. A score of 20–24 indicates an average self-concept. If you scored between 25 and 40, your self-concept appears to be in need of bolstering.

Components of Self-Concept

High self-concept is basic to all personal interactions. A healthy concept of self ensures confidence, worth, security, spontaneity, and other positive descriptors of the actualized person. Some use the terms *self-concept* and *self-esteem* interchangeably, but it would seem that total self-concept consists of many different components (including self-esteem), each necessary to complete the ideal self (Dusek and Girdano 1995). Six major components of self-concept—self-awareness, self-worth, self-love, self-esteem, self-confidence, and self-respect—are discussed here.

Self-Awareness Being self-aware is realizing that you have an impact in this world and that your presence and actions can and do influence others and vice versa. This does not mean that you are responsible for the reactions of others; they may choose to feel enhanced or

Table 6.1   Stages of Development (Erikson) and Self-Concept Characteristics

Stage 1:	Basic Trust versus Mistrust	Age: 1
	Positive Learning Results:	Trust, comfort, hope.
	Lack of Learning Results:	Mistrust, discomfort.
Stage 2:	Autonomy versus Shame and Doubt	Ages: 2–3
	Positive Learning Results:	Limits, willpower, separation, curiosity, exploration.
	Lack of Learning Results:	Fear of separation, shame, doubt.
Stage 3:	Initiative versus Guilt	Ages: 4–5
	Positive Learning Results:	Purpose and value, good feelings about self, healthy identity of being a boy or girl, imagination.
	Lack of Learning Results:	Feelings of guilt, being unacceptable, bad feelings about own sexuality.
Stage 4:	Industry versus Inferiority	Ages: 6–11
	Positive Learning Results:	Competence, self-boundaries, thinking, learning.
	Lack of Learning Results:	Feelings of failure, inferiority, and incompetence.
Stage 5:	Identity versus Role Confusion	Ages: 12–18
	Positive Learning Results:	Inner sense of self, uniqueness, faithful to another person or cause, sense of belonging, feeling of self.
	Lack of Learning Results:	Confusion, rebellion, lacks sense of belonging or having power of regeneration.
Stage 6:	Intimacy versus Isolation	Ages: 16–25
	Positive Learning Results:	Can love and receive love, can be close yet separate, intimacy with self and another.
	Lack of Learning Results:	Separate from others, isolated, not reassured of self by love from another, loss of self to others.
Stage 7:	Generativity versus Stagnation	Ages: 20–24
	Positive Learning Results:	Personal power to generate, create, or produce; committed to life; caring for others, society, planet.
	Lack of Learning Results:	Stagnation, feels life is boring, unexciting; feels incapable of caring for self, let alone family, neighbors, society, planet; lacks creativity.
Stage 8:	Ego Integrity versus Despair	Age 40 on
	Positive Learning Results:	Wisdom, accepts self completely and unconditionally, is one with all of life.
	Lack of Learning Results:	Has decided that life has been a waste, unmeaningful, and unproductive.
Stage 9:	Gerotranscendence	Age 70 on
	Positive Learning Results:	Acceptance of death, healthy withdrawal.
	Lack of Learning Results:	Nonacceptance of aging, disability, death.

Self-Assessment EXERCISE II

Choose the alternative that best summarizes how you generally behave, and place your answer in the space provided.

_____ **1.** When I face a difficult task, I try my best and usually succeed.
- a. almost always
- b. often
- c. seldom
- d. almost never

_____ **2.** I am at ease around members of the opposite sex.
- a. almost always
- b. often
- c. seldom
- d. almost never

_____ **3.** I feel that I have a lot going for me.
- a. almost always
- b. often
- c. seldom
- d. almost never

_____ **4.** I have a very high degree of confidence in my own abilities.
- a. almost always
- b. often
- c. seldom
- d. almost never

_____ **5.** I prefer to be in control of my own life as opposed to having someone else make decisions for me.
- a. almost always
- b. often
- c. seldom
- d. almost never

_____ **6.** I am comfortable and at ease around my superiors.
- a. almost always
- b. often
- c. seldom
- d. almost never

_____ **7.** I am often overly self-conscious or shy when among strangers.
- a. almost always
- b. often
- c. seldom
- d. almost never

_____ **8.** Whenever something goes wrong, I tend to blame myself.
- a. almost always
- b. often
- c. seldom
- d. almost never

_____ **9.** When I don't succeed, I tend to let it depress me more than it should.
- a. almost always
- b. often
- c. seldom
- d. almost never

_____ **10.** I often feel that I am beyond help.
- a. almost always
- b. often
- c. seldom
- d. almost never

_____Total Score

Scoring: Items 1 to 6: a = 1 point, b = 2 points, c = 3 points, d = 4 points
Items 7 to 10: a = 4 points, b = 3 points, c = 2 points, d = 1 point

Write your total score in the space provided, and on the Personal Stressor Profile Sumary Sheet located in Table Appendix 1 at the back of the book, and _then_ read the section _in this chapter pertaining to this Self-Assessment Exercise._

hurt by your presence, and this is their choice. Regardless of whether the smiles and intimacy, anger and criticism of others is intentional, every person has an impact on others.

What is the purpose of being self-aware? It is to see the interrelationship of all people and the part that you play in your own growth and development, and also in that of others.

Self-Worth   Some parts of the self-concept are inborn, and self-worth is one of them. A basic tenet of the founders of the United States (and other democratic nations as well) was that all citizens are created equal: No one person is worth more or less than any other human on this earth, and all have the basic rights to life, liberty, and the pursuit of happiness. This is an instance in which the written laws of the land paralleled the spiritual doctrine of the founding fathers. It assumed that all people come into this world and travel through it with a worth that is equal to that of all others. Nothing can be added to make one person worth more than another. Conversely, no horrible deed can reduce the basic human worth of a person. The only thing that reduces worth is when the individual assumes from life experiences that he or she has less than the 100 percent worth inherited at birth. The gravest mistake one can make with self-worth is trying to earn it. No one can get more than 100 percent, and everyone already has that. It can be unearthed or realized by an individual, but it cannot be earned from someone else.

Self-Love   Just as with self-worth, we all have an inborn capacity for self-love; it is not something one earns from others over a lifetime of struggle. Many believe that they have to earn self-love through sacrifice and punishment of self and through pleasing others. Those lacking in self-love must relearn compassion for themselves in all situations, through all emotions, and in all actions. This is done by letting go of judgments from outside: the self-judgments learned from parents, friends, teachers, and society.

Part of relearning self-love is learning self-forgiveness, which revolves around the basic belief that we all do the best we can with the skills we have at the time. This is not to say that we cannot learn more effective ways to behave; rather, it means accepting that "this is who I am, and this is the way I behaved in that situation. I'm learning to do it differently, but no matter how I do it and how it turns out, I love myself."

Self-Esteem   This is probably the most familiar component of self-concept, and many people use the two terms interchangeably. However, self-esteem is a compassion for self that is earned through one's actions (unlike self-worth and self-love, which are inherent). Because self-esteem is earned, it comes from success. Many earn self-esteem through their interpersonal relationships, academic accomplishments, sports, or successful job performance. Self-esteem that is rewarded internally is lasting, and it enhances the other self-concept components. However, self-esteem earned from the outside can be taken away at any time, which can be devastating. If an individual has earned esteem from the outside, the need for rewards and attention from others can become insatiable, and if that reward is removed or reversed (which happens from time to time within all relationships), feelings of powerlessness and of anger from being powerless result. It follows that internal resources are truer and more helpful for enhancement of self-concept than are pats on the back from others.

Self-esteem is itself built on some basic components: honesty, especially with oneself; responsibility for one's perception of what is real; trust; listening to intuitions and acting on them; and positive intent toward others.

Self-Confidence   Self-confidence is the earned or learned ability to cope with perceptions of the world (an individual's reality). Each person sets up his or her perception of the world and then handles those perceptions in a confident or not-so-confident manner. Success in this component comes from seeing planned outcomes develop into real outcomes by using past resources, trust, hope, and courage.

Self-Respect   Self-respect is the ability to honor, or appreciate, one's emotional nature: to express fear, happiness, anger, love, and joy appropriately when they are felt. This does not mean "dumping" these emotions on someone else but expressing them when the need is felt. Holding back from expressing an emotion not only blocks its energy but also shows lack of self-respect. When a person respects who he or she is, expression of emotions is natural and appropriate.

Effects of Self-Concept on Behavior

Researchers and clinicians have known for years that if, in a given situation, individuals devalue themselves and perceive themselves as helpless and certain of failure, this perception will virtually ensure failure in that situation. This concept has been referred to as the *self-fulfilling prophecy:* the likelihood of failure at some task will be greatly increased if you imagine yourself failing even before the task in question has begun. The converse of this relationship is true as well: if you imagine yourself succeeding at your task, your probability of success will be greatly enhanced. In his text *Self-Fulfilling Prophecies,* Russell Jones (1977) exhaustively reviews self-expectations (for example, the self-fulfilling prophecy) in terms of social, psychological, and even physiological outcomes. He concludes that interpersonal social success, psychological states such as depression and anxiety, and even physiological arousal (for example, stress) can all be dramatically affected by self-expectancies. In accordance with Jones, Seligman (1992) does not think that special intensive training will significantly raise a child's IQ or help the child talk three months early, but he is convinced that the social environment can produce a child who believes he or she is helpless and cannot succeed. When that happens, the child will under-perform, regardless of his or her IQ. However, if a child believes that he or she has control and mastery, that youngster may outperform more talented peers who lack such a belief. Byme (2000) studied the relationship between self-esteem and fear and anxiety. He found that in adolescents, as self-esteem scores raised, fear and anxiety diminished and positive active coping mechanisms increased. Young males had higher self-esteem scores than did females and showed better problem solving-skills which increased with age.

Self-perception also has its effect on hostility. People with low self-esteem are more vulnerable to interpersonal insult than those with high self-esteem, and those with low self-esteem become angrier than those with high self-esteem when they are unsuccessful in getting an apology (Goleman 1998; Ingram 1998).

Effects of Self-Concept on Disease

Not only are self-esteem and self-perception important both in the outcome of behavioral performance and in the severity of the stress experienced, but self-perception (especially the devalued, helpless, and hopeless image of self) may also play a significant role in the eventual onset of disease.

The bulk of research done with patients concludes that there may indeed be such a thing as "proneness." This tendency is characterized by gross self-devaluation, helplessness, and feelings of hopelessness. In effect, this personality style sees itself in a totally passive and dependent role within its environment. These individuals tend to see themselves as stupid, clumsy, weak, and inept even though their achievements are often enviable (Siegel 1990, 1999). This is as good a description of low self-concept as one is likely to find.

In summary, it should be emphasized first that perceptions of helplessness and self-devaluation can lead to increased stress. Second, a poor self-concept may also play a significant role in the onset of various diseases. It may be that a poor self-concept generally increases one's susceptibility to many disease forms. Third, by improving your perception of control and self-worth, you may begin to reduce and eliminate stress. You may find that as an added benefit, you begin to see your "luck" in all endeavors change as well. Finally, it is important to note that Self-Assessment Exercise 2 was not designed to give predictive insight into any particular illness; it merely gives you some feedback concerning your self-perception.

Enhancing Self-Concept

Everyone can work toward a more positive self-concept. Low self-concept is a result of negative beliefs about oneself, negative self-talk that fuels the old negative beliefs and the way life experiences are perceived. Until the negative spiral is broken, enhancement of self-concept is not possible. The following techniques present a number of levels of possible change.

List Your Resources   Write down all the resources that you have in your life. You are alive and have attained a certain number of years. What do you have going for you that has helped you get where you are now? In listing resources, remember to include physical and material resources such as income, clothing, housing, and money; social support resources such as family, friends, teachers, and counselors; internal resources such as empathy, tenacity, sense of humor, honesty, being a good friend to others, and so on.

Once you have listed as many items in each category as possible, write each resource on a three-by-five card, placing a new card on the top of the deck each day. On reading the daily resource, repeat several times to yourself or out loud that you possess this quality or resource. Merely reading the words on the card is not enough to enjoy how you feel about yourself and thus enhance your self-concept—you must internalize the resource and accompany it with a positive feeling.

Enlist Subpersonalities   Having listed internal resources, name them and then use them to help you in stressful situations. This concept was developed in the psychosynthesis movement of the 1960s and 1970s (Vargiu 1977). For example, a list of internal resources might be the following:

caring for others	intelligence	sense of humor
tenacity	reliability	risk taking

Give each of the characteristics an alliterative name, such as Connie Caring, Tony Tenacity, Ina Intelligence, Roy Reliable, and so on. Each of these "people" is part of your personal behavior style and has been hard at work to help you throughout the years.

When a stressful situation comes up, internally scan your cast of characters and call upon one or more to help you through the situation. Talk to the subpersonality (or write a script between you and the character), and let that part of you donate its expertise to the solution of the situation. At first this technique may seem a little silly, yet given time and serious thought, your subpersonalities can become very helpful.

Compliments

1. Practice giving compliments to others, and make a study of how they accept them. Do they just say "Thank you," or do they add on a statement of humility? Make your compliments "real" by commenting on something that you really like. Begin with your friends, then expand to others in your work or study space, sales clerks, service people, and so on.

2. Begin to accept compliments by giving a smile and a "Thank you." Period. Make no follow-up statement unless it is a positive confirmation of the compliment, for example, "Thank you. I really like it, too."

Assertiveness   Verbal assertiveness is saying what you like or dislike about someone or something without using degradation; it is getting what you want but not at the expense of someone else's self-esteem. Assertiveness is "feel good" communication. Some people confuse assertiveness with aggression. Aggression is demanding in a bossy and demeaning way that someone obey your wishes. It is an act of verbal pushing and shoving with no consideration for the other person's self-esteem. When the other person does not comply or agree, the aggressor insists that he or she is "dumb," "stupid," or "crazy" for not agreeing. When people respond to a situation aggressively, they often receive counteraggression, alienation, and defensiveness from the other person. Communication is virtually blocked, and all who are involved come away from the situation feeling anxious, angry, and misunderstood.

At the opposite end of the scale from aggression is nonassertive or passive behavior (see **Figure 6.1**). Many have learned in childhood to be passive placaters who do not have the skill to ask for what they want. Their mode of operation is to manipulate. They sit back wishing that someone would notice their needs and fulfill them, or they set up subtle and roundabout ways of getting what they want. Manipulators use guilt to get others to do what they want. They control others with shoulds, oughts, and ifs. Nonassertiveness is highly related to low self-concept. In becoming more assertive, it is important to know that you have certain inalienable assertive rights (Alberti and Emmons 1995), which include the rights to do the following:

- say no without feeling guilty
- change your mind
- take your time in planning your answer or action

Passive

This person is
- Shy
- Withdrawing
- Reluctant to assert rights and privileges
- Socially inhibited

Assertive

This person is
- Usually more extroverted
- Aware of rights and privileges and uses them constructively
- Socially productive

Aggressive

This person is
- Somewhat hostile
- A vehement defender of own rights yet often violates or usurps the rights of others
- Unmindful of where own rights end and the violation of others' begins
- Socially destructive

Figure 6.1 Assertiveness scale

- ask for instructions or directions
- demand respect
- do less than you possibly can
- ask for what you want
- experience and express your feelings
- feel good about yourself, no matter what

Assertiveness training in mainstream American culture involves operationalizing these rights.

The Assertiveness Ladder   (**Figure 6.2**) is a hierarchy of assertiveness exercises that you might attempt in your daily contacts with other people. The exercises are listed in order from least to most difficult. Start slowly at the bottom and progress up through the list. You might spend a week or two practicing each one before moving up to the next. If you begin to experience anxiety, drop back to the previous exercise for another week, and then try to move up again through the list.

Exercise 1: Greeting Others. Many unassertive people are too shy to greet others or initiate conversations. This exercise consists of initiating at least two exchanges or conversations per day with individuals whom you would not consider close friends. It may be difficult or seem "plastic" at first, but continue trying. You may meet some very interesting people.

Exercise 2: Complimentary Statements. This exercise involves giving others compliments. This is a social behavior that may lead to greater social horizons. Many unassertive people neglect to give compliments by rationalizing "Oh, that's dumb" or "Why would they care what I think?" Giving compliments is polite, and people probably do care what you think, so give it a try.

"Assertiveness"

Figure 6.2 Assertiveness ladder

Exercise 3: The Use of "I" Statements. Many unassertive people are hesitant or afraid to use the word "I." The reason is that the use of "I" shows ownership, and disagreement with an "I" statement by someone else is often seen by the unassertive person as a personal rejection. This is not usually the case, however. Do not be afraid to take a position. Let your preferences be known; if you do not, they will never be realized.

Exercise 4: "Why?" This exercise involves asking "why?" Many unassertive people feel that to ask why represents a challenge—but it does not. "Why?" simply asks for additional information. In this exercise, you should ask "why" at least two times a day from people you consider to be "above" you in status, position, or respect—your boss or a teacher, for example. If you think the word "why" may be too threatening to that person, substitute "What makes you think that?" or "How is that so?" or, finally, "Could you help me to understand that better?"

Exercise 5: Spontaneous Expression of Feelings. Unassertive people often repress feelings. This exercise consists of having you spontaneously react on a feeling level to someone else's statement or behavior. Repressed feelings are hazardous to your health and well-being; therefore, express them a little at a time. Try to express your emotional reaction at least two times a day. You will find it gets easier the more you practice. Remember, sometimes it is better to take the risk of hurting someone else's feelings than to keep your feelings bottled up. If that person is your friend, he or she will understand.

Exercise 6: Disagreement. This exercise involves disagreeing with someone when you feel that person is wrong. Many people take such disagreement personally, but that is a problem they must work out for themselves. If the other person is secure, he or she will know that disagreement can be a healthy and positive force for new ideas. Give it a try, but be sure not to be arbitrary—if you disagree with someone, make sure you really believe in what you are saying.

Exercise 7: Eye Contact. Maintaining eye contact is often one of the most difficult things for the unassertive person to do. You may find it awkward at first, but continue trying. The best way to attempt maintaining eye contact is to start with short intervals two to three seconds in length. Eventually extend it to four to five seconds, then nine to ten seconds. It is important that you not stare at people; this is too often interpreted as a challenge. Therefore, use this time interval technique. When you break eye contact, it is important not to look down; maintain your basic eye level. Do not look down!

When you can successfully climb up this Assertiveness Ladder, you will be well on your way to becoming an assertive individual and will have done much to improve your self-concept. Remember that not all assertive behaviors will result in rewards; other people may simply be defensive or aggressive. But do not allow their problems to hinder you. Feel good about yourself and your new assertive personality.

Interpersonal Effectiveness Training   One of the most useful tools you can find for enhancing self-perception may be referred to as Interpersonal Effectiveness Training (IET). Psychologists have used techniques for decades to help their patients improve their self-esteem and overcome dysfunctional passivity and the depression that may result.

IET is best understood within the context of helping people become more interpersonally effective and avoid the problems of passivity and of aggressive behavior (look again at Figure 6.1). As such, IET may also be thought of as a form of assertiveness training but far broader in scope. It should be used in any interpersonal situation in which you feel yourself pulled toward passive or aggressive behavior. It is critical to understand that the goal of such an exercise is not merely to "get your way." Rather, the primary goal is to avoid passivity or aggression toward others, both of which lead ultimately to interpersonal dysfunction. However, by avoiding passivity and aggression, you will find that your chances of obtaining what you seek will be enhanced and you will feel better about your own interpersonal effectiveness.

Any interpersonal situation in which you feel yourself pulled toward interpersonal passivity or interpersonal aggression is an appropriate situation in which to use IET techniques (refer again to Figure 6.1). The six steps of IET follow, in three stages: recognition, analysis, and action.

Recognition
1. Experience the presence of an emotional cue, for example, guilt, anger, loss of self-esteem, or even confusion.

Analysis
2. Analyze the situation:
   a. Has the other person done anything to violate your interpersonal rights?

      Try to see the situation from that person's eyes. If your rights have not been violated, do not continue this exercise. Similarly, do not continue if you decide it is really not worth discussion or if you feel it to be unwise from the "interpersonal politics" perspective. Otherwise, if your interpersonal rights have been violated and you feel the issue is worthy of discussion, then continue.

Action

3. Describe to the other person what they have done or what has happened that has violated your rights. Simply describe the facts.

4. Continue by telling the other person how the incident has made you feel, for example: "I felt . . . cheated, betrayed, stupid, foolish, angry, worthless, sad," and so forth.

5. Now inform the other person what you would like to see done to correct the situation, that is, to change it so that your rights are no longer violated. Use the principle of "minimal corrective action." This involves requesting that the situation be corrected but without making anyone else feel or look bad (for example, without punishing anyone). Be careful not to become aggressive here.

6. A final, optional step that you may employ if your wishes are not met and you feel your rights have still been violated is escalation. Escalation simply means that you inform, not threaten, the other individual of more action-oriented steps you will pursue if satisfactory action is not taken: For example, you may call someone of higher authority, and so on.

Remember, practice makes perfect, so start slowly at first. Also remember that no matter how interpersonally persuasive you may be, you cannot make anyone do anything that he or she does not really want to do. So, if after Step 6 you still have not gotten satisfaction, be proud of yourself; you have done all you could without resorting to passivity or aggression.

Common situations in which this exercise may be useful are the following:

1. Disputes with clerks while shopping

2. Disputes with repair people

3. Times when friends or family have hurt your feelings or violated your rights in some way (it is okay to ask for an apology for Step 5)

4. Encounters with "pushy" salespeople, and so forth

Assertive, Effective Complaints   A practical application of Interpersonal Effectiveness Training might be the following complaint exercise. Especially in our modern age of impersonal menu-driven phone trees and e-mail contact as the only way of communicating to solve problems, which are often a source of frustration and stress, it is important to know how to make an effective complaint, which is another form of assertiveness. Try the following steps:

Step 1: Is it really worth my time and energy to make this complaint? Sometimes the potential satisfaction is just not worth the aggravation. If you just cannot keep it out of your mind, then pursue it for your peace of mind.

Step 2: Put it in writing; it clarifies your thinking. If you actually reach a real person, follow it up with a letter or e-mail.

Step 3: Keep a record of who of you have talked to, when, and what they said.

Step 4: If you do not get satisfaction, go to the next layer up.

Step 5: Let them know what will make you happy. Often if they know what will make you happy and they can do it, its more expedient to give you what you want than take up their time.

Step 6: Know in advance what your next step will be so you can keep the process going and not start over. How often have you said after you hung up the phone "darn, I should have said..."?

Avoid Negative Self-Talk   Negative self-talk perpetuates negative feelings about the self and also continues to affirm negative self-beliefs. This exercise consists of the following steps:

Step 1: Monitor yourself for one day, and write down all the words and phrases you say to yourself that are negative. You might also enlist the help of others around you—have them identify statements they hear you say about yourself.

Step 2: For each negative phrase you have identified over the period of a day, write a positive follow-up. For example, a negative phrase might be: "You big dummy." Follow it with " . . . and I like you anyway."

Step 3: After this exercise, each time you hear yourself saying something negative about yourself, add something positive.

After mastering Step 3, each time you begin to say something negative about yourself, substitute a positive statement. Do not even bother to say the negative statement.

Examine Negative Beliefs   Negative beliefs are the basis for negative feelings and behaviors. What are the core self-concept beliefs on which you operate your life? Some possibilities that may stem from early childhood are as follows:

- I am an unlovable person.
- I do things so poorly that nobody could like me.
- No matter how hard I try, things always turn out badly.
- Nobody likes me, so why should I try?
- I am unworthy of the love and attention of others.

When you treat yourself in an unloving way or behave in a way that depreciates yourself, ask, "What must a person believe in order to behave in such a self-depreciating way?" Then turn the belief around to a positive statement that you repeat whenever you notice you are being unkind to yourself.

The beliefs that are the basis of your relationship with yourself are also the foundation for your beliefs about other people. This can be used to your advantage by changing your attitudes toward others and becoming more accepting, compassionate, and loving. As you release judgment of others, you may release judgment of yourself. A simple affirmation about others such as "Everyone does the best they can with what they have at any given time" allows you to let others be where they are without having to judge their actions. Such a statement does not mean that the person cannot grow and learn other ways of doing things; it merely says that they are doing the best they can. That affirmation can be extended to the self in stressful times: "I am doing the best I can with what I have right now."

This concludes the first part of this chapter regarding self-concept. Keep these precepts in mind as you apply them to stressful behavior patterns discussed in the second part of the chapter. Before we start on, this next part, stop and complete Self-Assessment Exercise 3. We will use the results to personalize the information in this section of the chapter.

Self-Assessment EXERCISE III

Place your answer to the following questions in the space provided before each number.

_____ **1.** I have no patience with tardiness.
     a. almost always   c. seldom
     b. often   d. almost never

_____ **2.** I hate to wait in lines.
     a. almost always   c. seldom
     b. often   d. almost never

_____ **3.** People tell me that I tend to get irritated too easily.
     a. almost always   c. seldom
     b. often   d. almost never

_____ **4.** Whenever possible, I try to make my activities competitive.
     a. almost always   c. seldom
     b. often   d. almost never

_____ **5.** I get aggressive when I have to wait.
     a. almost always   c. seldom
     b. often   d. almost never

_____ **6.** People tell me I'm a poor loser.
     a. almost always   c. seldom
     b. often   d. almost never

_____ **7.** I tend to lose my temper or get irritable when I'm under a lot of pressure.
     a. almost always   c. seldom
     b. often   d. almost never

_____ **8.** I tend to race against the clock.
     a. almost always   c. seldom
     b. often   d. almost never

_____ **9.** I become enraged when a car in front of me runs too slow.
     a. almost always   c. seldom
     b. often   d. almost never

_____ **10.** I catch myself rushing when there is no real need to do so.
     a. almost always   c. seldom
     b. often   d. almost never

                                                   _____ Total Score

Scoring: a = 4 points, c = 2 points, b = 3 points, d = 1 point

Write your total score in the space provided, and on the Personal Stressor Profile Summary Sheet located in Table Appendix 1 at the back of the book, and *then* read the section *in this chapter pertaining to this Self-Assessment Exercise.*

Stressful Behavior Patterns

We have known for years that specific patterns of behavior can adversely affect health. In other words, the choice of a particular health behavior can be the determining factor in the development of a disease. The prime example is the well-known list of cardiovascular risk factors, which include smoking, lack of exercise, obesity, and high-fat diets. It has been clearly demonstrated that the consistent practice of one or more of these behaviors will increase susceptibility to heart disease.

Is it possible that general behavioral tendencies can affect your health? Could it be that the way in which you generally interact with your environment may predispose you to stress and stress-related disease? The answer is a definite yes! Evidence strongly suggests that the manner in which you choose to interact with your surroundings can play a major role in determining whether you develop, for example, heart disease (Brown and Harris 1999; Eysenck 1995; Friedman 1996). These researchers have shown that specific patterns of behavior can adversely affect health. In other words, the choice of a particular health behavior can be the determining factor in the development of a disease.

Type A Behavior

Two cardiologists, Meyer Friedman and Ray Rosenman, in the normal course of treating their patients noticed some recurring behaviors among them, especially in relation to how they dealt with time. They noticed the extreme anxiousness of their patients in the waiting room and the constant focus of their conversations on time, work, and achievement. From their contact with coronary patients, Friedman and Rosenman, starting in the late 1950s, formulated a construct of action-emotion behavior patterns that seemed to embody the coronary-prone individual (1974). They referred to this construct as the Type A personality and included in it the following characteristics:

1. An intense sense of time urgency; a tendency to race against the clock; the need to do more and obtain more in the shortest possible time

2. An aggressive personality that at times evolves into hostility; high motivation, yet very easy loss of temper; a high sense of competitiveness, often with the desire to make a contest out of everything; the inability to "play for fun"

3. An intense achievement motive, yet without properly defined goals

4. Multitasking behavior—that is, the involvement in several different tasks at the same time

During a series of impressive research studies known as the Western Collaborative Studies, the Type A behavior pattern was shown to precede the development of coronary heart disease in 72–85 percent of the 3,411 men tested. These results strongly suggest that Type A action-emotion behavior patterns may be predictive of the eventual onset of heart disease (Friedman and Rosenman 1974).

Since the pioneering studies of Friedman and Rosenman, a wealth of research data on the Type A behavior pattern emerged. Physiologically oriented research has found Type A people to be more reactive in their sympathetic-nervous-system response when challenged or confronted by their environment than individuals who possess none of the Type A characteristics (Cooper 1995; Siegman and Dembroski 1989; Williams and Williams 1994). This sympathetic over-responsiveness has been suggested as the key pathogenic process leading to increased cardiovascular risk. By-products of chronic sympathetic activation include elevated serum-cholesterol levels, decreased vascular flexibility, increased blood pressure, and increased cardiac output—all of which, when chronic, can contribute to cardiovascular disease.

We have come far since the initial discovery in the late 1950s of the Type A pattern. There is evidence to suggest that as useful as the Type A construct is, it was never the intent of the primary researchers to develop a set trait profile, "you are it or not," label of an individual. They simply identified some traits in individuals who it turned out were at greater risk of cardiovascular disease. To some extent there is some danger in trying to identify an individual as a certain personality. Some factors are definitely more important than others. Having one of the more lethal characteristic may be very significant even though the individual scores low on the others and is thus not considered at risk because he or she does not score high on all of the items in the inventory (Smith and Gallo 2001). Instead of Friedman and Rosenman's four-component construct, we now believe anger, hostility, and to a lesser extent time urgency are the major pathogenic factors of the pattern.

Anger/Hostility

Research by numerous authors aimed at refining the Type A pattern and defining its specific pathogenic components has led us to believe the anger/hostility component to be the most toxic, pathogenic constituent in the Type A constellation (Williams and Williams 1994). Burg's (1995) review of anger, hostility, and heart disease develops a cogent argument for the disease-causing potential of anger and hostility. In a fascinating longitudinal study of midlife women, Adams (1994) found that hostility was correlated negatively with general health. This study extends the hostility research beyond heart disease. There is also some evidence that the time-urgent characteristic may be pathogenic as well, but the hostility trait seems to be the most pathogenic because of its high association with secretion of testosterone. Testosterone release is associated with atherosclerosis.

Take another look at Self-Assessment Exercise 3. It is a broad-ranged attempt at sampling the behavior pattern discussed in this section. We emphasized the dimensions of anger/hostility (Items 3, 4, 5, 6, 7 and 9) and time urgency (Items 1, 2, 8, and 10). A total score in excess of 24 may indicate presence of these behaviors and is not a measure of cardiovascular risk.

Fear and anger are the two emotions that, when chronically used, most negatively impact your health. The following exercise is intended to help you identify which emotions are your primary stress responses.

Fear is a lifesaving response, and anger can also be an appropriate response. However, when either of these emotions becomes a chronic response to life, it becomes inappropriate.

Fear is a "flight" stress mechanism; it is a constriction, a contraction, a pulling inward away from confrontation. All destructive emotions may be based on fear.

Anger is a "fight" stress mechanism that explodes outward. Anger is a family of feelings, varying in strength from annoyance to fury or wrath. Other members of this family are indignation, self-righteous anger, sulking, passive anger, and revenge.

Anger/Fear Recall Exercise In order to target these emotions for resolution, count how many times fear or anger is mentioned in the following list. If one response predominates, there is a message there for you.

1. Think of a situation that has occurred in your life recently that stirred up negative emotions in you (these are usually stressful situations). Now close your eyes and take yourself back into that situation. See in your mind's eye where this occurred and who was there; get a very clear picture of the situation; listen to what everyone was saying, including what you were saying to yourself; and allow yourself to experience the feelings you felt then and immediately afterward. Also remember what you were saying to yourself after the experience.

2. Now identify all of your feelings involved during and after the situation by putting a check in front of any or all of the following emotions that apply.

   "The situation that I am remembering made me feel . . ."

_____ Anxious	_____	_____ Hateful	_____
_____ Lonely	_____	_____ Insignificant	_____
_____ Submissive	_____	_____ Rejected	_____
_____ Confused	_____	_____ Stupid	_____
_____ Inadequate	_____	_____ Inferior	_____
_____ Frustrated	_____	_____ Rage	_____
_____ Irritated	_____	_____ Weak	_____
_____ Miserable	_____	_____ Critical	_____
_____ Discouraged	_____	_____ Guilty	_____
_____ Depressed	_____	_____ Bored	_____
_____ Foolish	_____	_____ Helpless	_____
_____ Bewildered	_____	_____ Furious	_____
_____ Embarrassed	_____	_____ Hostile	_____
_____ Insecure	_____	_____ Jealous	_____
_____ Ashamed	_____		

3. The two major negative emotions are anger and fear. On the line after each feeling you have checked, write in the basic emotion that best fits your feelings at the time.

   Example: ✓ Anxious <u>fear</u>   ✓ Stupid <u>anger</u>

4. Count the incidence of your responses, and identify which of the two basic emotions (anger and fear) you identify with most often in the list of feelings.

   Number of fear responses _____

   Number of anger responses _____

Anger is a natural emotional stress response that lets those around us know that we are displeased. In infancy, the displeasure may be hunger or wet diapers. Rather than lie in fear of not being fed, the infant screams for attention. Anger is an emotion of movement, sometimes the very forceful movement of outward hostility or violence. Warren (1983) describes anger as "a physical state of readiness . . . that internal happening which prepares us to cope with hurtful, frustrating, and fearful experiences." When a child learns that anger gets results, anger is used.

There are three basic beliefs or thoughts that tend to make us unnecessarily angry:

1. Unreasonable expectation: demanding or expecting too much from ourselves, others, or our environment. Whenever we use words like "should," "ought," or "must," there is a good chance our anger is due to unreasonable expectations.

2. Unreasonable evaluations: exaggerating the significance we attach to certain events. Whenever we find ourselves using words or phrases like "awful," "terrible," or "can't stand it," there is a good chance our emotional response is due to unreasonable evaluations.

3. Inaccurate appraisals: misinterpreting or mislabeling the behavior or intentions of others. Sometimes we get angry because we make errors in defining or interpreting the events around us.

Not all angry people are hostile, but all hostile people are angry. According to Dr. Redford Williams (1989), hostility means that you want to hurt or punish somebody. He defines three stages of hostility: (1) distrust of others, (2) feeling angry when you find somebody breaking "the rules," and (3) showing anger by saying something nasty, raising your voice, frowning or otherwise nonverbally showing displeasure, or making nasty gestures at the "cheater." A universal example of this is the line crasher (at the grocery, in traffic, or the theater line, for instance). Most of us are annoyed when someone drives up the side of the road and gets ahead of us in traffic, or sneaks into the "7 items only" line with a cart full of groceries. Clearly, they have broken the laws that we learned in elementary school: you must wait your turn in line and you must follow the rules. Hostile individuals look for people who are likely to break the rules. They hug the bumper of the car ahead of them so no one will cut in on them, and they count items in competitors' grocery carts. Hostile drivers are unveiled to all when they honk, gesture, yell, and perhaps even chase the offender to mete out justice, just as the hostile shopper snaps or yells at the full-cart offender. There are those individuals who have "free-floating hostility," which means that they are angry, or on the brink of anger, much of the time, with or without major cause.

Aggression and violence are striking-out behaviors of anger and hostility. These behaviors give us a true visual of anger: it is an explosion, a striking-out, a blowing up, an outward burst of energy. Warren (1983) describes four types of people who mismanage anger:

1. Exploders: these people are outwardly aggressive. They can't (don't) hold their tempers, and are easily recognized by others as hot heads.

2. Somatizers: these people turn their anger into somatic or body symptoms such as hypertension and boils. They think that this helps them not have to suffer the consequences of showing their anger.

3. Self-punishers: these individuals turn their anger on themselves in the form of depression, guilt, and low self-esteem.

4. Underhanders: these individuals try to hide their anger as sarcasm and dark humor. They insist that they are not angry. A major indicator of this type of person is the feeling of being put down, deflated, or verbally punched from their remarks.

Anger Management

Evidence points to the anger behavior pattern as being a learned behavior. As such, it can be unlearned or at least modified. If you are a anger reactor, that fact will be the hardest for you to face, but once you realize it, change can successfully occur. It means using behaviors that are more healthfully appropriate.

In the management of anger, the direction of motion must be borrowed one from the other. Rather than lash out, anger reactors must pull in their energy, reflect on their thoughts and beliefs about the situation. Brown and Schiraldi (2007), working with adolescents, suggest students be able to identify and describe their anger; express a desire to avoid unproductive anger responses; and demonstrate the ability to apply several of the many effective anger management techniques, such as the ones presented below.

Anger Management Techniques

In general, anger management techniques are ones that use energy for reexamining the situation and redirecting movement. Techniques that will help you get a handle on anger are covered in this section.

Anger Management Diary

1. Keep an anger diary for one week. On a three-by-five index card, for each incident jot down what precipitated the anger; how you reacted; how you felt before, during, and after the incident; what you expected from others in the situation; why you think others acted the way they did; your self-talk before, during, and after the incident; and how long the self-talk lasted.

2. Write a list of coping self-talk statements. Under the headings "Before the incident," "When physiologically aroused," "During the encounter," and "After the encounter," write four or five statements you can use to help you stay calm during that time. For example:

   Before: I don't need to get angry in this situation.
   Physiological Arousal: Relax now and stay centered. Breathe . . .
   During: What is my outcome here? Honey catches more flies than vinegar.
   After: I did the best I could. That could have been worse. I did a great job.

3. Choose the incident that provoked the least anger, and review it in your mind.

4. Use a relaxation technique that works for you (deep breathing, neuromuscular relaxation, and so forth), and while relaxed, mentally review the incident you have chosen. As you play through it, insert an appropriate positive coping self-statement at the four points outlined in Item 2.

5. When you can relive this incident with no feelings of anger, choose the next least stressful situation from your diary, and repeat the procedure using your positive coping self-statements.

6. When old incidents can be relived without anger, transfer the technique to future potential anger situations in your life.

Examine Beliefs Regarding Anger   An underlying cause of anger is not getting what we expect. Therefore, reducing the incidence of anger involves examining beliefs about expectations. Typical anger-inducing expectations are based on beliefs such as the following:

I know how to do it best and quickest.

If it's not done my way, it's done wrong.

If you can't do it quickly and excellently, get out of the way.

If I do everything "by the book," I'll be appropriately rewarded and live happily ever after.

If I hurry faster, I'll get everything done.

After an anger situation, review your thoughts and behavior. What must you believe in order to think and behave that way? On identifying an irrational or negative belief behind the anger, change it to a positive one such as "People have their own ways of doing things that are right for them."

Express your frustration. Frustration, a precursor to anger, is by definition inhibitive. Frustration impedes progress toward a desired goal or blocks desired behavior. Until alternatives that are as satisfying and immediate as the original goal are found, it is helpful to express frustration either by talking with someone else or by writing thoughts down on paper. As soon as possible after the event, sit down and write out what you experienced. Do not judge your writing. Just let everything come out, flowing freely. Write down what "they" said and what you said; write down how you felt, how you feel as you write, and you hope "they" feel. Write down what you wish you would have said, would have done, and will do next time. Write it all down—do not hold anything back; if you do, you have not released the emotional pattern.

After you have finished, put your journaling away for a few hours or overnight, then bring it out and read it objectively. Look for any insights or rethinking of the situation. Write down what you have learned from the situation that has helped in your growth. What might be the "gift" here? If none come to mind, put your journal away and come back to it in a week, a month, or longer to discover the learning from this situation.

If you fear that someone will read your journaling, burn it or otherwise release it after you have finished venting your emotion. If you choose not to keep it, release it with ceremony and finality.

Examine Attachment Involvement   Attachment means that the outcome of a behavior or a task will have a significant effect on the individual. You know you are too attached to the outcome when you ask yourself, "What will others think of me if I fail, if I don't do what they want, or if the project I'm completing isn't on time?" Extreme attachment involvement is often based on rewards from the system or from one specific person rather than from completing the job for the internal reward of a job well done. The "system," schools and jobs, usually rewards Type A behavior, and the Type A individual lives on those rewards. As long as the external rewards are the motivators for action, those who give out the rewards have control over the person seeking the rewards. Changing Type A behavior calls for gradual change to an internal reward system—that is, defining success according to individual outcomes, not outcomes set by outside institutions, family, or friends.

A basic technique here is to ask yourself, "Am I following a path with heart?" If so, the path will be more exciting than stressful. And if it is not a path with heart, try detaching, stepping back, and viewing stressful situations with objectivity:

- Am I the only one who can do this?
- Can I be the sole cause of failure at this task?
- Am I verifying others' reactions to me?
- Am I competing rather than cooperating?
- If I were an objective outsider, how would I view this situation?

The Reality Check presented in the category on control later in this chapter and the Goal Path Model discussed on the two previous pages may be helpful in reducing extreme attachment.

Anxiety and Fear Behavior

Fear is another innate emotion. It helps prevent our early demise by protecting us in dangerous situations, especially when the danger is overwhelming. Fear gets our attention by immobilizing us to some degree. If it cannot completely immobilize us, it constricts and contracts all the systems of the body to some degree.

Fear may take many forms, including the fear of the future, fear of others' opinions, fear of failure and inadequacy, and fear of success. It is present in all of us at some time or another, even in college professors (Nwadiani and Ofoegba 2006). Fear becomes a nuisance when we misread the seriousness of a potential threat or misinterpret an event. For people with low self-concept, negative beliefs about persecution, irrational interpretation of events, or a well-learned, childhood-ingrained fear response, nearly any situation or person may become a threat, and so fear is their constant companion. It keeps them rigid and constricted.

Fear has the opposite direction of energy in the body than that of anger. The direction of any movement in fear is inward. Fear is an implosion, a tightening, a drawing in, a contraction. The energy of fear constricts and strangles. The fear responder is often characterized as a "Don't push me" personality type. They will not move until they feel safe.

Anxiety is a basic component of stress. Anxiety may be thought of as fear, and in effect the two words may be used synonymously. The anxiety-reaction process begins when an individual perceives a stimulus (person, place, or thing) as challenging or threatening. This perception occurs in the higher (neocortical) regions of the brain and entails interpretation, or assignment of meaning to the stimulus, which makes the individual insecure or perhaps apprehensive.

These feelings of insecurity are transformed into physiological arousal of the endocrines and sympathetic nervous system. So now not only are the thought processes aroused, but the bodily processes are also.

Fortunately, this hyperaroused condition usually subsides shortly after the stimulus has been removed.

Most of us suffer from this form of arousal. It is quite common in this society to be occasionally faced with things that make us insecure and result in generalized anxiety. Ordinarily, the anxiety reaction represents no major threat to mental or physical health. As we discuss it here, anxiety is not only a symptom or manifestation of stress but also a cause of further stress. Chronic anxiety is another behavior pattern that appears to create excessive, chronic stress. If you are one of these people, you suffer from anxiety far more than most people because your reaction to a stressor results in a form of anxiety that seems to perpetuate itself. Therefore, the characteristic that makes you different from other people lies in the feedback mechanisms involved in the anxiety reaction. Most people experience anxious moments that quickly end when the stressor is removed. The **anxious-reactive** individual experiences stress that seems to persist, or increase, even after the stressor is gone.

The more severe form of anxiety does seem to represent a significant challenge to health and well-being by increasing the stress response. Indeed increased anxiety of no identifiable etiology was found to be associated increased physical symptoms and more numerous visits to health care facilities (Goodrich et al. 2005).

This self-perpetuating anxiety reaction, which persists or increases even after the original stimulus has been removed, means that the anxious individual suffers from a feedback "loop" that continues the anxiety reaction. The basis of this anxiety feedback loop is as follows: any arousal response to some perceived stressor can eventually assume the role of a stressor itself and, in turn, cause further arousal.

The feedback messages that further increase arousal can take three forms: cognitive, visceral (smooth muscle), and musculoskeletal (striated muscle). The first and perhaps most volatile feedback during stress reaches the body in the form of thoughts (cognitions) concerning the nature of the stressor and the possible outcomes. Fear-laden thoughts that follow the stressor are capable of inducing visceral arousal by way of the autonomic nervous system, and further thoughts may increase the musculoskeletal reaction of a stress response. These cognitions are perhaps the most harmful of the three feedback forms. Many individuals engage in what may be called "catastrophizing"; that is, they always perceive the stressor event as far worse than it really is. The catastrophizer often views all psychosocial stress in terms of life-or-death urgency. Catastrophizing is partly due to conditioning, but it is primarily a choice based on a belief. Consider the choice of paths in **Figure 6.3**. This tendency to consistently overreact may result in severe mental and physical incapacitation and trauma during a stress reaction and may increase the likelihood of psychosomatic disease.

Items 1, 2, 5, and 7 in Self-Assessment Exercise 4 concern catastrophizing tendencies. How did you score on them?

Other sufferers from cognitive feedback are those who relive any and all crises over and over in their mind for days or weeks after an incident. These "relivers" suffer from distress every time they relive the incident. Do you tend to relive stressful events? Items 3, 4, 8, and 10 in Self-Assessment Exercise 4 deal with that aspect. The "catastrophizer" and the

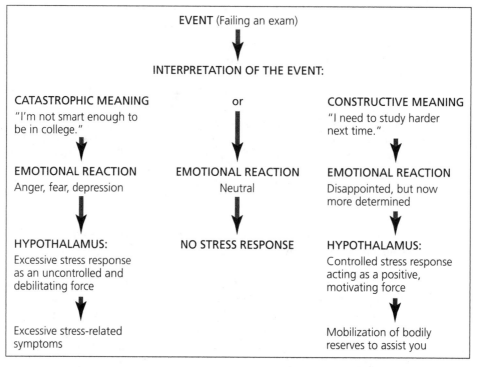

EVENT (Failing an exam)

INTERPRETATION OF THE EVENT:

CATASTROPHIC MEANING	or	CONSTRUCTIVE MEANING
"I'm not smart enough to be in college."		"I need to study harder next time."

EMOTIONAL REACTION	EMOTIONAL REACTION	EMOTIONAL REACTION
Anger, fear, depression	Neutral	Disappointed, but now more determined

HYPOTHALAMUS:	NO STRESS RESPONSE	HYPOTHALAMUS:
Excessive stress response as an uncontrolled and debilitating force		Controlled stress response acting as a positive, motivating force

| Excessive stress-related symptoms | | Mobilization of bodily reserves to assist you |

Figure 6.3 Choice of paths

Self-Assessment   EXERCISE IV

Choose the response that best summarizes how you usually react during anxious moments, and place the letter of that response in the space provided. When I'm anxious I . . .

_____ **1.** tend to imagine all of the worst possible things happening to me as a result of whatever "crisis" made me anxious to begin with.
   a. almost always   c. seldom
   b. often   d. almost never

_____ **2.** do everything I can to resolve the problem immediately; if I don't, I'll go crazy worrying about it later.
   a. almost always   c. seldom
   b. often   d. almost never

_____ **3.** will relive the crisis over and over again in my mind even though it may be over and resolved.
   a. almost always   c. seldom
   b. often   d. almost never

| **Self-Assessment** | CONTINUED |

_____ **4.** will be able to clearly picture the crisis in my mind hours or even days after it's over.

    a. almost always   c. seldom

    b. often   d. almost never

_____ **5.** get the feeling that I'm losing control.

    a. almost always   c. seldom

    b. often   d. almost never

_____ **6.** feel my stomach sinking, my mouth getting dry, or my heart pounding.

    a. almost always   c. seldom

    b. often   d. almost never

_____ **7.** tend to make "mountains out of molehills."

    a. almost always   c. seldom

    b. often   d. almost never

_____ **8.** have trouble falling asleep at night.

    a. almost always   c. seldom

    b. often   d. almost never

_____ **9.** have difficulty in speaking or notice my hands and fingers trembling.

    a. almost always   c. seldom

    b. often   d. almost never

_____ **10.** notice my thoughts "racing."

    a. almost always   c. seldom

    b. often   d. almost never

_____ Total Score

Scoring: a = 4 points, b = 3 points, c = 2 points, d = 1 point

Write your total score in the space provided, and on the Personal Stressor Profile Summary Sheet located in Table Appendix 1 at the back of the book, and _then_ read the section _in this chapter pertaining to this Self-Assessment Exercise._

"reliver" are forms of the anxiety characterized by prolonged feedback about the stressful event. This mechanism is depicted in **Figure 6.4** and is associated with excess worrying, which has been shown to be responsible for high scores on anxiety tests (Kelly 2004).

The second form of feedback involved in anxious behavior and the stress reaction is visceral, or smooth-muscle, activity. This involves the heart, stomach, gastrointestinal tract, and so on. The awareness of smooth-muscle activity, such as heart pounding or stomach gurgling, can increase stressful thought processes. In this way, visceral awareness can perpetuate further visceral activity. How responsive are your visceral mechanisms? Item 6 in Self-Assessment Exercise 4 concerns this issue.

Finally, anxiety feedback can occur in the musculoskeletal system. This involves overt movement of the striated muscles—those muscles attached to tendons and bones. In our own observations and research with public-speaking students, we have found that the awareness of trembling hands, awkward speech, or muscle tension can increase

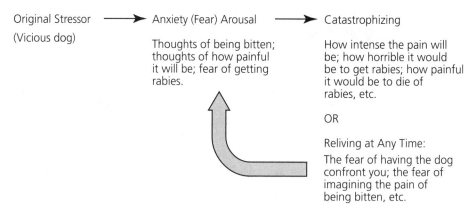

Original Stressor ⟶ Anxiety (Fear) Arousal ⟶ Catastrophizing
(Vicious dog)

Thoughts of being bitten; thoughts of how painful it will be; fear of getting rabies.

How intense the pain will be; how horrible it would be to get rabies; how painful it would be to die of rabies, etc.

OR

Reliving at Any Time:
The fear of having the dog confront you; the fear of imagining the pain of being bitten, etc.

Figure 6.4 Cognitive activity in the anxiety feedback loop

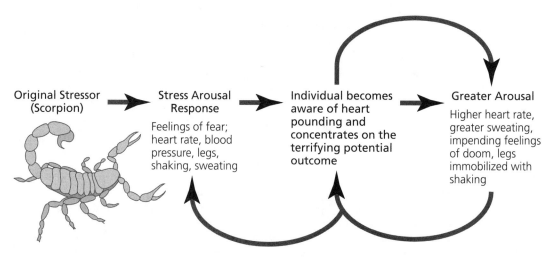

Original Stressor ⟶ Stress Arousal ⟶ Individual becomes ⟶ Greater Arousal
(Scorpion)   Response   aware of heart
                                        pounding and
Feelings of fear;   concentrates on the   Higher heart rate,
heart rate, blood   terrifying potential   greater sweating,
pressure, legs,   outcome   impending feelings
shaking, sweating   of doom, legs
                                                               immobilized with
                                                               shaking

Figure 6.5 Visceral and musculoskeletal activity in the anxiety feedback loop

visceral activity in the form of heart rate. Increased musculoskeletal activity has been found to lead to further increases in the same system. Item 9 in Self-Assessment Exercise 4 deals with how reactive this system is during stress. **Figure 6.5** is a diagram of the anxiety feedback loop at work in the visceral and musculoskeletal reactions.

In summary, the anxious individual is hypersensitive to stress reactions, which may occur on cognitive, visceral, and/or musculoskeletal levels. Once these reactions have been perceived by the individual, they form an automatic feedback loop that perpetuates and in some cases worsens the severity of the stress reaction. Perhaps the most severe form of this anxiety feedback is found in the catastrophizing individual, who consistently perceives problems (stressors) in the worst possible context. For these people, stress is a constant companion, affecting their daily behavior; catastrophizers are vulnerable to incapacitation from the slightest stressor and also to stress-related disease.

A total score of 25 to 40 in Self-Assessment Exercise 4 would indicate a high degree of anxiety reactivity. A score of 20 to 24 is average, and a score below 20 indicates low reactivity.

Anxiety and Fear Management Exercises

Fear reactors must learn to make outward movements to resolve the threatening situation. Fear is immobilizing them, so they must learn to move outward.

Thought Stopping   Thought stopping is a technique whereby an individual intentionally breaks the anxious cycle by abruptly leaving the obsessional thoughts. This can be done by two different methods. The more traditional technique of thought stopping involves shouting "STOP!" as soon as you become aware of the anxious reliving or catastrophizing. At first, the word may be shouted to yourself. If this is not forceful enough, shouting it aloud will successfully destroy the anxious cycle. You may then attend to other less-stressful thoughts. Another form of thought stopping is to switch abruptly to a pleasing, relaxing image or scene in your "mind's eye" as soon as you become aware of the anxious cycle. The scene should be the same one each time and should be a place, real or imagined, that you find aesthetically pleasing and relaxing. After dwelling on this place for thirty to sixty seconds, slowly reoccupy your mind with real-world demands. If no such relaxing image exists for you, counting backward from five to one will also work. Simply picture the numbers in your mind as large and bright images. By the time one is reached, the cycle will be broken, and you can begin thinking of other thoughts. If the cycle starts again, break it in the same manner. Continue doing so until the cycle remains broken, no matter how many thought-stopping maneuvers are necessary.

Fear History   Explore your fear history to learn more about responding in an anxious manner to stressful situations by writing your history of fear. When frightened as a child, how did you react? How did your parents react when they were fearful? Was there any one incident from which you seemed to learn the fear reaction? According to David Viscott (1997), the basic questions that reflect the predominant fears of most people are as follows:

- Am I good/am I bad?
- Am I lovable/am I unlovable?
- Am I strong/am I weak?
- Am I smart/am I stupid?
- Am I right/am I wrong?
- Am I worthy/am I unworthy

Whenever fear or anxiety experiences arise, even in adulthood we go back to these basic questions.

Choose an anxious situation from your childhood and identify the basis of that anxiety. It may have been a realistic reaction for you as a child, but is it still a realistic response now that you are an adult and have more knowledge and experience?

Take Action Fear constricts. The opposite of constriction is expansion or movement. When anxiety strikes, make an immediate plan of action so that you change the old, patterned response to fear. An example of this is the person lying in bed who hears a noise outside the window. An anxious reactor may become terrified and paralyzed in his or her bed. Making this situation nonstressful calls for getting up immediately, turning on the lights, and looking for the source of the noise. If the source is found to not be harmful, laughter and a pleasant goodnight to the source can end the incident. If the source is not found, an affirmation of "there is nothing here to be afraid of" can end the incident. If the source is found to be harmful, taking action to correct the situation is the only path to follow.

Give Away Fear

1. Write a lengthy, scary letter to yourself about your fear. Make it as fearful as possible. Catastrophize. Put it away for a day.

2. Come back the next day and make the letter even worse than it was. Follow the fearful feelings as deeply as you can. Again, put it away for a day.

3. Come back the third day with a red pen or pencil and identify the parts of your letter that have no rational basis.

4. After identifying which of your fears may be rational and which parts are not, release all the unrealistic, unfounded fear that you have put into the letter by burning it in a ceremonious manner.

5. Take action regarding the fear that is real; that is, if you really are going to lose your job, begin searching for a new one.

Examine Beliefs Regarding Fear What are your beliefs about what others can do to you and about your own strength and ability to maintain your security? What is the basis of such beliefs? Change the beliefs to positive statements, and begin to affirm that you are always safe and secure. Nothing can harm you. Try to summarize these beliefs. Write them down and analyze them as to where they came from, how they hold you back, and how they can be changed.

Stress and the Need for Control

Noted psychologist Albert Bandura (1997) states that it is mainly perceived inefficacy in coping with potentially aversive events that makes these events fearsome. To the extent that one can prevent, terminate, or reduce the severity of aversive events, we have little reason to fear from them. In other words, we could argue that the most powerful stressor of all is real or imagined loss of control. Indeed, what may contribute to all of the psychosocial and personality stressors examined in this chapter is a real or imagined loss of control over one's life. Consider these stressors:

- Lifestyle/environment change
- Frustration

- Overload
- Underload
- Low self-esteem
- Type A behavior (anger/hostility/cynicism, time urgency)
- Anxious reactivity

Contributing to each is clearly a real or imagined loss of control.

Self-Assessment   EXERCISE V

Answer each question, and place the letter of your response in the space to the left.

_____ **1.** How often do you find yourself feeling helpless or hopeless?
   a. almost always   c. seldom
   b. often   d. almost never

_____ **2.** How often do you find yourself in a situation that seems out of control?
   a. almost always   c. seldom
   b. often   d. almost never

_____ **3.** How often do you find yourself needing to have your life well planned and organized?
   a. almost always   c. seldom
   b. often   d. almost never

_____ **4.** How often do you find yourself feeling sad or depressed?
   a. almost always   c. seldom
   b. often   d. almost never

_____ **5.** How often do you find yourself fearful of losing control over your life?
   a. almost always   c. seldom
   b. often   d. almost never

_____ **6.** How often do you find yourself feeling insecure?
   a. almost always   c. seldom
   b. often   d. almost never

_____ **7.** How often do you find yourself needing to control the people around you?
   a. almost always   c. seldom
   b. often   d. almost never

_____ **8.** How often do you find yourself needing to control your environment?
   a. almost always   c. seldom
   b. often   d. almost never

_____ **9.** How often do you feel the need to have your daily activities highly structured?
   a. almost always   c. seldom
   b. often   d. almost never

Self-Assessment   CONTINUED

_____ **10.** How often do you feel secure?
      a. almost always   c. seldom
      b. often   d. almost never

_____ Total Score

Scoring: Items 1 to 9: a = 1 point, b = 2 points, c = 3 points, d = 4 points
Item 10: a = 4 points, b = 3 points, c = 2 points, d = 1 point

Write your total score in the space provided, and on the Personal Stressor Profile Summary Sheet located in Table Appendix 1 at the back of the book, and _then_ read the section _in this chapter pertaining to this Self-Assessment Exercise._

Richard Lazarus (1998) theorized many years ago that the more we perceive ourselves in control of a situation, the less severe the stress reaction will be. This conclusion certainly suggests that feelings of hopelessness and helplessness may be the fundamental cause of excessive stress. This point was clearly demonstrated during World War II. Psychiatrists observed that soldiers who could return enemy fire suffered fewer mental disorders than those who could not return fire but simply had to take shelter and hope that they would not be harmed. Similarly, it has been shown that just the expectation of control over stressors can reduce stress (Fisher 1995; Steptoe and Appels 1992).

Some researchers feel that the core of the negative emotional behavior patterns may be the need for control (Friedman 1996). This behavior is manifested by of competitiveness, time urgency, hostility, and low tolerance for frustration, all of which may be seen as conscious expressions of a need to control themselves and their environment. There is evidence that autonomic-nervous-system arousal may create a psychological discomfort that could increase the need to exert control. Hanton and colleagues (2003) observed that athletes who had the least confidence in their ability to control themselves and their environment experienced the most debilitating symptoms of anxiety.

On the positive side, such researchers as Lazarus (1998), Kobasa (1979), Bandura (1997), Cooper (1995), and Nuernberger (1997) all offer considerable evidence that a real or imagined sense of control over self or environment is a powerful stress-reducing mechanism. Classic studies of thirty years ago demonstrated that even animals (rats) that were given control over electric shock contingencies developed fewer ulcers than rats that had no control over the shocks.

It is clear that perceptions of personal control, that is, the perception that one can significantly alter events, figures prominently in most theories of how people respond to adversity, illness, and stress. A most fascinating demonstration of the influence of perceived control over physiology comes from David Barlow's laboratory. The research team administered 5.5 percent carbon dioxide (CO_2) to two groups of ten panic patients. One group was falsely informed that they could control the CO_2 levels, but the second group was not given that expectation. The group that falsely believed they had control over the CO_2 had significantly fewer symptoms of anxiety and panic. This study (Barlow 1988) once again demonstrates the power of the feeling of control, even if it is an illusion. Perception has consistently been shown to be a major factor in one's ability to see oneself in control and to in general manage the subsequent adverse stress arousal (Zautra 2003). Atchley (1999) stresses the importance of resilience, setting goals, self-confidence, and control in healthy adjustment to the aging process. **Figure 6.6** depicts the self-efficacy and stress-control process.

Now go back and examine your responses to Self-Assessment Exercise 5. Total scores in excess of 24 may indicate vulnerability to excessive stress due to feelings of impotency, for example, a sense of lack of control. Items 3, 5, 7, 8, and 9 indicate a need to control; Items 1, 2, 4, 6, and 10 indicate feelings of loss of control.

Control Exercises

The following exercises are designed to identify situations in which the need for control overshadows efficient use of time and energy. Learning to manage this overzealous need for control will reduce the stress in your life.

Keep a Journal   Whenever you experience the frustration of not being able to control all the things and people around you or you feel that parts of your life are out of control, write your experiences in a journal. Just expressing your feelings about the situation will help alleviate stress.

Figure 6.6 Control and stress

As we pointed out in the Introduction, journaling can be an effective way of working out stressful problems. Just writing down thoughts and feelings rather than keeping them unsaid is helpful in releasing emotions (Desalvo 1999). Journaling can be as simple as "keeping a diary" of daily stressors or as involved as writing down answers to a group of formal, leading questions. Ira Progoff (1992) has offered guidance in journaling for many years through books and workshops. Through the use of his techniques, we can look into the unconscious mind and unlock some of the motivations that create many of our stressful situations.

Calm Yourself   When your body is experiencing a state of stress arousal, you are likely to interpret the symptoms as a sign that you are losing control. One way you might begin to exert more control over your environment is to first regain control over your body. Several excellent breathing exercises are presented in Chapter 12.

Reality Check   With the Reality Check, when life seems out of control, take the following steps:

Step 1: Measure in numbers the difficulty of the situation. Get specific. If you cannot assess the difficulties in numbers, then give them quantitative ratings on a scale of one to ten. This causes the mind to think rationally instead of in terms of feelings.

Step 2: Rate your ability to do the job. Have you ever done this job or one like it before? How did you do? What resources do you have that have helped in the past? What new resources have you developed since that time that would help in this situation?

Step 3: Examine the consequences. What is the worst thing that could happen? What is the real likelihood (probability) of that actually happening? Rate this on a scale of one to ten.

Step 4: Release the irrational; develop an action plan for the rational.

Let Go of Judgments   If you can internalize that you are the only one responsible for your life, you must extend that to others around you. One person cannot make others do what they do not wish to do. Moreover, one individual does not have the right to manipulate the lives of others. The simple technique here is to say to yourself whenever you begin to judge others: "They are doing the best they can for themselves at this time."

Cognitive Restructuring   Cognitive restructuring refers to changing the meaning or your interpretation of the environmental stressors around you. Therapists such as Albert Ellis (1994, 1998, 1999), Aaron Beck (1999), and Beck and Beck (1995) argue strongly that the environment is not what causes most people stress, but rather it is their interpretations that actually cause the stress response to be triggered (see **Figure 6.7**). The source, then, of dysfunctional emotions and excessive stress is, in reality, irrational or maladaptive thoughts (ideation). Cognitive restructuring entails first identifying and then correcting these maladaptive thoughts.

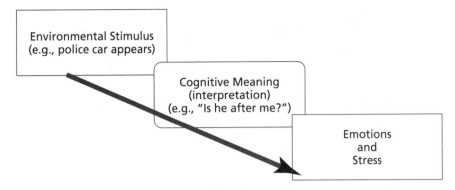

Figure 6.7 Cognitive interpretation

Some of the most common maladaptive, incorrect, or irrational interpretations of environmental events are listed here (based on the work of Ellis and Beck) along with their cognitive solutions/reinterpretations:

Problem: The tendency to jump to a specific conclusion without adequate confirmation (overgeneralization).

Solution: Search for more evidence that the conclusion is correct. If so, and if a problem exists, implement social engineering or problem-solving techniques.

Problem: The tendency to blame oneself for problems when little or no evidence exists for such a conclusion.

Solution: Search for other possible explanations to explain the problem.

Problem: The tendency to see things as "all or none" or "good or bad," that is, the tendency to see only extremes.

Solution: Begin to search for the "gray" areas, the in-between states. See that few things are all good or all bad.

Problem: The tendency to catastrophize about unpleasant events and to "make mountains out of molehills."

Solution: Assess the realistic chances of the catastrophe actually occurring. If chances are high, then begin social engineering or problem-solving strategies. If chances are low, ask yourself, "Couldn't I be using this energy in a better way other than wasting it in worry?"

Problem: The tendency to be limited in problem-solving alternatives, that is, an inability to see potential solutions.

Solution: Practice exercises in creative, nontraditional problem solving.

These are but a few of the major maladaptive cognitive patterns that often lead to excessive stress. Beck and Beck's book *Cognitive Therapy: Basics and Beyond* (1999) is an excellent guide to such problems, as is Ellis and MacLaren's *Rational Emotive Behavior Therapy* (1998).

In sum, by controlling your body's response to stressors through breathing exercises and by controlling your attitudes through exercises such as cognitive restructuring, you will gain far more control over stress, over health, and over life. You will find that at the same time you will become far less vulnerable to a dysfunctional need for control.

Examine Beliefs   Often the less we trust ourselves, the more we try to control others. As in the other discussions regarding beliefs in this chapter, people with a need to control the people and events around them must look at the irrational or negative belief system that is driving them. Some possible beliefs are:

- Everything will fall apart if I do not maintain control.
- The only way people will need me is if I am in control.
- No one who is not as bright or talented as I am has the right to be in control.
- If I don't control others, they will try to control me.
- Power is control.

Turn negative or irrational beliefs into positive ones; continue to affirm these positive beliefs by using them as the basis for noncontrolling behavior.

Practice Concentration   Excessive multitasking goes on because you allow it to go on. It has been shown that improving attention focus improves coping ability (Synder 2001). Time may be better spent by concentrating completely on one task, finishing it, and then going on to the next. Consider trying the following:

1. Read material that makes you concentrate—something with difficult concepts rather than simple ones.
2. When you are working on one plan and another pops into your mind, say "Stop it," and go back to the original plan.
3. Practice meditation, detailed visualization, progressive muscle relaxation, or other relaxation-training techniques in which you must focus on one thing at a time.
4. If a good idea about something else pops up in the middle of another project, and you can't "stop it," jot it down, and immediately go back to the original project.

Planning   Rushing into tasks without having adequately planned them results in stress that is highly preventable. The remedy is the Goal Path Model given here:

Step 1: Define the task:

Reasons for doing the task:

Step 2: Can the task be broken down into subtasks?

NO   YES

List each subtask and complete the rest of this form for each subtask.

Step 3: Evaluation or proofs of success (how will you know when you have succeeded with the task?). List proofs:

Step 4: What personnel or help will be needed? List:

What are possible resources for personnel?

Estimate costs and obstacles for getting personnel:

Step 5: What materials will be needed? List:

What are possible resources for materials?

Estimate costs and obstacles for getting materials:

Step 6: Estimate time required for each task in Step 2:

Step 7: Hypothesize all possible obstacles or blocks to success:

Step 8: For each obstacle, go back and develop at least one contingency plan:

Step 9: Evaluate your contingency plan:

Step 10: Begin.

Self-talk   Reduce negative self-talk as in Journal Entry 6.

Reduce negative self-talk using the technique presented in the previous category on self-concept within this chapter.

SUMMARY

The stress response is clearly linked to behavioral habits—it may be more important to understand the person who is under stress rather than the stressor itself. Consider the following points:

- Behavior reflects self-concept: We are as we act.
- Total self-concept is made up of self-awareness, self-worth, self-love, self-esteem, self-confidence, and self-respect.
- Poor self-concept plays a significant role in stress and disease.
- Anyone can improve their self-concept.
- How one communicates reflects self-concept.
- Assertiveness is not only positive and productive communication, but it is also stress reducing.
- Type A behavior is a pattern of behavior that is associated with cardiovascular disease.
- Anger, hostility, and perhaps time urgency are the major pathogenic (disease-causing) factors of the Type A personality.
- Behavior can be unlearned or at least modified.
- Anxiety, a basic component of stress, is not only a stress symptom, but also a further cause of stress.

- Anxiety may also be thought of as fear.

- Anxiety can cause further arousal by our thoughts, by smooth-muscle feedback, or by skeletal-muscle feedback.

- Perceived ability (efficacy) to cope relieves the fear of adversive events; the more we perceive ourselves in control of a situation, the less stressed we become.

SOURCES CITED

Adams, S. H. (1994). Role of hostility in women's health during mid-life. *Health Psychology,* 13, 448–95.

Alberti, R., and Emmons, M. (1995). *Your perfect right.* New York: Impact.

Atchley, R. C. (1999). *Continuity and adaptation in aging.* Baltimore: Johns Hopkins University Press.

Bandura, A. (1997). *Self-efficacy: The exercise of control.* New York: W. H. Freeman.

Barlow, D. H. (1988). *Anxiety and its disorders.* New York: Guilford Press.

Beck, A. T. (1999). *Cognitive therapy of personality disorders.* New York: Guilford Press.

Beck, J., and Beck, A. T. (1995). *Cognitive therapy: Basics and beyond.* New York: Guilford Press.

Bradshaw, J. (1992). *Homecoming.* New York: Bantam.

Brown, G., and Harris, T., eds. (1999). *Life events and illness.* New York: Guilford Press.

Brown, S. L., and Schiraldi, G. R. (2007). Helping adolescents understand and manage anger. *American Journal of Health-Education,* 38, no. 1, 44–50.

Burg, M. M. (1995). Anger, hostility and coronary heart disease: A review. *Mind/Body Medicine,* 1, 159–72.

Byme, B. (2000). Relationship between anxiety, fear and self-esteem. *Adolescence,* 35, 201+.

Cooper, C., ed. (1995). *Handbook of stress, medicine, and health.* Boca Raton, FL: CRC Press.

Dembroski, T., MacDougall, J., and Musante, L. (1984). Desirability of control versus locus of control. *Health Psychology,* 3, 12–26.

Desalvo, L. (1999). *Writing as a way of healing.* San Francisco: HarperSanFrancisco.

Dusek, D., and Girdano, D. (1995). *Emotional risk factors.* Winter Park, CO: Paradox.

Ellis, A. (1994). *Anger: How to live with it and without it.* New York: Citadel.

Ellis, A. (1998). *How to control your anxiety before it controls you.* New York: Citadel.

Ellis, A. (1999). *How to make yourself happy and remarkably less disturbable.* New York: Citadel.

Ellis, A., and MacLaren, C. (1998). *Rational emotive behavior therapy.* New York: Springer.

Engler, B. (1999). *Personality theories.* New York: Houghton Mifflin College.

Erikson, E. (1986). *Childhood and society.* New York: W. W. Norton.

Erikson, E. H., & Erikson, J. M. (1997). *The life cycle completed: Extended version with new chapters on the ninth stage of development.* New York: W. W. Norton.

Eysenck, H. (1995) Personality and cancer. In *Handbook of stress, medicine, and health,* ed. C. Cary. Boca Raton, FL: CRC Press.

Fisher, R. (1995). *Getting ready to negotiate.* New York: Penquin.

Friedman, M. (1996). *Type A behavior: Its diagnosis and treatment.* New York: Plenum.

Friedman, M., and Rosenman, R. (1974). *Type A behavior and your heart.* New York: Knopf.

Goleman, D. (1998). *Working with emotional intelligence.* New York: Bantam.

Goodrich, K., Kneuper, S., and Steinbauer, J. R. (2005). Stress perceptions in community clinic. *Journal of Community Health,* 30, 75+.

Hanton, S., Obrien, M., and Mellulieu, S. D. (2003). Individual difference, perceived control and competitive trait anxiety. *Journal of Sport Behavior,* 26, 39+.

Ingram, L. (1998). *Managing and coping with anger.* London: Royal House.

Jones, R. (1977). *Self-fulfilling prophecies.* Hillsdale, NJ: Lawrence Erlbaum.

Kelly, W. E. (2004). Examining the relationship between worry and trait anxiety in college students. *College Student Journal,* 38, 370+.

Kobasa, S. C. (1979). Stressful life events, personality, and health. *Journal of Personality and Social Psychology,* 37, 1–11.

Lazarus, R. S. (1998). *Fifty years of the research and history of R. S. Lazarus.* Mahwah, NJ: Lawrence Erlbaum.

Nwadiani M., and Oloegba, F. (2006). Levels of Perceived stress among lecturers in Nigerian universities. *Journal of Instructional Psychology,* 33, 66+.

Nuernberger, p. (1997). *The quest for personal power.* New York: Perigee.

Progoff, I. (1992). *At a journal workshop: Writing to access the power of the unconscious and evoke creative potential.* New York: J. P. Tarcher.

Seligman, M. (1992). *Helplessness.* San Francisco: W. H. Freeman.

Siegel, B. S. (1990). *Love, medicine and miracles.* New York: Harper & Row.

Siegel, B. S. (1999). *Prescriptions for living.* New York: HarperPerennial.

Siegman, A. W., and Dembroski, T. M., eds. (1989). *In search of coronary-prone behavior.* Hillsdale, NJ: Lawrence Erlbaum.

Smith, T. W., and Gallo, L. C. (2000). Personality traits as risk factors, in *Handbook of Health Psychology,* eds. A. Bawm, T. A. Revenson, and J. E. Singer, London: Lawrence Erbaum, 139–174.

Steptoe, A., and Apples, A. O., eds. (1992). *Stress, personal control and health.* New York: John Wiley and Sons.

Synder, C. R., (2001). Coping With stress. NY: Oxford University Press. 178.

Vargiu, J. (1977). Subpersonalities. *Synthesis,* 1, 51–90.

Warren, (1983). *Make anger your ally.* New York: Doubleday.

Williams, (1989). *The Trusting Heart.* New York: Times Books.

Williams, R., and Williams, V. (1994). *Anger kills.* New York: HarperPerennial Library.

Zautra, A. J., Emotions stress, and health. New York: Oxford University Press.

Journal Entry 5

Self-Talk

There is an axiom in psychology: "A person's mental health is directly related to the tone of voice in which he or she talks to him- or herself." Nobody likes to be criticized; it hurts, and it leads to feeling bad about yourself. Luckily you can usually manage to get away from those who criticize you too much. However, the one person you can never get away from is yourself, so self-criticism is your number-one worst mental health habit.

All the cells in your body hear your every word and every thought. Say only good things about yourself.

Self-Talk Exercise

In This Column	**In This Column**
List some of the negative comments you regularly say to yourself.	Change them to something positive.

For example:

I hate my body.	I like my body and I will work harder to make it better.
That was a dumb thing to do.	I didn't handle that as well as I might.

Your self-talk comments and positive changes to them:

Affirming

Affirmations are statements confirming that you already have what you envision having. They are written in the first person, present tense. They are positive statements accompanied with positive feelings: I am a wonderful person. Every situation is a learning experience. I deserve love and respect from everyone. I love myself as I am. Be careful not to use negative statements such as "I don't have anxiety."

Technique

1. Clearly get in mind what you want. Write an example here:

2. See yourself clearly in the situation, having obtained what you want. If you cannot see yourself having completely attained your goal, drop back to a point where you can see yourself succeeding and work forward from there. Do you have to drop back? To what point?

3. Experience the good feeling of having accomplished what you want. Can you close your eyes and really experience having what you affirm on a feeling level?

4. Make a meaningful statement regarding the accomplishment of getting what you want:

   It's easy for me to

   I enjoy having

   I'm becoming more and more

5. Write at least two affirmations for all aspects of your life: physical, social, emotional, spiritual, occupational, intellectual, other.

Physical

Social

Emotional

Spiritual

Intellectual, mental

Occupational

Other

Say your affirmations at least once a day, but preferably two, three, or more times. The times of day typically committed to affirmations are upon rising and before going to sleep. Remember, negative self-talk perpetuates negative feelings about yourself and also continues to affirm negative self-beliefs. Positive self-talk (affirmations) does just the opposite and is perhaps the most potent stress management technique.

 Write a positive word or short phrase about self-talk that will be useful to you in future situations.

Demands and Expectations

Stressors originate in the complex interaction between socialization and perception. That is, they are sociological events we may perceive as undesirable on the basis of our experiences or other learning processes. People and our relationship to them, along with our perception of the relationships, construct a fascinating mosaic that greatly affects our stress, health, and happiness. This chapter examines the stressful impact of the expectations that society in general, and people in particular, have on all of us.

Five life processes appear to have strong connections with stress; they are as follows: (1) change and our relationship to our ever-changing life; (2) overload, or expectations accelerating out of control as we attempt to keep up with the fast-moving people and events in our lives; (3) frustration, or our inability to gain satisfaction from the people, events, and institutions in our lives; (4) boredom and loneliness, the failure of our relationships; and (5) the relationship interdynamic itself. We will examine these potential sources of distress and look at examples of how each touches our daily lives. Before you read each section, be sure to complete the self-assessment exercise that precedes it. These exercises help clarify the material that follows. Each section is followed by several effective stress management tools for you to try if you are vulnerable to any of these stressors.

Change

We are simultaneously experiencing a youth revolution, a racial revolution, a sexual revolution, a colonial revolution, an economic revolution, a war on terror revolution, and the most rapid and deep-going technological revolution in history. "Era of change" could be the single most descriptive phrase for the twentieth century. It appears that the twenty-first century can see only continued change, and at an even faster rate!

Most of us have been reared with the belief that change is good and desirable, as it usually denotes an easier and more productive life. However, in his book, *Future Shock*, Alvin Toffler (1970) foresaw that even though change is a necessary element in societal behavior, if it is too intense or too massive, the participants may cease reaping its rewards and begin realizing how devastating it can be. Although Toffler spoke somewhat as a philosopher and social critic, the scientific literature strongly supports his contentions.

Adaptive stress occurs when life situations demand that change occur and we must try to keep up with it. In the modern industrial world, change is seen as "the end" of a period of stability or security of some kind and is therefore related to fear. Even when change is desired, movement from the old situation in which comfort and security have been established is somewhat stressful. The philosophical concept of change is that it is the only constant and is to be expected, not feared. In our society, in which change occurs quickly, there is little emphasis on the transition between the old and the new. Cultural anthropologist Angeles Arrien (1994) reminds us to look at a culture's literature to find what is most and least important to that culture. She then points out that in the United States, very little literature on transformation and transition exists. There are few major rites of passage and few ceremonies that honor the change process. The new is prized and the old is discarded. In this culture, there is an expectation that we should make changes quickly and get on to the next item.

Birth and death are excellent examples of the "instant change" mentality. After a woman gives birth, she is expected to get right back into her predelivery routine. Likewise, upon the death of a loved one, the bereaved may show their grief perhaps through the time of the funeral rites but are then expected to get back to the usual lifestyle.

Your health, and even your very survival, is based largely on your body's ability to maintain a healthy balance of mental and physical processes. This equilibrium is called **homeostasis.** It has been suggested that excessive change is harmful to health because it tends to destroy homeostasis and thereby force the body to restore homeostasis through adaptation.

Homeostasis: equilibrium in the internal functions of the body

Adaptation: the body's tendency to fight to restore homeostasis in the face of forces that upset this natural bodily balance

Life Events

In the early 1960s, Thomas H. Holmes and Richard H. Rahe attempted to discover whether change had major effects on human health. Generic change—that is, change having either positive or negative consequences—was the focus of their research. Based on earlier work by Adolph Meyer with "life charts" (paper-and-pencil tools for creating a medical biography), Holmes and Rahe compiled a list of positive and negative life events that seemed to contribute to the stress reaction. From these efforts emerged the Social Readjustment Rating Scale (SRRS), first published by Holmes and Rahe in 1968. This scale originally listed forty-three life events, and each carried a weighting indicating the amount of stress to be attributed to it. The weightings were determined by the sample populations they tested, and the weighting units were called life-change units (LCUs). The most highly weighted life event was the death of a spouse (100 LCUs), and the lowest-weighted event was a minor violation of the law (11 LCUs). Interestingly enough, outstanding personal achievement was weighted with 28 LCU, only one point

Self-Assessment   EXERCISE VI

The following are events that may occur in the life of a college student (Rahe 1967). Check each event that has happened to you during the last twelve months.

Life Event	Point Value
_____ Death of a close family member	100
_____ Jail term	80
_____ Final year or first year of college	63
_____ Pregnancy (to you or caused by you)	60
_____ Severe personal illness or injury	53
_____ Marriage	50
_____ Any interpersonal problems	45
_____ Financial difficulties	40
_____ Death of a close friend	40
_____ Arguments with your roommate (more than every other day)	40
_____ Major disagreements with your family	40
_____ Major change in personal habits	30
_____ Change in living environment	30
_____ Beginning or ending a job	30
_____ Problems with your boss or professor	25
_____ Outstanding personal achievement	25
_____ Failure in a course	25
_____ Final exams	20
_____ Increased or decreased dating	20
_____ Change in working conditions	20
_____ Change in your academic major	20
_____ Change in your sleeping habits	18
_____ Several-day vacation	15
_____ Change in eating habits	15
_____ Family reunion	15
_____ Change in recreational activities	15
_____ Minor illness or injury	15
_____ Minor violations of the law	11

Score: _____

Add up the point values for all the items you checked. Write your total score in the space provided, and on the Personal Stressor Profile Summary Sheet located in Table Appendix 1 at the back of the book, and *then* read the section *in this chapter pertaining to this Self-Assessment Exercise.*

less than trouble with in-laws! This points to one of the more important aspects of this study of life events: it concentrated on generic change, a force that causes stress through the destruction of homeostasis.

Remember, change, or the disruption of homeostasis, produces stress and adaptation, whether the event is desirable or undesirable. Negative or distressful events are usually the most harmful, for they are more disruptive for a longer period. They have a secondary effect in that they stimulate fear, self-doubt, catastrophic imaginings, and other negative thoughts that linger in the mind. However, positive events can likewise be stressful in that they also initiate change that necessitates adaptation. Usually, though, positive change does not produce the secondary effect of the negative event and thus is given fewer points in the weighting of life events.

One question that always arises in weighting life events is "Doesn't a specific event exert differing amounts of stress on different individuals?" Technically, the answer is yes because everyone's perception of the events in their lives differs. How you perceive an event in your life is tempered by your past experiences. For example, knowing what to expect is a great help in overcoming stress. Someone who has not lived through an event will anticipate the event as being more stressful than someone who has already experienced it. Novelty is always stress arousing, but that new situation becomes tempered through subsequent experiences. Nevertheless, some events are stressful no matter how many times you experience them, and as such they are only minimally less stressful through experience.

Consider moving, for example. The first move is the most difficult, and you become more efficient with experience, but each move still requires much adaptation. If you own a house, the process of finding a realtor, negotiating prices, being displaced during showings, trying to live in a perpetually clean house for weeks or months, finding a new residence, securing new loans, and countless other details is a source of constant stress. Packing, accumulating records, taking care of making the move itself, and finding a new physician and dentist and new stores, schools, and friends are additional stressors. Thus, even if the move is to a better job in a nicer place, and even if moves have been made before, moving still causes much change and much adaptation. Moving is therefore considered a stressful event.

With this concept of generic change as a stressor in mind, Rahe and Holmes amassed data from their Social Readjustment Rating Scale. The SRRS is administered by asking respondents to indicate how many of the items they have experienced over the past twelve months. A total LCU score is then obtained by adding up the LCUs for all of the items that have been checked. This scale has proved to be a remarkable predictor of physical and mental illness for a two-year period after the accumulation of the stressors. This scale has also been modified and designed for various populations, such as college students, and Lazarus (1998) also designed a "hassle scale" that was made up of smaller daily-life stressors such as concerns about body weight or not getting enough sleep.

An important concept here is susceptibility. A high score does not mean that the individual will definitely become ill. It means that the individual is more susceptible to illness than those with lower scores. However several studies have found stressful life events to be related to increased incidence of breast cancer (Ollonen et al. 2005); increased incidence of breast cancer with decreased life satisfaction scores as an intervening variable (Golden-Kreutz et al. 2005); and an association between high-stressful life events and relapsing, reoccurring multiple sclerosis. There are many intervening variables, the most important of which might be the stress intervention techniques the individual currently practices. A study on individuals with high life event scores found that the group of subjects participating in a program utilizing stress reduction techniques had lower incidence on myocardial infarction (Haldar et al. 2005)

If you have not yet done so, go back and add up your score on Self-Assessment Exercise 6. If your total score for the year was less than 150 points, your level of stress, based on life change, is low. If your total was between 150 and 300, your stress level is moderate; you should minimize other changes in your life at this time. If your total was more than 300, your life-change level of stress is high; you should minimize any other changes in your life and work more vigorously at instituting some of the stress intervention techniques presented in this book.

Now that you have determined your life-change score, let us see how life change may lead to illness. Remember that change, whether favorable or unfavorable, requires adaptation. Change disturbs the equilibrium, inducing a temporary destruction of homeostasis. Such disequilibrium is met by the body with attempts to restore homeostasis. Selye (1976) points out that adaptation stresses the body by requiring a concerted effort on its part to restore balance. This effort to restore homeostasis requires adaptive energy, and, unfortunately, adaptive energy will eventually diminish if the disequilibrium becomes highly intense or chronic. When a person's adaptive energy is drained, dysfunction can occur on a localized, or specific, level. When the body is totally depleted of adaptive energy, general bodily exhaustion may result in death.

Richard Lazarus (1998) proposes that stress usually depends less on life events than on the cognitive processes involved in the individual's perception of those events. He notes that although life events can indeed predict illness, some individuals with high life-change scores simply do not get ill. Conversely, many individuals have low life-change scores but do get ill. These noteworthy observations led Richard Rahe to suggest that future research focus on moderating variables such as factors that allow people to tolerate high levels of change without suffering illness. Rahe (1979, 3) states:

> [T]he qualities of life change events are qualities of the individual rather than aspects of the environment. It should be clear to investigators that when they gather sentiments of upsettingness, desirability. . . and what have you, they are measuring a variety of subjective responses to the environment which confound objective estimates of life change.

Life change is a complex construct. Most studies show a relationship of life events to others though others did not. Some of the factors that seem to moderate the process whereby life events lead to illness are considered below.

Hardiness

Researchers turned their attention away from those who got sick to those with a high life event score who remained well. Besides the perception issue previously discussed, they isolated several variables that seemed to promote wellness in the face of adversity. Kobasa and her colleagues (1979) have called these three moderating factors (control, challenge, and commitment) hardiness. Hardiness seems to be a powerful force that protects us from the potentially harmful effects of high life change.

Control   Albert Bandura (1997) argues that it is mainly perceived inefficacy in coping with potentially aversive events that makes them fearsome. To the extent that one can prevent, stop, or diminish the severity of stressful events, there is little reason to fear them. In other words, situations in which we perceive ourselves as being helpless or trapped or feeling out of control will be far more stressful than situations over which we believe we have some control. In addition, when we feel in control we are trying to influence outcomes or act rather than react.

Challenge   Challenge identifies the personality factor of "change as perceived challenge," meaning that one tends to believe that change is a normal process of living and can be an incentive for personal growth. The Challenge attitude is viewing stressful changes as opportunities for new learning (Khoshaba and Maddi 2001).

Commitment   Kobasa (1979) and Maddi (2002) also identify the personality factor of commitment, or the tendency to involve oneself in life experiences, rather than to be alienated or threatened by them or to passively observe them. For years, Kobasa's work was the major investigation into the concept of hardiness, or stress resistance. Others have also investigated the concept and reported similar results. Based on the Stress Resistance Project at Boston College, Ray Flannery Jr. has added to our insight regarding how people withstand the adverse effects of stress. Studying more than 1,200 men and women, Flannery (1993) was able to move beyond Kobasa's original findings. He describes stress-resistant individuals as having these eight specific characteristics:

1. take personal control in their lives
2. are task involved and focused
3. consume few dietary stimulants
4. exercise aerobically

5. practice relaxation exercises
6. seek social support systems
7. have a sense of humor
8. claim religious values

Another analysis of this notion of stress resistance came from Ken Pelletier (1994). Pelletier conducted a five-year investigation of fifty-one prominent individuals who showed an unusual ability to cope with stress and to grow in spite of it. A key finding was the discovery of an altruistic theme that was consistent among those interviewed. But the altruism discovered was not an inherently self-sacrificing altruism as we typically think of it. Rather, it was an altruism that seemed to make these altruists healthier by engaging in the process of giving to others. Pelletier referred to it as "enlightened selfishness." An altruism through which one reaches for the deeper meaning of being human may be the most powerful stress buffer of all.

When changes must occur, three main elements are involved: (1) the present situation, (2) a picture of what the changed situation will be like, and (3) the transitional time between those two situations. What we call change is the transition time that it takes to get from situation A to situation B, as **Figure 7.1** shows.

Adaptive stress may occur at various points in Figure 7.1. It may occur at point A, when an individual is asked or expected to change, and that person does not aspire to change. It may also occur at A, when an individual is tired of or bored in the present situation but doesn't know what else to do. It may occur when an individual no longer wants the old situation and aspires to a new situation, but doesn't know how to go

Figure 7.1 The Components of Change

about getting there. Then, once a new, attainable situation is desired and the individual steps into the transition area, there may be the stress of learning new skills, meeting new people, and so on. Even when the new situation is reached, adaptive stress may occur if the individual feels uncomfortable with the change. The question is what influences the perception of that change and how do the personality constructs under discussion determine the outcome in situation B.

Whether these factors are behaviors or personality traits, they are conceptualized in terms of appraisal and problem representation. Take the tendency to perceive life change as a challenge rather than a threat or another component control which has been discussed for years as internal locus of control. This construct involves the belief that factors influencing the outcomes of experiences reside within the person, and are potentially controllable. If the appraisal process is positive, it is reasonable to expect positive outcomes that characterize optimistic individuals and a tendency to form stress reducing thoughts in demanding situations. The pessimistic style is likely to promote negative appraisals of life events; that is, cynical beliefs lead to stress-inducing appraisals. In light of the information on emotion and plasticity discussed in Chapter 5, is a positive thinking optimist one who has trained their emotional development and altered the brain function accordingly? Can you learn to be a challenged optimist or the opposite? Despite the general criticism of trying to develop all-encompassing profiles as discussed in the section on Type A personality, hardiness or a least its components points to how intense or negative a life event will be. Its chronic impact on health will be negative as you perceive it to be or how you have trained your emotions to react.

In summary, change can be a positive force for growth or a negative force that may lead to mental and/or physical deterioration. The key lies not so much in whether the change is positive or negative, a major life event or a minor hassle, but rather in how intense and chronic its impact is; and the impact of life changes will be as intense and chronic as you perceive and allow them to be. Regardless of the point at which one feels adaptive stress, there are techniques that can help resolve or eliminate the problem.

Adaptive Stress Exercises

The following exercises have been found to be helpful in adaptive-stress situations.

Establish Routines If you are happy in your present situation but don't like surprises in your schedule, establish predictable patterns in your life. Write them down. For each routine, give ten minutes or more for transition time from one set of activities to another.

1. Establish daily routines at home, work, and school.

2. Establish a regular eating and physical-activity program.

3. Establish set sleep patterns.

4. Establish rest and relaxation times and places. You might establish certain hours of the week as a mental-health getaway. Make sure they are times when you engage in truly relaxing behavior. A vacation during which you travel is usually not free from adaptive stress, so do not count vacations as mental health days unless they are truly relaxing to you.

Avoid Change   If your life-change points in Self-Assessment Exercise 6 totaled over 300 and if you are in a position to choose whether or not change is going to occur in your life, avoid change at this time. Some individuals who are going through a great deal of life change choose to stop smoking or go on a diet while their anxiety levels are high. It is usually better to wait until life settles down to engage in new ventures.

Plan for Change   Adopting the belief that change is one of the constants in life can get one ready emotionally and psychologically for change. When change comes, it is expected. Some changes, such as a new boss entering the company or new professors or advisers in place of the old, can be small reminders that change is constant. Other changes, such as an unexpected death, may be much more serious but are also reminders that change constantly occurs.

An exercise for this technique is to say to yourself, "Change is constant," or "I expect things to be constantly changing," whenever you note any kind of change, even a bud turning into a flower or a sunny day being interrupted by storm clouds and rain.

A second exercise is to learn to say what you prefer without being addicted to the "old" way: For example, "I prefer to have Dr. Jones teach this class, but since she is gone, I'll take it from someone else."

Action Plan   This involves completely thinking through the process shown in Figure 7.1 and then committing to writing a specific plan of action for change. To do this, follow these steps:

1. Get a good picture of the present situation. Write or even draw it on a piece of paper.

2. Get a good picture of the situation as you would like it, making sure that it is a picture that you can achieve on your own. We are often confronted with divorced men or women whose ideal picture is of the partner returning and the two of them living happily ever after. Their real need is to paint a picture that they can achieve themselves. Once a realistic picture is clear in your mind, write or draw it on paper.

3. Prepare a detailed, sequential plan to get from your present situation to your ideal situation.

   a. Define the ideal situation so that it is clear in your mind.

   b. List the main subtasks in sequential order—what must be done first, second, and so on.

    c. Under each subtask, identify what resources (both people and materials) will be needed, what skills (new and old) will be necessary, what proof you will insist on in order to know that each subtask is complete, what may block your action at each subtask, and how to get around those blocks.

    d. Identify activities that must be ongoing throughout the transition period (for example, assertiveness training, relaxation training, or exercise program).

    e. On one large sheet of paper (or smaller ones taped together), diagram your transition process, using Figure 7.1 as a model. Draw each subtask as a stepping stone. When the path between situation A and situation B is familiar and active, it becomes less fearful and thus less stressful.

Frustration

Do you ever get uptight because the car in front of you was going too slowly? Have you ever stood in a long line and become antsy because it didn't move fast enough? If you've experienced these or similar situations, then you know what it is like to be frustrated. Complete Self-Assessment Exercise 7 to see how much of a stressor frustration is in your life.

    Frustration: the thwarting or inhibiting of natural or desired behaviors and goals. Frustration occurs when we're blocked from doing something we want to do, whether that something is a behavior we wish to perform or a goal we wish to attain. Emotionally, we respond to frustration with feelings of anger and aggression and with the nervous and hormonal responses that accompany them. Frustration, then, causes the stress response, and in a highly technological, urban society this source of stress should be recognized so that it may be dealt with. Four major sources of everyday frustration in the urban and suburban society are overcrowding, discrimination, socioeconomic factors, and bureaucracy.

Overcrowding

As our cities slowly grow into mass urban corridors, or megalopolises, social scientists wonder about the effects of such increasing human density on the overall quality of life. The definition of crowding includes the space allotted per organism, or the sensation or perception of being crowded. The latter part of the definition makes the way we perceive a situation the determinant of whether crowding exists. Crowding, then, becomes a function not solely of space and people but also of an individual's perception or feeling of being crowded. Such a perception is highly relative. Three could be a crowd in one situation, and thirty-three might not be a crowd in a different situation. If you perceive yourself as being crowded (inhibited in your behavior or goal attainment by the presence of others), then overcrowding exists, and it is a stressor for you.

    Many good studies have been conducted with interesting results. A review of experiments with animals has shown that crowding produces excessive stress-hormone secretion, excessive adrenaline secretion, atrophy of the thymus gland (which involves the immune system) and of secondary sexual characteristics, and elevated blood pressure. Researchers conclude that there is abundant evidence that among animals, at least, crowded living conditions and their immediate consequences impose a stress that can lead to abnormal behavior, reproductive failure, sickness, and even death. The impaired health status of

| Self-Assessment | EXERCISE VII |

Choose the most appropriate answer for each of the following statements, and write the letter of your response to the left of the question. How often do you . . .

_____ **1.** feel stifled or held back in your personal or professional life?

    a. almost always   c. seldom

    b. often   d. almost never

_____ **2.** feel a need for greater accomplishment?

    a. almost always   c. seldom

    b. often   d. almost never

_____ **3.** feel as though your life needs guidance or direction?

    a. almost always   c. seldom

    b. often   d. almost never

_____ **4.** notice yourself growing impatient?

    a. almost always   c. seldom

    b. often   d. almost never

_____ **5.** feel you are in a "rut"?

    a. almost always   c. seldom

    b. often   d. almost never

_____ **6.** feel disillusioned?

    a. almost always   c. seldom

    b. often   d. almost never

_____ **7.** feel frustrated?

    a. almost always   c. seldom

    b. often   d. almost never

_____ **8.** feel disappointed?

    a. almost always   c. seldom

    b. often   d. almost never

_____ **9.** feel inferior?

    a. almost always   c. seldom

    b. often   d. almost never

_____ **10.** feel upset because things haven't gone according to plan?

    a. almost always   c. seldom

    b. often   d. almost never

_____ Total Score

Calculate your total score as follows:

a = 4 points   b = 3 points

c = 2 points   d = 1 point

Write your total score in the space provided, and on the Personal Stressor Profile Summary Sheet located in Table Appendix 1 at the back of the book, and *then* read the section *in this chapter pertaining to this Self-Assessment Exercise.*

stressed mice was also reflected by a significantly lower survival rate after termination of the crowding. The findings demonstrate that chronic intermittent exposure to a psychosocial stressor results in adrenal insufficiency, increases in the severity of the acute inflammation, and impairs the healing phase (Reber et al. 2006).

This research on animals seems conclusive, but there is still doubt whether these findings apply to humans. The problem in research on humans is that a feeling of crowding depends on our perception, which is a function of complex sensory and thought processes in addition to the more basic lower-brain processes that we share with the so-called lower animals. In addition, this complex integration of perceptual processes may be different for different types of people or different ethnic groups. However, in general, research supports the theory that when individuals feel inhibited or frustrated due to overcrowding, the stress response results.

Early research was done by Tanner (1976) and Singer (1975), who studied train commuters in Stockholm and found that the first passengers on a commuter train experienced less stress than those who boarded the train after the halfway point. This was true even though the earlier boarders had to tolerate the crowding for twice as long. He concluded that the resultant stress was not a function of crowding alone, but came more from the later arrivals being inhibited from gaining a seat and from stowing their coats and briefcases. Koslowsky et al. (1995) found similar results and added that the stress of crowding was exacerbated by the feeling of competition with other people in the crowd for places, seats, and so on. When shortness of time was added to the equation, stress became severe.

The popular press has taken this research and applied it to the situations that seem to be more important to our modern lifestyle. Nance (2006), extrapolating from the animal studies and applying the principle to airline travel, reports that airline executives are indeed worried about the impact of crowding aboard airplanes especially considering the trend toward the new generation of jumbo passenger planes. Add the out-of-control nature of the experience, time pressures, and being thwarted by long lines at security, and you have the potential for the perfect air rage storm or a least the perfect pressure-cooker milieu for stress-related body responses. Again these situations involve the stresses of lack of control over our environment, overcrowding and violation of personal space, noise, delays, and unwelcome interaction with other travelers. In Chapter 9 on relationships, we will discuses in depth interaction energy among people occupying the same intimate space. Our sensitive human organism picks up the energy of others around us and it takes a super calm body-mind to fight off the tense, angry energy that can exist in overcrowded environments. Even when we travel by car, then we can experience stress from congestion, physical discomfort, air pollution, and noise. The frustration caused by congestion augmented by time pressure can be an intense source of frustration: many studies have tracked the direct physiological effect of traffic congestion in raising blood pressure and releasing stress hormones into the body. When two stressed individuals with anger and hostility issues get together in a frustrating traffic jam, an all too often a dangerous road rage incident results. Some commonsense deterrents are presented below (Trapp 2006):

- Leaving earlier for work so we beat the rush
- Checking on a map to see if there is a better way around regular congestion spots

- Making sure that we adjust the controls of our car so that our driving position is as comfortable as possible
- When using public transport, reading or distracting ourselves in some other way
- Playing calming music when frustrated
- Using relaxation techniques to manage stress; some can even be done in a traffic jam
- Using the power of positive thinking to think about the current frustrating situation in a more positive way

In summary, don't underestimate the significance of overcrowding as a source of stress: as with congestion (a form of crowding), it becomes a problem when it interferes with our ability to achieve our goals. This is often the case when we need to get somewhere quickly. Crowding also forces us into closer contact with strangers than we would often like, triggering all of the social taboos associated with unwanted physical contact and invasion of personal space. The studies on animals and humans indicated that there is an innate, biological mechanism that links overcrowding with stress. However, as we have learned, perception is very important in the manifestation of stress. We know that in some highly populated cultures, overcrowding does not appear to produce the level of excess stress that is seen in lower-density population areas. Perhaps this represents a healthy adaptation, or it may be an example of Hans Selye's concept of a disease of adaptation. While less of an issue in the United States except in situations of urban poverty or migrant worker camps, people report excessive, unwanted social interactions, insufficient privacy, and are observed to be more socially withdrawn under crowded living conditions. If people socially withdraw from one another as a way to cope with crowding, this could lead to an unintended side effect of breakdowns in socially supportive relationships. A breakdown in socially supportive relationships could, in turn, account for some of the pathological consequences of chronic, high-density living conditions.

Discrimination

Discrimination may be the most widely destructive form of frustration-caused stress. Discrimination refers to unfavorable actions taken against others because of religion, race, social status, gender, sexual preference, physical characteristics, national origin, or even general lifestyle. Although it is widely denounced as inhumane, discrimination appears to be ingrained in much of our social fiber and has been the basis of many social and occupational attitudes and practices (Burnback 1998; Stith 1998; Welch and Gruhl 1998). Discrimination taken to its extreme in the form of "ethnic cleansing" has been responsible for the death and torture of millions of people around the world throughout history, including the present. Religious discrimination, while never really absent, has reared its ugly head in the extreme in the last decade.

Prejudice and discrimination can stifle anything from simple day-to-day activities to long-range goals and dreams (Heilbroner 1993; Young-Bruehl 1998). As long ago as 1969, the National Institute of Mental Health reported that prejudice and discrimination result in the retardation of intellectual functioning and a decreased probability of healthy personality development, particularly in children. The report indicted prejudice as a potential cause of increased violent tendencies and a general distrust of democratic institutions and systems. Finally, it concluded that prejudice harms the development of self-concept in children. This is as true today as it was then. In one study, many researchers found a relationship between the perception of racial discrimination and decreased coping ability, stifled problem-solving ability, and increased stress, which further correlated with decreased life satisfaction (Barnes and Lightsy 2005).

Reverse discrimination has appeared in the United States as a means of compensating for the discrimination injustices of the past. All the same, it too is discrimination and involves essentially the same stress reactions for those discriminated against. Therefore, reverse discrimination is just as harmful to health as the discriminatory practices it was designed to correct.

Socioeconomic Factors

Stress may also be caused by frustrating socioeconomic conditions. Inflation, unemployment, excessive taxation, and general economic recession or depression can create stress on massive social scales, as was apparent in the Great Depression of the 1930s. During periods of economic turmoil, ambitions may be shattered. Maintaining financial security may become a day-to-day endeavor. Sending one's children to college, retiring early, owning a house—all of these aspirations may be frustrated by financial insecurity. The stress of such realities can be as detrimental to the health of the frustrated individual as it is to his or her finances. It has been shown that mental disorders, suicide, crime, and disease increase significantly during socioeconomic hardship, and family and marital relationships seem to be strained as well.

The effects of poverty on those at the lowest socioeconomic levels may lead to personal insecurity. Many of those living at the poverty level have a sense of powerlessness and hopelessness, and many suffer from a general personality disorientation in which they believe their role in life is meaningless. Such conditions are clearly harmful to the health of these people and of society in general. This is not "brain surgery"; it's logical common sense and probably does not personally apply to most readers of this book, except perhaps for those going into social work. What does apply is the new economic reality of the modern consumer. Those with money enough to be the new superconsumers, those who fuel the fires of global capitalism, are the one spending most of their money on nonessential goods and services such as larger houses, expensive cars, and all the advanced technological gadgets we can't seem to live without, not to mention all the personal and professional advisers, manicurists, massage therapists, coaches, and therapists. The fact is we spend more money on nonessentials than essentials and then all too often end up deeply in debt in the process. Psychologically we are in the same boat as the financially burdened mentioned above. In spite of our relative affluence, personal debt, foreclosures, and bankruptcies are ever increasing. Benjamin Barber in his book *consumed* (2007) describes these obvious pitfalls and resultant stressors but goes deeper into the psychology of the modern consumer as having childlike judgment and swallowing the advertising bait hook, line, and sinker. On some level, this new consumer seems to value the unneeded, but on a deeper level feels vaguely guilty, especially in light of the plight of so many less fortunate around the globe. If this subtle level of stress, born out of basic humanitarian responsibility, exists at all, it is most likely buried deep in some spirtual/philisophical pain pocket, covered by layers of psychological defense mechanisms. What we have learned about stress so far is that someday the subconscious, which is the body and noncommunicating brain, will deliver the message.

Overcrowding, prejudice and discrimination, and adverse socioeconomic conditions are sources of frustration, or the inhibition of human behavior, in modern urban society. Such inhibition can produce stress reactions that are expressed in anger, aggression, increased sympathetic nervous activity, and increased mental trauma.

Now that you have reviewed some of the causes of frustration stress, return to Self-Assessment Exercise 7. The highest score possible is 40, and the lowest is 10. The higher your score, the greater your perception of frustration and the more stressful frustration would appear to be for you. General guidelines are 25–40 = high frustration/high stress; 20–24 = moderate frustration/moderate stress; and 10–19 = low frustration/low stress.

Frustration Alleviation Exercises

Frustration is a stressor because it is by definition inhibitive. Frustration impedes progress toward a desired goal or blocks desired behavior. The techniques given here present ways that action can be continued, even though you are being thwarted in some part of your life.

Express Your Frustration   Until alternatives as satisfying and immediate as the original goal are found, it is helpful to express frustration either by talking with someone else or by writing thoughts down on paper. This helps release the stress buildup and may give insights about the situation.

Determine Your Real Outcomes   Using the Outcome Model (Girdano and Dusek 1988), follow each step beginning with stating what you want to a concrete action plan. The steps are as follows.

What Do I Want?   Although frustration is caused by blocks of progress, many blocks occur because we are not really sure what we want in the first place. If the outcome is not clear, the path is not direct, and we tend to wander off course, letting relatively minor obstacles block our path and cause frustration.

How Will Things Be Different and Better in My Life When I Get What I Want?   This is the "heart" question. If the path does not have meaning in the first place, it is easy to surrender to frustration. If the outcome is stated in the positive, the human mind will work harder to achieve that outcome. Thinking of one's life in negative terms expands negative energy around the outcome, and the body automatically defends itself against negative events. The ego does not want to face negative inputs, so defenses are built up against the activity. Thus, sometimes the block that frustrates us is of our own creation so that we will not pursue activities that make us feel bad about ourselves.

What Will I Take as Proof That I Have Been Successful in Reaching My Outcome? Sometimes our frustrations and subsequent stress are the result of actually meeting our real goals but not knowing it. We have what we wanted but do not realize it. It is important to set up concrete and countable signposts that will indicate when we are nearing our goal and when we reach it.

What Are My Useful Resources?   This will be specific to each project, although after several projects, common resources (especially positive personality traits) will begin to emerge. List all of your internal and external resources. Remember your family, friends, financial ability, and inner resources that have gotten you to where you are now.

What Has Kept Me from Reaching This Outcome Before?   If you have attempted to reach this outcome before or have tried for success in a similar endeavor, what stopped you? Past blocks will almost certainly be blocks in the future unless they are discovered and removed. Spending time analyzing and correcting blocks may be the single most effective frustration management technique.

What Am I Willing to Do as a Plan of Action to Get to My Outcome?   Although this is a specific project, you will probably use old successful patterns to help you get to this outcome. If your style works, find a way to adapt it to your new situation. If your old plan does not work, change it by increasing your resources and diminishing your blocks. Formulate a specific plan much like that used in the Goal Alternative System presented next.

Examine Beliefs   The beliefs that we hold regarding our relationship to the rest of the world have been formed very early in life and therefore are deeply ingrained. Old, buried beliefs are sometimes difficult to unearth so that we may look at their logic in light of our present development. Beliefs formed during childhood are based on the beliefs of significant others and also on the skills and knowledge that the child possessed. The beliefs that worked for a certain period of time may no longer be useful because the individual has new knowledge, skills, and experiences as an adult. The steps that can be used to examine beliefs are as follows:

Step 1: *Question:* When frustration occurs, say to yourself, "What would a person have to believe in order to become frustrated in such a situation?"

Step 2: *Answers:* Examine some possible answers to your questions. The beliefs listed here (Girdano and Dusek 1988) may provide a starting point.

- I must not change my beliefs, attitudes, or actions because they have gotten me this far.
- I must understand the universe before I can live happily in it.
- I will be seen as an inferior person unless I do well and win the approval of others.
- I cannot exist without sincere and constant love and approval from everyone who is in my life.
- I must be able to do at least one thing with thorough competence.
- Justice, fairness, and equality must prevail, or life is too unbearable.
- I must not experience or show negative emotions because they make me perform badly and others don't like them.
- I must control or change people who I consider dangerous.
- I must not question or doubt the beliefs that authorities hold. If I do, I should be punished.

- I should get what I want when I want it, regardless of what others think or do.

- Others must not unjustly criticize me.

- Others should not behave in a stupid or incompetent manner.

- Others will treat me the way I think I should be treated.

Turning Beliefs Around.   After identifying the belief on which the frustration is based, turn the belief around so that it becomes positive. For example: "I cannot buy the computer I want because my father says it is an inferior machine and I could get a better price on a model that I don't really want. I identify that my frustration stems from my belief that my father knows what is best for me. I turn the belief around to 'I am the only one who knows what is best for me,' or 'I can choose to take the advice of others, especially when I honor their expertise, but I must make my own choices.'"

Take Action.   Act on the positive belief. Continue to affirm that belief. Write it down on a card, and place the card in a conspicuous place in your house or car.

Behavioral Skills.   Acting on new positive beliefs may call for the learning of new skills such as assertiveness. Telling others that they are no longer expected to control your behaviors may call for preparatory skills that you must be willing to learn.

Overload

Have you ever felt that the pressures of life were building up so that you could no longer meet their demands? Perhaps you felt as though there simply wasn't enough time in the day for you to accomplish all the things you needed to do. During this time, you may have noticed a decline in your social life and an increase in "self-centeredness." Perhaps you lost sleep and so became tired and irritable. You may even have become more susceptible to colds and flu. If any of these things sounds familiar, chances are you were a victim of overload.

Overload, which means the same as overstimulation, refers to the state in which the demands around you exceed your capacity to meet them. Some aspects of your life are placing excessive demands on you. When these demands exceed your ability to comply with them, you experience distress.

> Overload: a level of stimulation or demand that exceeds the capacity to process or comply with that input; overstimulation

The four major factors in overload are

1. time pressures,

2. excessive responsibility or accountability,

3. lack of support, and

4. excessive expectations from yourself and those around you.

Any one or a combination of these factors can result in stress from overload. Overload is one of the most pervasive stressors in modern society. It encompasses the city, the occupational environment, the school, and even the home.

Overload at Home, Work and at School

Toward the end of the 1970s, predictions were that the forty-hour workweek would fade into memory, and the remainder of the century would see workers with more and more free time. New disciplines such as leisure counseling were being developed to help people sort out how best to use this newfound free time. These predictions were not all wrong. The forty-hour week is indeed a thing of the past. It has been replaced with the forty-five-plus-hour workweek. Demand for higher productivity (especially in high-tech industries) has made overload in the workplace a virtual certainty. Deadlines (time pressure); excessive responsibility and accountability; lack of managerial or subordinate support; and excessive role expectations from self, supervisor, and subordinates can all create overload. Task overload occurs when the work environment places demands that are beyond a person's resources. In our time- and money-oriented society, it is not surprising that many jobs are deemed more stressful than is healthy for employees. This is especially true in this age of increased organizational accountability. Think of the tasks that are creating (or have created) overload for you. Make a list of them for further reference as you read the intervention techniques presented later.

The effects of time pressure on workers have been known to researchers for almost a half century. Friedman, Rosenman, and Carroll (1958) studied tax accountants at the peak season (just prior to April 15). Analysis of blood samples revealed significant increases in serum cholesterol and blood-coagulation times. Both of these signs indicate excessive stress, which may eventually contribute to the development of heart disease.

Perhaps the best example of occupational task overload is seen in air-traffic controllers (ATCs). They are faced with a combination of excessive time pressures, life-and-death responsibility, often insufficient support (managerial and/or technical), and a virtually damning expectation for perfection from themselves and others. Research on these workers clearly demonstrates the stressful outcome of task overload. For example, at Chicago's O'Hare Airport researchers found that ATCs were under greater stress than pilots flying ten-hour flights in simulators. This conclusion was reached by measuring secretions of the adrenal medullae and the adrenal cortex (the main stress hormones). Compared with telecommunication operators, ATCs showed considerably stronger stress reactions on the job, based on analysis of their blood. Research has revealed that ATCs are occupationally predisposed to certain stress-related diseases, the most significant of which is hypertension, followed by peptic ulcers, and finally diabetes.

These studies demonstrate the devastating effects of task overload as a stressor. The important point here is not that work is stressful but rather that certain intrinsic elements of a job task may be highly stressful if the occupational demands are hyperstimulating and exceed an individual's resources.

The academic environment is also becoming increasingly stressful for students. This society's demand for higher education has created a highly competitive academic environment reaching back even to the primary grades. Children are pressured to do well academically to ensure college admission. Once in college, the student is exposed to the possibility of graduate or professional schooling, but many graduate and professional schools demand "honors status" for a student to even be considered for admission. Added to the grade battle are admissions tests, which are stressors in themselves. Little wonder that test anxiety is becoming a major problem in the academic world. Test anxiety may lead to inaccurately low evaluations of a student's scholastic achievement or potential.

Self-Assessment EXERCISE VIII

Choose the most appropriate answer for each of the following ten statements, and write the letter of your response to the left of the question. How often do you . . .

_____ **1.** find yourself with insufficient time to do things you really enjoy?
   a. almost always   c. seldom
   b. often   d. almost never

_____ **2.** wish you had more support/assistance?
   a. almost always   c. seldom
   b. often   d. almost never

_____ **3.** lack sufficient time to complete your work most effectively?
   a. almost always   c. seldom
   b. often   d. almost never

_____ **4.** have difficulty falling asleep because you have too much on your mind?
   a. almost always   c. seldom
   b. often   d. almost never

_____ **5.** feel people simply expect too much from you?
   a. almost always   c. seldom
   b. often   d. almost never

_____ **6.** feel overwhelmed?
   a. almost always   c. seldom
   b. often   d. almost never

_____ **7.** become forgetful or indecisive because you have too much on your mind?
   a. almost always   c. seldom
   b. often   d. almost never

_____ **8.** consider yourself to be in a high-pressure situation?
   a. almost always   c. seldom
   b. often   d. almost never

_____ **9.** feel you have too much responsibility for one person?
   a. almost always   c. seldom
   b. often   d. almost never

_____ **10.** feel exhausted at the end of the day?
   a. almost always   c. seldom
   b. often   d. almost never

_____ Total Score

Calculate your total score as follows:

a = 4 points   b = 3 points

c = 2 points   d = 1 point

Write your total score in the space provided, and on the Personal Stressor Profile Summary Sheet located in Table Appendix 1 at the back of the book, and *then* read the section *in this chapter pertaining to this Self-Assessment Exercise.*

For many students, the academic grind has led to dropping out of school, poor self-concept, and more severe mental disturbances (the most severe of which has been suicide). In response to the growing pressures of education, many schools have increased their funding for counseling and mental health services; this is especially true in higher education. Schools have initiated programs to help students learn to study, reduce test anxiety, and generally improve coping skills.

The home has always been a potential source of overload stress. The small, comparatively low-cost "first home" of many couples with children is easily outgrown, and space is at a premium. In addition to perceived crowding, a multiplicity of electronic gadgets around the home—televisions, radios, CD players, DVD players, computers, and cell phones—contribute to overload stress. Never-ending home repair, yard work, and everyday household chores round out a picture of the home as an overload stressor; and especially when both the adults are working long workweeks, little time is left for shopping, laundry, and basic cleaning. Unfortunately, it seems that no matter where you go or what you do, you become a prime candidate for this society's far-reaching stressor: overload.

Overload is not only imposed by the outside; it is also often self-initiated. The Internet and television have influenced a heightened susceptibility to advertising. Buying the latest stuff, which keeps getting better and faster and more convenient, has increased consumerism and fuels our fast-growing economy. Wanting more and more demands more money, which of course comes from more work and more self-imposed overload. In the old mining communities in Appalachia, workers would have to buy all of their goods from the company store. At the end of a hard week's work, they often owed the company instead of walking away with money. As the song went, "Another day older and deeper in debt." Today the "company" is the consumer economy fueled by advertising that keeps the people working harder to buy the latest, fastest, trendiest (and often unnecessary) items. The cost is excessive stress, stress-related illness, and overall less satisfaction with life.

Self-Assessment Exercise 8 was designed to assess your level of stress due to overload. Total your points and see how stressed you are by overload. Roughly speaking, a total of 25 to 40 indicate a high stress level, one that could be psychologically and physiologically debilitating. You suffer from overload when faced with excessive demands to the point where your stress response is aroused.

Burnout   Excessive overload over a prolonged period of time leads to a state of mental and/or physical exhaustion known as burnout. The three stages of burnout appear in **Table 7.1.**

Fortunately, burnout is not permanent—it is reversible. Furthermore, it is preventable (Kompier and Cooper 1999). Relaxation, proper diet, and physical exercise not only help you recover from burnout but can also prevent this problem from occurring in the first place. These topics are discussed in depth later in this book.

Exercises to Alleviate Overload Stress

Overload is a function of four major factors: (1) time pressure, (2) excessive responsibility or accountability, (3) lack of support, and (4) excessive expectations imposed by you or by others. Consider the following techniques for alleviating the stress of overload.

Table 7.1 The Stages of Burnout

Stage 1: Stress Arousal (includes any two of the following symptoms)

1. Persistent irritability
2. Persistent anxiety
3. Periods of high blood pressure
4. Bruxism (grinding your teeth at night)
5. Insomnia
6. Forgetfulness
7. Heart palpitations
8. Unusual heart rhythms (skipped beats)
9. Inability to concentrate
10. Headaches

Stage 2: Energy Conservation (includes any two of the following)

1. Lateness for work
2. Procrastination
3. Needed three-day weekends
4. Decreased sexual desire
5. Persistent tiredness in the mornings
6. Turning work in late
7. Social withdrawal (from friends and/or family)
8. Cynical attitudes
9. Resentfulness
10. Increased alcohol consumption
11. Increased coffee, tea, or cola consumption
12. Apathy

Stage 3: Exhaustion (includes any two of following)

1. Chronic sadness or depression
2. Chronic stomach or bowel problems
3. Chronic mental fatigue
4. Chronic physical fatigue
5. Chronic headaches
6. The desire to "drop out" of society
7. The desire to move away from friends, work, and perhaps even family
8. Perhaps the desire to commit suicide

Note: These stages usually occur sequentially, from Stage 1 to Stage 3, although the process can be stopped at any point.

Source: Everly, 1986. Occupational Stress Management. In G. Everly and R. Feldman, eds. Occupational Health Promotion, New York: Wiley, 1985.

Express Your Feelings   Talk with someone or write down your feelings on paper. Do not allow your emotions to get bottled up. For detailed instruction, see the suggestions regarding assertiveness in Chapter 6.

Negotiate   If you perceive that your feelings of overload are being brought on by a person, negotiate with that person to reduce the load or the deadline.

Some sound rules of negotiation include the following (Fisher, Ury, and Patton 1991):

1. Focus on the benefits that will come from your position, such as value, results, and recognition rather than standing for or against certain positions, such as time or price.

2. Separate the personal relationships from the problem you are negotiating.

3. Handle emotions as legitimate but unrelated to the substance.

4. Let people blow off steam and do not take it personally.

5. To be understood, speak purposefully. Speak about yourself, not about "them," which promotes defensiveness.

6. Build a relationship so that you may prevent future negotiation problems.

7. Focus on common elements, values, and interests rather than differences.

8. Invent options for mutual gain. Brainstorm for new ideas.

9. If they are more powerful, recast an attack on yourself as an attack on the problem.

Manage Time   Understandably, students and employees are in a position that what they do and when they do it are dictated by outside demands; thus freedom is limited. As you move up the ladder of success in work and in school, more latitude is given as to when tasks can be completed. Learning to use this freedom is synonymous with learning how to manage time. Take the example of being asked to write a term paper or a report at work. If it is going to take sixty hours to complete, and if you wait until the last minute, you must continually work on the project. Your time is dictated; thus you have no freedom. If you decide to work on the project, for example, for three hours every Tuesday and Thursday afternoon, you remain in control of your time.

There is freedom in structure; and in order to structure, you must prioritize. Working under a deadline is the most obvious form of time overload, but much of this stress can be controlled by effective time management.

Three Steps to Time Management:

Step 1: Establish long-term goals (three to six months) and develop a plan of action.

Step 2: Establish intermediate goals or priorities (one to four weeks) and develop a plan of action.

Step 3: Develop a weekly habit of setting short-term priorities and an action plan for the coming week. Once you have completed the weekly plan, use the same steps to plan for your intermediate and long-term goals.

Use these steps to plan the coming week:

1. Make a list of things you need to do this coming week.

2. Prioritize your "things to do" as listed above by assigning them to one of the following categories:

   A = Top-priority tasks that must be completed by the end of this week. (What is top priority for you?)

   B = Medium-priority tasks without urgent deadlines.

   C = Tasks that really can wait.

A Tasks	Time	B Tasks	Time	C Tasks	Time

3. Estimate and record on the above chart the time required to complete each task—be realistic. Then go back and increase each of the time estimates by 10 to 15 percent. This provides some cushion for error or for unexpected problems.

4. Transfer your "things to do" to a weekly calendar. First, place all "A" tasks in the best time slots for you. If there is time available, add B tasks. List C tasks at the bottom of your calendar; when all A and B tasks are taken care of, do a C task or two.

Remember to get the important tasks done before taking care of less important tasks that might be easier, but fill up your valuable time. Sometimes a less important task can be dropped off the list completely as it loses its importance. You'll be glad you didn't waste your time doing that one!

As you list and prioritize your tasks, be aware of tasks that might best be delegated to the helpers around you. If you must be a perfectionist, be selective about it. It is reasonable to shoot at perfection on your A tasks, and maybe some B's, but don't get sidetracked by doing your low-priority tasks perfectly. Maybe your helpers don't do the job exactly as you would, but while they are getting it done you have time to accomplish your top priorities.

If you find yourself overwhelmed by a monster task, break it into parts. Chapters are easier to write than novels. Learn to say "no" to free up your time. People will learn to respect your time as you learn to manage your time.

Remember that the object is to get where you want while also staying happy and healthy. Be sure to schedule "play time" and relaxation time: not only do these times reward you, but they also reenergize you.

During your busiest, most hectic times, taking the time to plan can be most beneficial.

As you are planning and doing your tasks, remind yourself that although some tasks are unpleasant, most are enjoyable and rewarding. If not, you may want to rethink your long-term goals. If joy is the end, then joy must be the means.

Say What You Want   When you feel that someone is imposing more work or responsibility on you than is appropriate at the time, tell that person that the timing is inappropriate. If you do not wish to do a task, say no. Ask for help from others. Sit down and objectively look at your load in relation to those around you. If you get up and make breakfast for everyone before you go to work, cook dinner, straighten the house, and put everybody to bed after you come home from work, then do the laundry on your day off, look at the responsibilities of everyone else in the household. If the responsibilities are out of balance and the expertise of others is sufficient to carry out some of your duties, ask for a family meeting. Discuss the inequities and reassign some of the duties.

Delegate   As in the preceding technique, duties can be shared when you learn to delegate some of the tasks and responsibilities. This is more than asking for what you want; it is giving up some control over how things will be done by completely giving a task to someone else. The connotation of delegation is that you are in a position of authority and that others are there to help you complete certain tasks. Be thoughtful when you delegate, and take into consideration the workload of others so that you do not overload them. Also, when you give a task to someone else, either give them detailed instructions or give them the authority to do it their way.

Expectation History   Where did your levels of expectation originate? What kind of expectations did you learn from your mother and father? What do (did) your parents and other significant people in your life expect from you? From themselves? From others? What is a reasonable expectation level? There is an old equation:

$$\text{Happiness} = \text{what you get} \div \text{what you expect}$$

If you get \$100 but you expected \$1,000, your quotient is less than 1. If you get \$100 but expected that amount or less, the quotient is 1 or more. When unrealistically high expectations are set, they result in overload stress. When expectations are kept to a minimum and are realistically set, they result in foundational goals rather than system overload.

Examine Beliefs   Using the discussion on beliefs given in the previous section on frustration, think about your long-held beliefs regarding what you expect from others, which is a good reflection of what you expect from yourself. If others cannot please you with their performance, you probably cannot please yourself with your performance. Some of the negative beliefs that may arise here are as follows:

- Work is not done until it is done perfectly.
- I must always perform at the 90 percent level of effectiveness, creativity, and intellectual excellence or I will be considered a sloppy person.
- Others cannot do the job as well as I can.
- If you want it done right, you have to do it yourself.
- The world has no room for a person who performs at less than maximum effort all the time.

When you find that you hold negative beliefs about perfection and expectations, reverse that belief and continue to affirm it until it is the basis for your expectations.

Example: "I must perform with perfection, or I will not be accepted (loved) by others." This belief might be turned around to: "I will do the best I can within reason. Pleasing me is more important than pleasing others."

Decision Making and Problem Solving

There are a few events in our lives that are almost guaranteed to cause stress, and one such event is making a decision. Making decisions encompasses the stress of change and the stress of overload exacerbated by the fear of making the wrong choice. Making decisions can be so stressful and anxiety producing that many people make a lifestyle out of avoiding making choices and putting off the ones they do until the last possible minute. That is why there are so many undeclared majors among college juniors and even seniors. The stress risk in decision making is most pronounced when one becomes obsessed with the details of decision making and insists that one must always find the "right answer." During a crisis, the ability to handle difficult tasks requiring intensely focused attention is decreased.

Traditional decision-making theory says that the decision maker should do the following:

1. Thoroughly examine a wide range of alternatives.

2. Take into account the full range of objectives to be fulfilled and the values implicated by the choice.

3. Carefully weigh both the costs or drawbacks and the benefits of the alternatives.

4. Intensively search for new information relevant to alternatives.

5. Conscientiously take account of any new information or expert judgment that may or may not support previously held preferences.

6. Reexamine positive and negative consequences.

7. Make detailed provisions for implementing the chosen course of action with a contingency plan for dealing with known risks (Janis and Mann 1976).

In real life, the process goes more like this:

The consideration of the problem and potential solutions is time and pressure dependent. In other words, the hunt for the best solution loses intensity when you uncover an acceptable solution. An increase in stress caused by time constraints or worry over being wrong leads to premature closure. The greater the stress, the greater the tendency to make a premature choice of alternatives for a correct response. The greater the stress, the greater the likelihood that a decision maker will choose a risky alternative (Russo 1990).

Prejudiced feelings or subconscious preferences guide the "full range" of objectives, which systematically eliminates alternatives as they emerge instead of bringing all facts to the table and scrutinizing them. Key factors are enhanced or inhibited, and alternatives are prematurely colored for choice or rejection at this stage. The greater the stress, the greater both the distortion in perception of threat and poor judgment. Under increasing stress, productive thoughts decrease and distracting thoughts increase.

Focused problem solving includes seeking preliminary information and then more information and input from others. Problem-solving action includes making alternatives, taking specific action, and learning new skills, especially how to negotiate a compromise.

The emotional focus is on affective regulation, or control of emotion. This is often done with suppression—trying not to think about it, denying feelings, and withholding immediate action; by resigned acceptance—waiting for time to solve the problem, or submitting to fate; or by using emotional discharge—letting off steam, crying, smoking, overeating, or acting out.

Here are some known patterns of decision making:

1. Unconflicted inertia—complacently continuing the status quo and ignoring the risk of deciding;

2. Unconflicted change—uncritically adopting whatever is suggested with preparation for setbacks, accepting reality, or redefining the situation to find something good (that is, things could be worse);

3. Defensive avoidance—doing nothing, denying fear or anxiety, trying to forget the whole situation, and engaging in fantasy rather than thinking about the problem;

4. Hypervigilance—panic, searching for a way out, shifting back and forth between alternatives, taking almost anything for relief, cognitive construction, repetitive thinking, and emotional excitement; and

5. Vigilance—searching for relevant information, assimilating it in an unbiased manner, appraising it, looking at alternatives, and deciding (Clemen 1996; Golub 1996).

The goal is to select the best solution from among the alternatives you have considered while at the same time controlling excess stress that is detrimental to good decision making and to your health (Keeney 1996). You can usually eliminate poor solutions by recognizing they won't work or require skills and resources you don't now have. Other choices can be eliminated because they might involve too high a price—some kind of potential disaster.

Even more important to the discussion of decision making as a stressor is the impact the process has on health. The philosophical take on decisions is to accept the best choice and stop obsessing about the decision. Let go of the unselected options. After making a decision, it takes a little time to reprogram your thinking and to fully commit yourself to the chosen course of action. It may be helpful, especially when the decision is hard to make, to remember that in many cases there is very little difference among the alternative solutions. Give up the notion of finding the one right answer. All your options will probably work out about equally well. We are faced with decisions every day even though most of them are minor. On even the major ones, you cannot "should have" yourself to death. Just get on with making your decision work for you. Although you cannot do everything right, you can make something right out of everything you do.

An Exercise in Healthy Decision Making   When faced with a decision, first clearly delineate the choices. Write down the pros and cons for each alternative choice, and assign a weight (0 to +10) to each pro and a weight to each con (0 to −10), indicating how important that factor is. By adding up the pros and cons separately, you get a total score for each alternative. Next, compare the totals for each alternative course of action. This should usually reveal the best choice. This is a cost–benefit analysis that involves weighing the eventual effectiveness of the solution in solving the problem.

This process is used mostly with big decisions and should save your emotional well-being during and after the decision. Unfortunately, many decisions become exceedingly complex, because there are either several alternatives or many pros and cons to consider. Moreover, the weight you would assign a pro or a con will probably vary from time to time and may actually be prejudiced by feelings one way or the other. Indeed, optimists tend to overemphasize the opportunities in certain choices, whereas pessimists exaggerate the possible dangers of certain alternatives. Usually, if the decision is a major one, you need to weigh the pros and cons, and get a second opinion to double-check your judgments. With the ever-increasing reliance on computers, it is not surprising that computer-supported decision models are becoming popular. Even though complex data can be handled with computer assistance, defining issues and selecting responses are still subject to human bias (Smith 1998).

Boredom and Loneliness

The idea that overstimulation of your mental and emotional processes can result in stress and ill health probably did not surprise you. But now consider the notion that understimulation of these very same processes can result in the same stress response and the same deterioration of your health. We call this state deprivation stress.

Deprivation Stress: the psychophysiological stress response caused by states of boredom and/or loneliness

Deprivation stress was defined over fifty years ago as "the internal bodily reaction to cognitive understimulation"—that is, our body's response to boredom (monotonous, unchallenging tasks) and loneliness (emotional deprivation) (Galdston 1954, 45). Nothing has changed since then to alter the perception of monotony. In affluent societies, advanced technology relieves humans of many tasks, but the human time and interest in those tasks are often replaced with the boredom of watching a machine do the work. Highly repetitive or insufficiently challenging tasks can result in distress. There is certainly nothing wrong with having machines do monotonous work provided you can find more stimulating things to do with the time.

Even with hundreds of channels on TV, video games, and the Internet, boredom appears to prey quite heavily on adolescents. Some psychologists suggest that as many as 20 percent of adolescents in the United States are psychologically handicapped by boredom and depression. Such a handicap may lead to loss of self-esteem and eventually to self-destructive behaviors such as drug abuse and even suicide, one of the leading causes of adolescent death. As a result, billions of dollars are spent each year on entertainment and diversions for adolescents. All of these signs appear to indicate that massive technological advances are serving to bore many Americans to death! The critical factor seems to be how creative, active, or challenging an activity is. Without these factors, no matter how much time is spent in the activity, it is still boring.

Loneliness can also be a devastating stressor. Children who are not given adequate, caring attention are known to suffer from stimulus deprivation. Such emotionally deprived children may suffer a decreased production of growth hormones and subsequent retardation of growth and development. But when these children are placed in an emotionally supportive environment, their growth returns to normal. Nevertheless, psychological scars may persist for a lifetime.

For the major causes of death in the United States (heart disease, cancer, and automobile accidents), mortality is higher among single, widowed, and divorced individuals of all races and both sexes than among married individuals; and interpersonal unhappiness, the lack of love, and human loneliness appear to be the root of physical problems (Bruno 1997; Sanders 1998). In a further discussion in Chapter 9 on relationships, we make a distinction between being alone and loneliness. Once again the difference lies in one's perception and has a large impact on how one tolerates or thrives on being alone.

How well do you tolerate deprivation stress? Self-Assessment Exercise 9 was designed to help you find out. If your score is 25–40, you are vulnerable to deprivation stress; you seem to need stimulation to avoid stress. If your score is 20–24, you are average. If your score is 10–19, you have a high tolerance for low stimulation.

Self-Assessment   EXERCISE IX

Choose the most appropriate answer for each of the following statements, and write the letter of your response to the left of the question. How often do you . . .

_____ **1.** feel that your work is not stimulating enough?
  a. almost always   c. seldom
  b. often   d. almost never

_____ **2.** lose interest in your daily activities?
  a. almost always   c. seldom
  b. often   d. almost never

_____ **3.** become restless during your daily routine?
  a. almost always   c. seldom
  b. often   d. almost never

_____ **4.** feel "insulted" by the simplicity of your work?
  a. almost always   c. seldom
  b. often   d. almost never

_____ **5.** wish your life were more exciting?
  a. almost always   c. seldom
  b. often   d. almost never

_____ **6.** become anxious from a lack of stimulation?
  a. almost always   c. seldom
  b. often   d. almost never

_____ **7.** become bored?
  a. almost always   c. seldom
  b. often   d. almost never

Self-Assessment   CONTINUED

_____ **8.** feel that your usual activities aren't challenging enough?
      a. almost always   c. seldom
      b. often   d. almost never

_____ **9.** daydream during your work?
      a. almost always   c. seldom
      b. often   d. almost never

_____ **10.** feel lonely?
      a. almost always   c. seldom
      b. often   d. almost never

_____ Total Score

Calculate your total score as follows:

a = 4 points   b = 3 points
c = 2 points   d = 1 point

Write your total score in the space provided, and on the Personal Stressor Profile Summary Sheet located in Table Appendix 1 at the back of the book, and *then* read the section *in this chapter pertaining to this Self-Assessment Exercise.*

Exercises to Help with Deprivation Stress

As overload is a stressor because of excessive stimulation, deprivation or boredom is one because of insufficient stimulation. Like all of the stressors discussed here, deprivation is an idiosyncratic and relative phenomenon. In general, deprivation is alleviated by increasing the level of stimulation. The techniques given here present various ways of increasing stimulation and interaction.

Keep a Journal   Writing your feelings about loneliness, boredom, or lack of involvement helps alleviate deprivation stress in two ways: (1) it is an active process that may also include creativity, and (2) the expression of negative emotions helps to release these feelings.

Physical Activity   Become active in a preset or self-originated activity program. Larger cities have YMCAs offering activity courses for small fees. Also available are spas and health clubs, although these are usually more expensive. Every college has a physical education department and campus recreation. Collect catalogs and/or call these establishments to compile a list of possible activities, and then choose one or two that you have always wanted to do. Joining activity classes is also a very good way to meet people with interests similar to yours.

If you have the expertise and desire to set up your own activity program, sit down and plan how you will carry it out for the first month. (A plan for starting a physical activity program is presented in Chapter 17.) Write your activity plan on a calendar. Also, try to get a friend to join you; motivation is usually enhanced by performing activities with others.

Join a Social Group   Using the references to institutions that offer physical activities, obtain information from them regarding other activities such as men's or women's support groups, single-parent groups, reading groups, and so forth. Your city may have a formal listing of social-support groups available in the community. If you have a special interest but there is no established group, consider starting such a group by placing a notice in your apartment building or dorm or by placing an advertisement.

Ask for Human Contact   This technique calls for learning assertiveness skills discussed in the self-concept section in Chapter 6. Please read that section.

Examine Beliefs   What would a person have to believe to remain unhappily in isolation or boredom? Possible negative beliefs:

- I do not deserve the company of fun and interesting people.
- I cannot disclose who I am to others, or they won't like me.
- People will only hurt me and take advantage of me.
- It takes too much effort to make friends.
- I am perfectly happy being by myself.
- If I do make friends, they will just abandon me.

As in past discussions of beliefs, the technique here is to not only examine the negative beliefs that keep you in isolation or boredom but also to turn the belief into a positive statement and begin to live by the new belief. Example: "It takes too much effort to find something exciting to do." This belief can be turned around to: "Getting involved in activities I really like to do is becoming easier and easier."

SUMMARY

Change, overload, frustration, boredom, and loneliness have strong connections with stress. Consider the following points:

- Adaptive stress occurs when situations demand that we change.
- The Social Readjustment Rating Scale measures the impact of change on an individual and predicts the likelihood of resultant stress-related illness.
- Control, challenge, and commitment help prevent or alleviate adaptive stress.
- Frustration (being inhibited from attaining desired goals) is a major stressor in society.
- The frustration of overcrowding produces the stress response in those who feel that their space has been invaded.
- Discrimination and prejudice may be the most widely destructive form of frustration-caused stress.

- Burnout is a common product of overload—being asked to carry a continuously heavy workload, especially in a bureaucratic atmosphere.

- Not having enough stimulation can also cause stress.

SOURCES CITED

Arrien, A. (1994). *The four-fold way.* San Francisco: HarperCollins.

Bandura, A. (1997). *Self-efficacy: The exercise of control.* New York: W. H. Freeman.

Barnes, B. W., and Lightsy, O. R., Jr. Perception of racial discrimination coping, problem solving and life satisfaction. *Journal of Multicultural Counseling and Development*, 33, 48.

Barber, B. R. (2007), *Consumed: How markets corrupt children, infantilize adults and swallow citizens whole.* New York: W. W. Norton.

Bruno, F. (1997). *Conquer loneliness.* Foster City, CA: IDG Books Worldwide.

Buljevac, D., Hop, W. C., Reedeker, W., Janssens, A. C., van der Meche, F. G., van Doorn, P. A. and Hintzen, R. Q. (2003). Self reported stressful life events and exacerbations in multiple sclerosis: Prospective study. British Medical Journal, 327, 646.

Burnbach, J. (1998). *Job discrimination.* Ojai, CA: Voir Dire Press.

Clemen, R. (1996). *Making hard decisions.* Pacific Grove, CA: Duxbury Press.

Fisher, R., Ury, W., and Patton, B. (1991). *Getting to yes: Negotiating without giving in,* 2nd ed. New York: Penguin.

Flannery, R. B. (1993). *Becoming stress resistant.* New York: Continuum.

Friedman, M., Rosenman, R., and Carroll, V. (1958). Changes in the serum cholesterol and blood clotting time in men subjected to cyclic variation of occupational stress. *Circulation,* 18, 852–61.

Galdston, I. (1954). *Beyond the germ theory.* New York: Health Educational Council.

Girdano, D., and Dusek D. (1988). *Changing health behavior.* Scottsdale, AZ: Gorsuch.

Golden-Kreutz, D. M., Thornton, L. M., Wells-Di, G. S., Frierson, G. M., Jim, H. S., Carpenter, K. M., Shelby, R. A., and Andersen, B. L. (2005). Traumatic stress perceived global stress and life events: Prospectively predicting quality of life in breast cancer patients. *Health Psychology,* 24, 288–300.

Golub, A. (1996). *Decision analysis: An integrated approach.* New York: John Wiley and Sons.

Haldar, A., Saha, S., Mandal, S., Haldar, S., Mundle, M., and Mitra, S. P. (2005). Life events as risk factors for myocardial infarction: A pilot case-control study in Kolkata, India. *Journal of Health, Population and Nutrition* 23, 131–36.

Heilbroner, R. (1993). Stereotypes, prejudice and discrimination. In *Experiencing race, class, and gender in the United States,* ed. V. Cyrus, Mountain View, CA: Mayfield, 144–45.

Holm, J., and Holroyd, K. (1992). The daily hassles scale revised. *Behavioral Assessment,* 14, 465–82.

Holmes, T. H., and Rahe, R. H. (1968). The social readjustment rating scale. *Journal of Psychosomatic Research,* 11, 213–18.

Janis, I. L., and Mann, L. (1976). *Decision-making.* Riverside, NJ: Free Press.

Keeney, R. (1996). *Value-focused thinking.* Boston: Harvard University Press.

Kobasa, S. C. (1979). Stressful life events, personality, and health. *Journal of Personality and Social Psychology,* 37, 1–11.

Kompier, M., and Cooper, C. (1999). *Preventing stress, improving productivity.* New York: Routledge.

Koslowsky, M., Kluger, A., and Reich, M., eds. (1995). *Commuting stress: Causes, effects, and methods of coping.* New York: Plenum.

Lazarus, R. S. (1998). *Fifty years of the research and history of R. S. Lazarus.* Mahwah, NJ: Lawrence Erlbaum.

Maddi, S. R. (1996). *Personality theories: A comparative analysis.* New York: Brooks/Cole.

Khoshaba, D. M. & Maddi, S. R. (2001). *HardiTraining.* Newport Beach, CA: Hardiness Institute.

Maddi, S. R. (2002). The story of hardiness: Twenty years of theorizing, research and practice. *Consulting Psychology Journal,* 54, 173–85.

Malkin, M. (2002). *Invasion.* Chicago: Regnery Publishing.

Nance, J. J. (2006). *A refresher on etiquette at 35,000 ft.* ABC News report, January 11.

Ollonen, P., Lehtonen, J. and Eskelinen, M. 2005. Stressful and adverse life experiences in patients with breast symptoms; a prospective case-control study in Kuopio, Finland. *Anticancer Research,* 25, 531–36.

Pelletier, K. R. (1994). *Sound mind, sound body.* New York: Simon & Schuster.

Rahe, R. H. (1967). Life crisis and health change (Report No. 67–4). Annapolis, MD: U.S. Navy Bureau of Medicine and Surgery.

Rahe, R. H. (1979). Life change events and mental illness: An overview. *Journal of Human Stress,* 5, 2–10

Reber, S. O., Obermeier, F., Straub, H. R., and Neumann, I. D. (2006). Chronic intermittent psychosocial stress (social defeat/overcrowding) in mice increases the severity of an acute DSS-induced colitis and impairs regeneration. *Endocrinology* 147, no. 10, 4968–76.

Russo, J. E. (1990). *Decision traps.* New York: Fireside.

Sanders, J. (1998). *Facing loneliness.* New York: Discovery House.

Selye, H. (1976). *The stress of life.* New York: McGraw-Hill.

Singer, J. (1975). Commuter stress. *Science Digest* (August), 18–19.

Smith, C. L. (1998). *Computer-supported decision making: Meeting the decision demands of modern organizations.* Norwood, NJ: Ablex.

Stith, A. (1998). *Breaking the glass ceiling: Sexism and racism in corporate America.* New York: Warwich.

Tanner, O. (1976). *Stress.* New York: Time-Life.

Toffler, A. (1970). *Future shock.* New York: Random House.

Trapp, J., (2006). Road rage ranks as top highway safety issue. Spokesman magazine, (October).

Welch, S., and Gruhl, J. (1998). *Affirmative action and minority enrollments in medical and law schools.* Ann Arbor: University of Michigan Press.

Young-Bruehl, E. (1998). *The anatomy of prejudices.* Boston: Harvard University Press.

Journal Entry 7

Time

One concept of freedom is doing what you want to do when you want to do it. If you are obligated for whatever reason to do something or be somewhere, then your freedom is compromised. A good place to start to look at freedom is to look at how much of your time is obligated and to whom. Complete the following exercise.

How Much Time Is Obligated?

In the left-hand column, estimate what percent of your time (consider all of your waking hours) is obligated to other things and people. In the right-hand column, estimate on a scale of 1 to 10 how much you enjoy the time you spend at this activity or with these people. Give the highest degree of enjoyment a 10 and the lowest a 1.

_____ Peers at school/work   _____

_____ Supervisor at school/work   _____

_____ Clients/instructors   _____

_____ Other Work   _____

_____ Friends   _____

_____ Lover/spouse   _____

_____ Children   _____

_____ Relatives   _____

_____ Agencies/organization/religion   _____

_____ Plants/animals   _____

_____ Self-care   _____

_____ Domestic affairs   _____

_____ Free time with no agenda   _____

_____ Other _____   _____

Spend a few minutes analyzing your time commitments. You might use this circle to slice up the pie according to your different commitments.

What kind of balance are you striking? How you do think this affects your stress levels?

Now look at the right-hand column. Are there more low numbers than highs? How often does a low number (say 5 or lower) appear next to an activity that occupies a high percentage of your time?

Although it may be unrealistic to be totally relaxed while writing a term paper or long report, if you do not enjoy the time spent writing, then it is doubtful you will enjoy your work life if you choose writing or the law as a career. Or if you do not enjoy your science classes, perhaps choosing medicine would not be a good idea.

 Journal about your insights into your obligated time and your enjoyment of how you spend your time. Spend a little time reflecting on how much you enjoy the time you spend with the people in your life.

 Write a positive word or short phrase about balancing time commitments that will be useful to you in future situations.

CHAPTER 8

Stress and the Human Environment Interaction

Human relationships may be responsible for most of our excess stress, but there is also a great potential for excess stress arising from our relationship with the environment. Although environmental stressors act through innate biological mechanisms, such as sound perception and basic metabolism of foods, this is rich soil for personal growth and choice making that decreases stress on the body.

Five classes of environmental stimuli that may play a role in distress are (1) body rhythms; (2) eating and drinking habits; (3) drugs, including alcohol and nicotine; (4) noise pollution; and (5) changes in climate and altitude. We discuss each of these in this chapter.

Time and Body Rhythms

Time has always been recognized as a major stressor. Most people think of deadlines as the only cause of time-related stress. There are, however, other stressful aspects of time. The natural world also runs on time. Solar or light time, lunar time, and seasonal time are but a few examples. The human body also runs on time—temperature time, metabolic time, energy time, and hormonal time (DeHaro & Panda 2006; Yamaguchi et al. 2003). As social, cultural, and technological beings, we have arrogantly ignored our biological time or rhythm for the sake of convenience and conformity. However, we need to synchronize work and recreation schedules with what is socially and economically efficient. Therefore, we utilize artificial light, and we speed through time zones. All of these things affect the body's natural tempo and rhythm. Undue irritability, emotional instability, and increased susceptibility to illness are the price we pay for being out of phase with the body.

Circadian rhythms are regular changes in mind and body that occur in the course of a day (*circadian* is Latin for "around a day"). Most of these rhythms are controlled by the body's biological "clock," specifically the *suprachiasmatic nucleus* or *SCN*. This is actually a pair of tiny brain structures that contain thousands of neurons. The SCN rests in the hypothalamus (again, turn back to Chapter 2 if you've forgotten just where the hypothalamus is). Light that reaches photoreceptors in the retina of the eye creates signals that travel along the optic nerve to the SCN. Then, signals from the SCN travel to several brain regions, including the *pineal gland,* which responds by switching off production of the hormone melatonin. The body's level of melatonin normally increases after darkness falls, making people feel drowsy. The SCN also governs functions that are synchronized with the sleep–wake cycle, including body temperature, hormone secretion, urine production, and changes in blood pressure.

This is important not only for adapting to the changing seasons but also for adapting to socially imposed environmental changes such as lighting, travel, and shift work. The Industrial Revolution, maximal production, efficiency, war, and around-the-clock police, fire, and medical attention have all prompted the shift- or night-work concept. The studies conducted on shift workers have shown an increase in accidents between two and four in the morning, accompanied by a decrease in work performance, and police officers are more apt to sleep on duty during these hours. Airline pilots exhibit their quickest reaction time and best psychomotor coordination between two and four in the afternoon and their poorest performance between two and four in the morning. Radar operators are more likely to make errors and have a harder time staying awake during the hours they would normally be asleep. (Have you ever wondered why the airlines offer reduced rates for overnight flights?)

It is not that the body cannot adjust to changes in lighting or time zones; rather, it cannot make the necessary adjustment in the short time usually allowed (Shiftwork Alert Editors 1998). For example, a night worker's body temperature cycle would be expected to be opposite that of a day worker's yet it usually is not, unless the night-shift schedule is maintained for several weeks—long enough for the body to adapt to a new schedule. In many companies, a worker may rotate shifts each week, one week working nights and the next week working days. Such rotation does not allow the worker adequate time to adapt. Jet lag is an ultimate example of what results from speeding through time zones without time to recover.

Jet Lag

Jet lag is attributed primarily to the body's need to resynchronize its circadian rhythm to the night and day cycle of the new environment. There are, however, other factors believed to exacerbate the symptoms of jet lag:

- being tired, stressed, ill, or hung over at the start of the journey
- the dryness and sometimes the staleness and lack of air in the airplane
- alcohol consumption on the flight, which can exacerbate dehydration
- restricted physical mobility during the flight
- pressure changes from rapid climb to and descent from cruising altitudes

The recent interest in jet lag has spurred several studies that have found a syndrome of symptoms that have been humorously described as a sickness that makes you feel like your passport picture looks. This syndrome includes:

- headache
- blurred vision

- GI problems, including loss of appetite
- increased sweating
- alteration of sleep patterns (nightmares, insomnia)
- menstrual difficulties for female flight attendants

This seems to be the price one must pay for making several phase shifts in a short period. These studies have shown that adaptation differs with each body rhythm. For example, it takes five days for urinary electrolytes to adjust to a new schedule, eight days for heart rate, ten days for urinary steroids, and six days for temperature. Concerned and forward-looking companies have increased layover time for airline crews and business travelers, correctly reasoning that the extra cost of room and board is a good investment when weighed against the potential costliness of accidents, poor business decisions, or illness.

Stop here and complete Self-Assessment Exercise 10 before reading the next section.

Self-Assessment EXERCISE X

Choose the most appropriate answer for each of the following ten statements, and place the letter of your response in the space to the left of the question.

_____ **1.** How many cups of caffeinated coffee do you drink in an average day?
  a. 0 or 1   c. 4 or 5
  b. 2 or 3   d. more than 5

_____ **2.** How many cigarettes do you smoke in an average day?
  a. 0 or 10   c. 21–40
  b. 11–20   d. more than 40

_____ **3.** Do you add salt to your food?
  a. yes   b. no

_____ **4.** How many cups of caffeinated tea do you drink in an average day?
  a. 0 or 1   c. 3 or 4
  b. 1 or 2   d. more than 4

_____ **5.** How many soft drinks do you consume in an average day?
  a. 0 or 1   c. 3 or 4
  b. 1 or 2   d. more than 4

_____ **6.** How much alcohol (liquor, wine, or beer) do you consume during an average week?
  a. 0–7 drinks   c. 15–21 drinks
  b. 8–15 drinks   d. more than 21 drinks

_____ **7.** Do you eat a nutritionally balanced diet?
  a. no   b. yes

_____ **8.** All together, how many pastries, pieces of pie, pieces of cake, donuts, or candy bars do you eat in an average day?
  a. 0   c. 3 or 4
  b. 1 or 2   d. more than 4

Self-Assessment   CONTINUED

_____ **9.** Do you eat a well-balanced breakfast most mornings?
   a. no   b. yes

_____ **10.** How many slices of white bread do you eat during an average day?
   a. 0   c. 3 or 4
   b. 1 or 2   d. more than 4

                                            _____ Total Score

Calculate your total score as follows:

For Questions 3, 7, and 9:
a = 4 points   b = 0 points

For all other questions:
a = 1 point   c = 3 points
b = 2 points   d = 4 points

Place your total score in the space provided here and on the Personal Stress Profile Summary Sheet in Table Appendix 1. Then read the sections "Eating and Drinking Habits" and "Drugs."

With jet lag, it is estimated that it takes about twenty-four hours to adjust to each one-hour time difference. Jet travel alters more than sleep–wake cycles it also affects heart rate, blood pressure, respiration, body temperature, urinary output, hormone secretion, and mental functioning because these are all regulated on a twenty-four-hour cycle. To beat jet lag, it helps to manipulate your blood chemistry by providing proteins that affect the brain's biochemistry in the direction of wakefulness and alertness and by providing carbohydrates that tend to calm the mind and damp out distractions (Anderson and Vail 1998; Fairechild 2004). The following routine is suggested for the day of departure:

Flying west to east:
   Exercise in the morning
   Breakfast and lunch high in protein
   Dinner and evening snacks high in carbohydrates

Flying east to west:
   Carbohydrate breakfast
   Protein lunch and dinner
   Exercise in the afternoon

Plan your arrival for the morning so that you have all day to acclimatize by eating and exercising in the manner just given. Exercise raises the body's temperature, so when you arrive in the east in the morning, vigorous exercise helps you wake up. Vigorous exercise in the afternoon when you arrive in the west helps you stay awake past what would be your bedtime at home. Eating fatty foods within the first day or two after your arrival counters the effects of a dietary regimen of protein and carbohydrates; alcohol exacerbates the fatigue of jet lag, so it is best to drink alcohol only in the evening, if at all.

Another way to alleviate the stress caused by jet lag is to schedule a buffer day after you arrive at your destination. Use that day to relax and adjust your internal clock.

Eating and Drinking Habits

Everyone knows that good nutrition contributes to healthful living, but few realize the extent to which our eating and drinking habits contribute to our daily stress levels. The consumption or lack of consumption of certain foods and the consumption of some kinds of beverages can add to the stress of everyday life by stimulating the sympathetic stress response directly or by contributing to its stimulation through creating a state of fatigue and increased nervous irritability (Sizer & Whitney 2003). Either condition lowers your tolerance to the common stresses of day-to-day living. There are several eating and drinking habits that may be involved in stress. Some of the more common ones are examined in this section.

On Self-Assessment Exercise 10, if you scored between 30 and 40 points, your eating and drinking habits definitely make you more vulnerable to stress. Scores below 15 points show low vulnerability.

Sympathomimetic Agents

Sympathomimetic agents are chemical substances that mimic the sympathetic stress response. Many foods naturally contain these substances. When consumed, they trigger a stress response in the body, the severity of which will depend on how much of the chemical was consumed. The most common of these sympathomimetic stressors in the modern diet is caffeine, a chemical that belongs to the xanthine group of drugs. Xanthines are powerful amphetamine-like stimulants that increase metabolism and create a highly awake and active state. They also trigger release of the stress hormones that, among other actions, are capable of increasing heart rate, blood pressure, and oxygen demands on the heart. Extreme, prolonged stress-hormone secretion can even initiate myocardial necrosis—that is, destruction of the heart tissue.

Coffee (*Coffea arabica*) is the most frequently consumed source of caffeine. Americans over the age of fourteen consume an average of three cups of coffee a day! The average brewed six-ounce cup of coffee contains about 108 milligrams of caffeine. Caffeine consumption of more than 250 milligrams per day is considered excessive and will have an adverse effect on the human body. A lethal dose of caffeine could be consumed in the form of twenty cups of coffee if drunk all at once! Frequent side effects of excessive coffee drinking are anxiety, irritability, diarrhea, arrhythmia (irregular heartbeat), and inability to concentrate, in addition to a host of symptoms characteristic of the stress response. Coffee may also stimulate the secretion of the digestive enzyme and other biochemical substances necessary for arousal and adaptation responses (Nawrot et al. 2003)

During stressful times, high levels of certain vitamins (such as vitamin C and B vitamins) are needed to maintain proper function of the nervous and endocrine systems. They are also called on to help carry out carbohydrate metabolism and gluconeogenesis (the process whereby the body forms glucose for more energy). Vitamin C and choline are necessary elements in the production of adrenal hormones, which are secreted during the stress response. Deficiencies of these vitamins lower tolerance to stressors and ability to cope with them. In turn, excessive stress over prolonged periods may deplete the body of these vitamins, making an individual more prone to vitamin deficiency.

Table 8.1 Sugar in Common Foods

Food	Portion	Tsp. Sugar*
Chocolate bar	1 average size	7
Chocolate fudge	$\frac{1}{2}$ square	4
Marshmallow	1 average size	$\frac{1}{2}$
Chocolate cake	$\frac{1}{12}$ cake (2-layer, icing)	15
Angelfood cake	$\frac{1}{12}$ cake	6
Doughnut, plain	3″ diameter	4
Brownie	2″ × 2″ × 3/4″	3
Ice cream	$\frac{1}{2}$ cup	5–6
Sherbet	$\frac{1}{2}$ cup	6–8
Apple pie	$\frac{1}{6}$ medium pie	12
Cherry pie	$\frac{1}{6}$ medium pie	14
Pumpkin pie	$\frac{1}{6}$ medium pie	10
Sweet carbonated beverage	12 oz.	9
Ginger ale	12 oz.	7

*100 grams sugar = 20 teaspoons = 1/2 cup = 1/2 ounces = 400 calories.

One common dietary component implicated in depletion of the B-complex vitamins is refined white sugar. Another is refined white flour. Sugar—and therefore sugar products such as cakes, pies, cookies, and candy (see **Table 8.1**)—is a good source of energy but has no other redeeming feature. For sugar to be utilized for energy, however, the body must have B-complex vitamins. Natural foods that need these vitamins for their metabolism contain the necessary vitamins, but because sugar contains none of them, it must borrow them from other food sources. This may create a B-complex debt in the body. If this borrowing occurs frequently or if the body does not have sufficient sources of B vitamins from nutritious foods or supplements, the result may be a B-vitamin deficiency and symptoms such as anxiety, irritability, and general nervousness. This vitamin depletion may be exacerbated by stress because of the increased utilization of these vitamins in the stress response.

Hypoglycemic Stress

Another way in which diet may predispose an individual to distress is through **hypoglycemia**, or low blood sugar (Nadler 2003). Symptoms may include anxiety, headache, dizziness, trembling, and increased cardiac activity. These symptoms may cause normal stimuli to become severely acute stressors by making the individual highly irritable and impatient. In effect, they lower the individual's stress tolerance. This is routinely seen in people who get "crabby" when they are hungry. Although there are numerous causes for hypoglycemia, we are most interested in the two directly related to dietary behaviors. **Reactive hypoglycemia** is caused by high intake of sugars within a limited amount of time. Eating a meal high in sugars or even snacking on foods high in sugars may cause a hypoglycemic reaction in individuals prone to this disorder.

Functional hypoglycemia occurs when meals are missed, and it may be exacerbated by sugar intake that results over time in a lower overnight (or fasting) blood-sugar level than would be considered normal.

The process by which such dietary behaviors lead to hypoglycemia is somewhat paradoxical because hypoglycemia is preceded by a state of high blood sugar (hyperglycemia). The high intake of sugar first raises the sugar level in the blood. This high blood-sugar level stimulates the release of insulin (almost instantly), which allows the excess sugar to enter all the body's tissues. Therefore, the blood sugar is not selectively saved for the central nervous system, whose function and vitality depend on it. Generally, if blood-sugar levels drop below 60 milligrams of glucose per 100 milliliters of blood, symptoms such as irritability, anxiety, and fatigue occur.

In extreme cases of high sugar intake, the symptoms of hypoglycemia may occur within a short period and may be so severe as to cause nausea, staggering, slurred and mixed speech, and fainting. Extreme hypoglycemic shock can result in coma and death, but in this situation there is generally some underlying cause, such as a pancreatic tumor or insulin shock, as seen in diabetics. Whether due to perpetual high sugar intake or other physiological conditions, a low blood-sugar level due to hypoglycemia may be responsible for "midmorning slump" and continual hunger that seems to be sated only with sugar products such as cookies, sweet rolls, candy bars, or soft drinks. Because many people eat only a jelly roll, doughnut, or bowl of highly sweetened cereal for breakfast, it is to be expected that low midmorning blood sugar will bring about increased response to stress situations and diminished ability to perform. The same situation may occur in midafternoon or at any other time of day after high sugar intake—or merely from not eating. The best way to avoid the stresses of hypoglycemia and its glucocorticoid stress response is to eat well-balanced meals (the size of which should be determined by the energy demands for the next few hours) containing a minimum of sugar and processed foods.

Sodium Intake and Fluid Retention

Salt (sodium chloride) is the mineral most responsible for regulating the body's water balance. The sodium ion in salt causes retention of water within the body; therefore, high levels of table salt or of foods naturally high in sodium may result in excessive fluid retention. Excessive fluid retention has the effect of increasing nervous tension (through edema, an abnormal accumulation of fluid) in the general nervous tissue and cerebral tissue (de la Sierra 2003).

On average, the higher the salt intake, the higher the blood pressure. Nearly all Americans consume substantially more salt than they need (USDA 2005). The natural salt content of food accounts for about 10 percent of total intake; salt added at the table or while cooking provides another 5–10 percent; and about 75 percent is derived from salt added by manufacturers. **Table 8.2** lists foods high in sodium. The body has the ability to store salt, so daily survival needs are relatively low (less than 1 gram). However, the average person consumes 4 to 8 grams per day (an average shake of salt from the salt shaker is 100 milligrams). Dietary Guidelines for America recommends that we consume less than 2,300 mg (about 1 tsp of salt) per day.

Some people tend to be more salt sensitive than others, including those with hypertension, blacks, and middle-aged and older adults. It is recommended that these individuals

Table 8.2   Foods High in Sodium

Most Canned Foods	Cheeses	Baking Soda
meats	processed cheese	(sodium bicarbonate
soups	cheese dips	contains about 1,000 mg
stews	snack cheese spreads	of sodium per level teaspoon)
sauerkraut		

Pork Products	Seasonings	Most Fast Food
ham	prepared mustard	
bacon	catsup	
sausage	Worcestershire sauce	
hot dogs	soy sauce	
	pickles	

Snack Foods	Relishes	
pretzels	meat tenderizers	
popcorn	peanut butter (most brands are	
potato chips	heavy in sodium additives)	

Note: As a rule, processed foods contain more sodium than fresh foods.

consume no more than 1,500 mg of sodium per day and meet the potassium recommendation of 4,700 mg/day with food. A good, nutritious diet provides the necessary daily intake of sodium (USDA 2005).

In many people, increased blood pressure is the most common manifestation of the stress reaction. However, if a person's blood pressure is already high due to excessive fluid retention, the pressure elevation during distress may reach a danger point. It may become high enough to increase the risk of stroke or heart attack or perhaps become chronically elevated.

Many salt substitutes are becoming popular, the most frequently-used one being potassium chloride. You can switch to one of the commercial substitutes and derive some of the same taste benefit without risking stress. However, the USDA (2005) warns that although substitutes containing potassium chloride may be useful for some, they can be harmful to people with certain medical conditions. These folks should consult a health care provider before trying salt substitutes.

An individual's preference for salt is not fixed—taste for salt tends to decrease as one adapts to a lower-salt diet. The conscious manipulation of eating behavior to provide the nutrients essential for fighting stress is called nutritional restructuring, and it can be a powerful addition to the holistic pattern for stress control.

Eating Guidelines

To combat everyday stressors and prevent further stress from the foods you have chosen to include in your diet, it is important to develop healthful eating habits. In 1990, a major study in epidemiology (the branch of science that studies the causes and control of diseases) disclosed some important nutrition research facts to the public, all of which relate to the effect diet has on stress levels. This study, called the China Health Project (CHP), began in 1983 and tracked the daily living habits of 6,500 Chinese in sixty-five counties across rural China. The study (Chen, Campbell, Li, and Peto 1990) has been called "The Grand Prix of Epidemiology" because of its longitudinal nature (the same people are studied over a period of years), its breadth (it studied a wide range of dietary, environmental, and health factors), and its validity (a very stable population in each of the sixty five counties). The people were genetically quite similar within each province, and there was a great deal of ethnic variation from region to region.

The researchers of this study, who were from Cornell University in the United States, Oxford University in England, and two Chinese academies, have confirmed some nutrition-disease relationships that American nutritionists have been hedging on for years. Some of the general results and recommendations of particular importance to stress and disease are the following:

- A high cholesterol level is a major predictor of disease, especially cardiovascular disease.
- Diets high in protein, fat, calories, and calcium are good for early childhood growth but are related to higher breast cancer rates among women later in life.
- A diet high in fiber can protect against colon cancer (a major killer in more affluent societies).
- A vegetable-based diet is completely safe and much healthier than an animal-based diet.

The following recommendations should help make your diet more healthful and less stressful (Harris 1996):

1. Replace some animal-based protein with plant-based protein and carbohydrates such as whole grains, beans, and tofu or with look-alike foods such as vegetable- or soy-based burgers and hot dogs.

2. Cut down on dairy consumption by substituting soy beverage for milk, tofu for cheese, soy- or fruit-based desserts for ice cream, and fruit preserves for butter.

3. Shop more frequently, and buy fresh foods. Buy locally grown foods when possible.

4. If you have to eat in a fast-food restaurant, choose salads, vegetables, and soups rather than the high-fat foods.

5. Eat smaller meals evenly spaced rather than loading up on dinner (or any one other meal).

6. Plan your daily menu each morning, and save time by preparing ahead for dinner, including such tasks as soaking beans.

7. Change your eating habits slowly, incorporating one thing at a time. Note how your health changes with your dietary changes.

8. Buy a good vegetarian cookbook and/or take a cooking class featuring vegetable-based foods. Eat at least one cruciferous vegetable per day (broccoli, cauliflower, cabbage, and so on) and at least one vegetable that is high in beta carotene (broccoli, tomato, carrots, and so on).

9. Eat fresh fruits in season, preferably raw rather than canned in syrup or cooked as a sauce. Red and orange fruits are high in beta carotene.

10. In the milk, yogurt, and cheese group, choose low- or no-fat dairy products.

11. In the red meat, poultry, fish, dried beans, eggs, and nuts group, avoid fatty red meat and poultry, prepare meats by broiling or grilling rather than frying.

12. In the fats, oils, and sweets group, use vegetable oils in moderation, remove animal fats from the diet as much as possible, and don't load up on sweets at any one time.

In 1992, the U.S. Department of Agriculture published a Food Guide Pyramid that soon came under fire and eventually developed into the USDA's MyPyramid program (USDA 2007). This program can be accessed at www.MyPyramid.com, where if offers everyone a personalized eating plan with foods and amounts that are right for the individual.

The Stress of Overnutrition

The advent of the twenty-first century has brought with it the fear of terrorism, loss of jobs, loss of retirement funds in the stock market, lack of affordable health insurance, a demand that we work longer and harder and live in credit card debt, and other deep-seated fears. Many of the fearful turn to food for nurturance. After the terrible events of September 11, 2001, the consumption of sweets and fatty foods increased. While the market price of Fidelity Magellan tanked, Krispy Kreme donuts were selling like, well, donuts.

America is getting fatter and fatter, which is reflected in soaring rates of weight-related death and disease (see **Table 8.3**); and with that goes the emotional and social pain of being overweight or obese. If a person has a Body Mass Index (BMI) of 25–29.99 or is 25–30 pounds over their recommended weight for their height they are considered *overweight*. If they have a BMI over 30 or are 30 pounds or more over this limit, they are considered *obese*. Body Mass Index is computed by dividing body weight in kilograms by height in meters squared. A BMI table is provided in Chapter 17.

Anyone who ever watches Oprah knows that being overweight or obese has emotional roots. Overeating and underexercising is not a simple lifestyle problem. We have explained in the earlier chapters of this book that behavior is a reflection of our emotions, our self-concept, our beliefs, and the thoughts that emanate from them. The key to being at a healthy weight and staying there is dependent on these background issues that surround eating. We contend that a weight management program should be a good stress management program that also focuses on food and fitness. Food is intended to nourish our bodies, not allay loneliness, anger, boredom, or anxiety. There are psychological, emotional, even spiritual behaviors that will truthfully allay these dysphoric conditions. Food just cannot solve these problems. So, the stress of being overweight or obese in a thin-demanding society is not resolved here by merely suggesting a proper eating style or a good fitness program. The answer is in solving the emotional, mental, and spiritual blocks that motivate one to overeat and do nothing about weight gain and unhealthy body composition.

Just as in any high-risk health behavior, the overweight/obese person must consider the risks versus the benefits of overnutrition. If the benefits are immediate and certain,

Table 8.3 Overweight and Obese Individuals Are at Increased Risk of these Physical Ailments

High blood pressure, hypertension

High blood cholesterol

Type 2 (non-insulin-dependent) diabetes

Insulin resistance, glucose intolerance

Hyperinsulinemia

Coronary heart disease

Angina pectoris

Congestive heart failure

Stroke

Gallstones

Gout

Osteoarthritis

Obstructive sleep apnea and respiratory problems

Some types of cancer (such as endometrial, breast, prostate, and colon)

Complications of pregnancy

Poor female reproductive health (such as menstrual irregularities, infertility, irregular ovulation)

Bladder control problems (such as stress incontinence)

Psychological disorders (such as depression, eating disorders, distorted body image, and low self-esteem)

Source: National Institutes of Health (2002).

one is more likely to engage in the behavior than if the consequences are delayed and uncertain. Immediate gratification from food is a sure reward. Will weight loss somewhere down the road be as satisfying? What kind of motivation is necessary to bank on that future?

Losing weight is not an easy task because it calls for a fairly complex change in lifestyle. Where the overweight have been eating as much of the kinds of foods that nurtured them, they are asked to give up "biggy" portion sizes and foods they love. Where they have been accustomed to not much more exercise than walking to the refrigerator, they are asked to participate in regular physical activity or exercise programs on a daily basis. Where they have used food as an answer to the daily stressors in life, they are asked to learn to manage stress in healthy ways such as meditation, journaling, exercise, or muscular relaxation.

Here are some of the more current statistics that should be throwing up red flags for the entire population and encouraging them to maintain a healthy weight:

- Nearly 40 million American adults are obese, up almost 8 percent since 1991. That means that one in five American adults is obese. One in fourteen is diabetic.

- More than half of Americans—56.4 percent—are overweight (up from 45 percent in 1991).

- Overweight people are more likely to develop heart disease, stroke, diabetes, certain types of cancer, gout, and gallbladder disease. Being overweight is also likely to cause sleep apnea and osteoarthritis.

- All of these conditions can be reversed to some degree with weight loss, especially if caught early enough.

- Older fat people are twice as likely to have a stroke than thin people; the chance of stroke rises 6 percent with each 6–7 pounds gained.

- Diabetes alone accounts for $100 billion in health care spending each year—and the costs are climbing. Most cases are likely adult-onset diabetes.

- Obesity-related diseases are the second-leading causes of premature deaths (next to smoking-related diseases) (CDC 2007; NIH 2003).

The USDA Food Guide Pyramid mentioned earlier had to be revamped (USDA 2007) because it encouraged the population to place six to eleven servings of pasta, potatoes, bread, rice, and cereal on their plates each day without stressing the drawbacks to these foods, especially how they contribute to the obesity epidemic (Weil 2001). Most of these foods that Americans prefer are white potatoes, French fries, breads made with white processed flour, white rice, processed breakfast foods high in sugar, and other starchy products that create carbohydrate intolerance and insulin problems (as discussed early regarding reactive hypoglycemia).

The emotional and physical stress of being overweight or obese can be helped with good nutrition and exercise, but a stress management lifestyle program to go along with them is a *must*. For weight reduction and maintenance:

1. Examine the emotional and psychological ramifications of food in your life and motivation for eating, and then develop a stress management program that alleviates problematic eating,

2. Follow the suggestions in this chapter regarding dietary guidelines, and

3. Develop a fitness program that allows you to exercise away more calories than you eat.

Exercise is more than a calorie-burner—it uses up stress products in the body that, if left at high levels, can create health hazards. We devote the whole of Chapter 17 to physical activity as a form of stress management. Take it seriously. The guidelines suggested there are also pertinent to weight loss and maintenance.

Drugs, Alcohol, and Tobacco

Although people smoke and take drugs (including alcohol) for various reasons, a common motive is to alter their state of consciousness in an attempt to reduce emotional and mental stress. Just as we saw in the case of overeating, overweight, and obesity, the taking of substances must be examined at the level of motivation. Most smokers, drinkers, and drug takers are knowledgeable about the dangers of their chosen substance. The dangers of smoking (both tobacco and marijuana) have been well laid out by the scientific community; mind-altering drugs from alcohol (as a depressant) to cocaine (as a stimulant) are well known. Why, then, do individuals continue to take something that can cause greater problems to not only themselves, but others around them—their friends, family, society at large?

As we mentioned regarding the stress of being overweight or obese, one thing that determines the use of any substance is the balance between perceived risks and benefits associated with a substance. The *benefits* associated with drug use tend to be more immediate and certain whereas the *risks* tend to be more distant and uncertain; for example, the stimulation of nicotine is immediate and certain, while the threat of cancer is more distant and uncertain—the negative effects may or may not happen so they have less control over current behavior. We know from behavioral theory that immediate and certain consequences elicit greater behavioral control than uncertain and delayed ones do.

There are three major influences on drug taking or abstinence: biomedical, social, and individual. Biomedical facts include genetic susceptibility to certain substances, such as Native American susceptibility to alcohol. Genetics affect metabolism of drugs, responses to them, and one's vulnerability to dependence. Alcoholism is considered a disease, not merely a result of bad behavior choices.

Social influences include those of people, events, or consequences *outside* the individual. Here we are talking about peer pressure and the rewards or punishments from those around us. Individual influences are those inherent within a person's psychology and belief system. Although there is little besides abstinence that can be done about the biomedical influences, the other two have a great deal to do with stress management as it has been presented so far. The misuse and abuse of alcohol and other drugs strongly reflect one's strength of character, self-concept, emotional quotient, interpersonal communication abilities, and spiritual individuality.

Drugs

The sense of unreality and lack of self-awareness that result from some forms of drug use may be calming in the sense that the drug temporarily blocks one from actively thinking about a problem. Unfortunately, the problem still exists. It is stored in parts of the brain and is producing feelings and other body alterations even though the drug taker is not actively aware of them. Problems are still present and continue to stress the system. The only difference is that the flow of active, here-and-now thoughts has been temporarily blocked. The feelings of self-transcendence vanish once the drugs wear off and can be regained only by repeated use of the drug. There is little positive carryover, little is learned in the drug state, and few people experience long-term positive change from the drug experience. Their world, their problems, and their coping mechanisms are the same as before. Drugs have fulfilled a limited goal, an altered state of consciousness, but they have not fulfilled the dream—that the experience would somehow grant the user greater insights and the ability to naturally transcend the ego and live a calmer, more relaxed and enlightened life.

The passivity of the drug experience is in itself a drawback. Experiences in which the individual just rides along, seeing, feeling, and experiencing, are somehow not as satisfying as those in which the individual is the active, creative center of the experience. Creative activities increase one's self-esteem and in a circular pattern increase motivation and readiness for future unknown ventures.

An altered state can also be induced through such activities as meditation and daydreaming or by hypoarousal or hyperarousal of the central nervous system. It is healthier to induce these states by mind direction than by using drugs. There are many popular techniques for inducing a self-transcendent, altered state of consciousness through mind direction or control. Yoga, meditation, muscle relaxation, autogenic training, and biofeedback are but a few examples. These constitute a more positive approach than drugs, not only because they are less dangerous, more socially acceptable, and more controllable but also because they are active and creative, requiring and promoting self-control and self-discipline. They are learning exercises that result in temporary feelings of self-transcendence, thus providing the foundation and motivation to reeducate one's thoughts and coping processes. If mastered, they lead to an even higher state—that of conscious self-transcendence, a less conscious, more self-expanded state in which boundaries are infinitely extended. This is a health-promoting state because it is integrated with ongoing life and provides benefits to the individual, society, and humankind in general.

Research in the 1990s has offered strong evidence that two common "oral" habits, cigarette smoking and extensive caffeine consumption, may be highly deleterious to health, either singly or when combined, and that much of this effect is attributable to excessive stress.

Go back to Self-Assessment Exercise 10 and examine Items 1, 2, 4, and 5 (if the soft drinks contain caffeine). If you responded with c's or d's for those items, your diet could be hurting your health, regardless of your total score on the exercise.

Throughout history, people have used drugs and become dependent on them. During the twentieth century, however, drug use and abuse reached epidemic proportions. No one reason can be offered as an explanation. However, the most often mentioned reason was a way to cope with stress. Hoffman and Carbone (2002) reported that low self-esteem was associated with drug use, as was parental substance use disorder and the risk of adolescent drug abuse. Others have reported that there was a significant association between drug dependence in young adults and stressful life events, emotional abuse by caretakers, and physical abuse by partner or spouse (Turner and Lloyd 2003).

Whatever the reason, researchers have found that each type of drug produces a specific psychological state, or an altered reality, and that chronic users choose a specific drug because of the state it induces. From the first experience of an altered state, the person may or may not seek that experience again. If the reason is "just to see what it's like," the person's motivation is experimental or curiosity. If the altered state is sought repeatedly, the motivation changes. It may be for perceived pleasure, for escape from a world that seems stressful, or to satisfy physical and psychological addictions. Compulsive users find that virtually every aspect of their lives revolves around obtaining, maintaining, and using the drug. These individuals, described as being drug dependent, are controlled physically, psychologically, and socially by their drug habit. Although that does not seem like competent coping to most of us, it actually is a coping mechanism to those in the cycle because it is predictable and makes many stressful decisions for the individual.

Drug rehabilitation research has documented lack of self-identity as a deep-seated cause of drug abuse. This is a common theme for individuals who also experience excess stress as well. In contrast, people who are comfortable with themselves are less inclined to try to alter their self-perception through drugs. Many drug and alcohol rehabilitation programs are aimed specifically at the formation of a positive identity (Gerstein and Lewin 1990; Sales 1999).

Alcohol

The human organism does not require alcohol, yet throughout history alcohol has been an integral part of life in most parts of the world. Alcohol has gained the reputation as the ultimate stress-relieving drug, and relaxation and recreation are the most often cited reason for consuming it. Political leaders celebrate important agreements with a toast. Glasses are raised to toast the bride and groom and the New Year. Elaborate establishments are built to provide places to gather and consume alcohol. The average household contains some form of alcoholic beverage. In the United States, a temporary prohibition of alcohol from 1920 to 1933 produced the largest episode of civil disobedience in U.S. history. Alcohol is not consumed only when one feels deviant or defiant. It is not used only to mask stress, insecurity, or depression or to give a person courage. It is a cultural adjunct. To some extent and for some people, alcohol consumption is pleasant and pleasurable. For many others, however, especially people with emotional problems and those who overindulge, alcohol presents a problem—a self-inflicted, individual problem for which society as a whole pays a great price (Malone et al. 2004).

In 2002, 55 percent of U.S. adults were current drinkers. Forty-five percent of U.S. adults do not drink any alcohol at all. Fewer Americans consume alcohol today as compared to 100 years ago (USDA 2005). Alcohol may have beneficial effects when consumed in moderation. The lowest coronary heart disease mortality occurs at an intake of one to two drinks per day. Sickness and death are highest among those drinking large amounts of alcohol (USDA 2005). The USDA's Dietary Guidelines for Americans suggest:

- Those who choose to drink alcoholic beverages should do so sensibly and in moderation—defined as the consumption of up to one drink per day for women and up to two drinks per day for men.

- Alcoholic beverages should not be consumed by some individuals, including those who cannot restrict their alcohol intake, women of childbearing age who may become pregnant, pregnant and lactating women, children and adolescents, individuals taking medications that can interact with alcohol, and those with specific medical conditions.

- Alcoholic beverages should be avoided by individuals engaging in activities that require attention, skill, or coordination, such as driving or operating machinery.

You can protect yourself from alcohol abuse in several ways. Best advice: Don't drink at all if you have any reason to suspect that you are prone to alcohol abuse. Second best: Drink in moderation. Don't glorify alcohol or your ability to consume it. Learn to recognize the signs of overdrinking and use these as a signal to slow down. Common signs are loud talking, slurred speech, walking unsteadily, dropping things or spilling drinks, perspiring, and turning red or pale in the face.

Don't drink and drive. Carpool, select a designated driver who will not drink, call a friend, take a taxi, or stay the night. Don't let your friends drive if they've been drinking. Stay in control. Learn how to keep track of your blood alcohol level by knowing your weight, the amount of alcohol you've consumed, and your drinking time. Keep yourself busy with interesting and active pursuits. Avoid friends who do little else besides drink for their recreation.

If you find that you are:

- drinking, even in moderation, every day
- in a habit of constantly talking about your drunken exploits
- arriving late at work or missing early classes because of hangovers
- getting drunk regularly
- drinking to dull the hurt of loneliness and to counteract frequent depression
- driving after drinking
- needing to brag constantly about your ability to drink,

you should seriously consider cutting down on how much and how often you drink, for you are developing an addictive behavior pattern. If cutting down is difficult for you to do alone, seek help. NOW. Talk to your doctor or a counselor about the possibility that you are drinking too much. Be honest. If you aren't comfortable in doing this, look up the telephone number for Alcoholics Anonymous (AA) and call. Ask how you can tell whether you are drinking too much and whether AA can assist you in finding help (Acker and Tracy 2004; Brown and Lewis 1999; Meyers and Smith 1999).

To avoid slipping past a pleasurable social interaction into intoxication for you and your guests at parties and other recreational functions, try some of these suggestions:

- The party atmosphere should be relaxing, and whatever can be done to make everyone mix should be done. One reason people drink too much at social gatherings is that they cannot seem to get conversations going.
- The volume of music should be low enough to allow people to socialize. Again, when you cannot talk, you drink more.
- Food should be served. It not only slows down the absorption of alcohol but also satisfies some oral needs to supplant the continual sipping of drinks. Good food also takes some of the spotlight off alcohol. Foods that have some protein content are best: for example, cheese and crackers, Swedish meatballs, hard-boiled eggs, cheese fondue, pizza, and bite-size cold cuts.
- Activities should be going on, with some effort to get everyone involved. Dancing, games, sports, and good conversation quickly become the focus, and drinks become supplementary only.

Tobacco

The final consideration in this section is the use of tobacco products. The harmful effects of smoking and chewing tobacco are well known (USDHHS 2004). Less advertised is how the drug nicotine contributes to distress. Nicotine stimulates the adrenals, which release hormones that elicit the stress response—increased heart rate, force of cardiac contraction, blood pressure, respiration rate, and release of fatty acids and glucose into the blood, among other body reactions. More people die from the nicotine effects of tobacco (cardiovascular complications) than from carcinogenic tars.

Tobacco contains nicotine. Like caffeine, nicotine is a sympathomimetic chemical, and as such it is capable of stimulating all the adverse effects of the arousal response noted earlier. It causes a stress response each time it is taken into the body, whether by smoking a cigarette, inhaling the smoke of others, or chewing tobacco. The smoker and the person facing almost any everyday stressors exhibit the same physiological state. One difference is that the chronic smoker's physiological functioning is continually elevated to the point where this arousal state becomes the "normal" state. Being without the stimulating effect of nicotine creates a mild depression and a generally uneasy feeling that lead to the desire for additional nicotine for a pickup. As the chronic smoking habit develops, the stress tolerance to nicotine is increased, and the adverse stress-related effects become somewhat reduced, but the smoke continues to affect the smoker's respiratory system. They also affect the nonsmoker. Because the nonsmoker has developed little if any tolerance to nicotine, the smoke can cause decreases in work performance. A smoky working area can irritate the nonsmoker's eyes and nose, impeding detail work, concentration, and tolerance for more difficult work tasks.

Scientists have long known that nicotine, like other addictive drugs, attaches to neurons of the brain's reward system, where beneficial behaviors are rewarded and reinforced. These reward neurons, called dopaminergic neurons, trigger release of the neurotransmitter dopamine in a nearby brain region. When nicotine attaches to these neurons they increase their activity, flooding the region with dopamine, which produces pleasure and a disposition to repeat the behaviors that led to it, creating the process of addiction (Zickler 2003).

Following alcohol, the nicotine present in tobacco is the second most widely used drug in the world. The American Cancer Society tells us that 48 million Americans smoke, yet since 1965 more than 40 percent of all adults who ever smoked have quit (ACS 2007). Nicotine meets the established scientific criteria for classification as a dependency-producing drug. Tobacco use, like use of other abused drugs, often is peer initiated, and the primary reason given for its use is again pleasure and relief from stress. Social support for tobacco use allows for tolerance and habitual patterns to develop with repeated use. Tobacco use may produce both psychological and physical dependence. Smoking is one of the more difficult dependencies to end, perhaps because smoking was acceptable for so long, and smokers developed the dependency early and continued it for decades. Smoking cessation treatment results in short-term success rates as high as 70 percent, but these rates decrease significantly to an average of between 6 percent and 15 percent one year later. The reasons some people succeed and others fail are not well understood, but many researchers believe that success is a result of a combination of personal motivation, an effective plan of action, and not trying to quit during periods of high stress.

Successful smoking cessation programs tend to include the following core elements (Girdano and Dusek 1988):

1. *Healthful lifestyle.* An essential component of an effective program often is not included in smoking cessation programs, and this oversight undoubtedly contributes to the high failure rates. This phase focuses on psychological needs that smoking traditionally has satisfied. The goal is to extinguish these needs and develop lifestyle skills that will help the nonsmoker remain a nonsmoker. The basic components are as follows:

2. *Relaxation and stress management skills.* Part of almost every smoker's habit is the use of cigarettes to control one or more of the following factors: excess anxiety, low self-esteem, excess anger, depression, a stressful lifestyle, and the inability to relax.

3. *Diet.* Many smokers are nervous eaters who have substituted smoking for eating because often, when smoking stops, eating and weight gain problems emerge. This creates fear in weight-conscious smokers. Close attention to diet and weight management counseling are essential to the success of most smoking cessation programs.

4. *Exercise.* Exercise not only is integral to a healthful lifestyle but also may be essential to smoking cessation programs because it builds confidence and self-esteem, reduces anxiety and excess stress, burns calories, and is antithetical to the physical deterioration caused by smoking.

Noise Pollution

Briefly, the ear is made of three parts: outer ear, middle ear, and inner ear. The first two parts conduct sound coming in toward the inner ear. These outer parts convert high-amplitude and low-pressure vibrational sound into low-amplitude and high-pressure vibrations needed for transmission in the inner ear. The cochlea of the inner ear, a snail-shaped organ buried in the temporal bone, contains cilia-like hair cells that convert sound waves into nerve impulses. These impulses make their way into the auditory portion of the brain cortex, where the actual sensation of sound occurs and the auditory signal is decoded. Hair cells are very minute and delicate (thousands of them would fit in 1 centimeter). They are easily damaged by loud and prolonged noise, and once destroyed they do not reproduce themselves. The damage to these cells might be compared to walking across a lawn. If you walk carefully and don't damage the grass, it rebounds. If you continue to tromp across the grass again and again, it cannot rebound and thus dies.

The study of noise as a stressor is somewhat complex because noise, more than the other environmental stressors examined in this chapter, has a strong social component (Dooley 2005). Noise can produce a stress response by doing one or more of the following:

1. stimulating the sympathetic nervous system

2. being annoying and subjectively displeasing

3. disrupting activities

Noise also has a psychological aspect: it may be perceived as unwanted or somehow inappropriate. This reaction—and the accompanying stress response—can occur at any frequency level. For example, a conversation at a distance of 3 feet generates only about 60 decibels, far below the pain threshold; yet if you are trying to figure out your income tax or study for a final exam, this conversation could be highly stressful because it disrupts your activity. Similarly, what may be music to you may be noise to someone else. Thus, the music you play every day and find relaxing might be very annoying, and thus stressful, to another person.

Whether noise has a predominantly physical or psychological effect, it is clearly capable of producing the stress response. Research has demonstrated that noise can produce cardiovascular changes. Studies of the effects of noise on blood circulation found that acute exposure to moderately high noise frequencies was capable of decreasing circulation to the arms, legs, hands, and feet. A more recent study discovered that repeated exposure to noise may result in a permanent rise in blood pressure due to structural adaptation of the heart and blood vessels. Finally, studies in an industrial environment demonstrated that workers exposed to moderate and high levels of noise had higher blood levels of the stress hormones. Such findings prompted the National Institute for Occupational Safety and Health (NIOSH) to go on record stating that noise is capable of stimulating changes in essential physiological functioning suggestive of a general stress reaction (1977). Workers under noisy conditions tend to suffer from shorter concentration spans and a lower frustration threshold. The U.S. Department of Labor (1992) has stated that government employees should not be exposed to steady noise levels in excess of 90 decibels per eight-hour day. **Table 8.4** gives the noise level of various activities.

Finally, we should consider adaptation to noise. Adaptation requires energy and therefore can deplete the body of biological and psychological stamina. Selye (1976) notes that, although humans can adapt to stressors, they ultimately pay the price in biological depletion and, should the exposure become chronic, in eventual breakdown. It appears that prolonged exposure to noise can have physiologically and psychologically damaging effects on the human organism. Prolonged loud noise results in the diminished capability to hear.

Learning to avoid loud, obnoxious sounds is an effective stress management tool. There are several ways to remove yourself from the harm of noise: (1) remove yourself from the noisy environment, (2) protect yourself with earplugs while staying in the

Table 8.4 Noise Levels (in Decibels) of Various Activities

Sound	Decibel Level
Jet takeoff from 200 feet	140 dB
	120 (painful to humans)
Rock music	110
Automobile horn from 3 feet	110 (extremely loud)
Motorcycle	100
Garbage truck	100
Pneumatic drill	90
Lawn mower	90 (hearing loss after repeated 8-hour exposures)
Heavy traffic	80
Alarm clock	80
Shouting, arguing	80 (very loud; evidence of a stress response)
Vacuum cleaner	75 (loud)
Freight train from 50 feet	70
Freeway traffic	65
Normal conversation	60
Light automobile traffic	50 (moderate; disruption of conversations)
Library	40 (sleep disturbed)
Soft whisper	30 (faint)

noisy environment, (3) avoid noisy environments whenever you have a choice, and (4) assert your right to have a quiet environment when others are encroaching on your boundaries.

Music Therapy

Sound has a major impact on all of us. Soft ballads soothe us; anthems stir us; heavy metal sends some into a frenzy. It is natural that therapists have adopted sound and music for a variety of therapeutic uses.

Music therapy can reduce heart rate, blood pressure, pain, and anxiety. In hospitals, music is used to help alleviate pain, improve patients' moods, counteract depression, promote movement during physical rehabilitation, calm or sedate, induce sleep, counteract fear, and reduce muscle tension. In nursing homes, it is used to boost the residents' level of physical, mental, and social functioning. In education, it is successfully used for calming and concentration (Press 2006).

There has been little if any scientific testing of music therapy, and the few available reviews are quite mixed. The treatments are unlikely to cause harm unless they are used as substitutes for proven therapies. However, they may not be extremely helpful, either.

Music therapy ranges from listening to music to improvising tunes, writing songs, discussing lyrics, performing compositions, using music and imagery, and learning through music. Because music therapy is used in so many different ways, there is no one typical approach. Music intended for relaxation should have about seventy to eighty beats per minute, similar to the heart rate. A faster beat may create tension. It should be low in pitch because a high pitch also fosters tension. Volume should be kept low because high volume can cause pain. When used to reduce anxiety, music should have a slow, steady rhythm; a low pitch; liberal orchestration; and relaxing melodies. Instrumental selections are considered more effective than vocal music because patients may focus on words and their meaning rather than on relaxing with the music.

Climate and Altitude

When the body is exposed to changes in temperature, humidity, and altitude, it responds with stress arousal and then goes into the resistance phase, which readies it for prolonged exposure to the stressor. Carrying the concept of the general adaptation syndrome to completion, if the exposure to the stressor is too extreme or continues too long, the body can no longer protect itself, and the individual perishes. Every winter in the mountains, hunters, snowmobilers, skiers, and others become lost, disabled, or caught in an avalanche and suffer from frostbite or hypothermia as a result of the low temperatures, the altitude, or both. Likewise, fall football practice may take its toll in heat prostration or heat stroke.

Many skiers or summer vacationers from the "flatlands" arrive at high altitudes and want to perform the same as they do at home. Oxygen is not as available to the cardiovascular and muscular systems at these higher altitudes, so demands on these systems must be reduced. Preparing both of these systems before vacation time helps alleviate some of the altitude stress.

The sun is also a factor, especially when rays are reflected off snow or water. A total sunblock or high-sun-protection-factor lotion is a must, especially for winter vacationers who have not exposed their skin to the sun since the previous summer.

Altitude sickness also hampers many mountain visitors. It is especially exacerbated by sudden changes to a higher altitude and by drinking alcohol.

Ask an athlete from the Colorado mountains what it is like to compete in the summer heat and humidity of Florida. Just as change in altitude causes stress, so does change in climate (to a hotter, colder, drier, wetter, more humid, or less humid place).

Cold climates demand special clothing. Down-filled or other insulating outerwear, polypropylene or wool underwear, and wool outerwear are especially suited to cold weather. Dress in layers with wool or some other "wicking" material next to the skin to take the perspiration away from the skin and the material next to the skin. (Winter sports enthusiasts know that cotton kills through hypothermia.) A warm hat, a good pair of gloves or mittens with glove liners, and insulated boots are also necessary for comfort in cold climates. If the weather is bitterly cold (either ambient temperature or because of added wind-chill factor), a scarf and/or face mask may also be helpful in staying safe and comfortable while outside.

Hot and humid climates are especially stressful to those who are not acclimated to them. When traveling in these conditions, slow down activity until some acclimation occurs. Because of fluid loss, drink ample liquids, especially good, clear water. Some water-soluble vitamins are lost through sweating, so it is best to maintain adequate intake of the B vitamins and vitamin C. Because potassium and sodium are necessary for water balance in the body, intake of these minerals should also be monitored. A good, balanced diet of fresh fruits and vegetables, calcium-rich foods, whole-grain products, and fish or lean meats normally provides the vitamins and minerals needed for maintaining water balance in the body.

Dry climates also demand that one focus on water balance and care of the skin. However, dry skin does not necessarily mean that low humidity is the culprit. Healthy skin protects itself with natural oils, the production of which is at least in part dependent on the presence of the water-soluble vitamins A, D, E, and K. When the skin cannot lubricate itself, a good natural moisturizer is called for.

SUMMARY

The environment presents many potential stressors and stress management choices. Consider these points:

- Identifying which choices are yours and which are deeply influenced by others around you can be a step toward stress management.

- The body is stressed when natural body rhythms are thrown off by shift work, jet lag, and other time-shift activities.

- Certain foods and beverages are sympathomimetic in nature, causing the stress response to occur. The stress response further robs the system of vitamins and minerals needed for the normal maintenance of organs and tissues.

- Sugar and starches that quickly enter the bloodstream can create carbohydrate intolerance, which may lead to diabetes and other diseases.

- Excessive salt intake can lead to hypertension and increased nervous tension.

- Overeating is a serious physical and emotional stressor for many overweight and obese Americans.

- Although many people take drugs, including alcohol, to combat stress, chemical substances contribute little to self-improvement, self-concept, or self-responsibility, thus exacerbating mental and emotional stress.

- Chronic use of nicotine results in a prolonged stress response related to death and disease.

- Noise can cause physical damage to ear structures, deplete the body of biological and psychological stamina, and result in diminished productivity.

- Prolonged climatic or altitude stress may result in diminished function leading toward death.

- All of the environmental stressors mentioned in this chapter can be avoided or alleviated with educated personal choices.

SOURCES CITED

Acker, C. J., and Tracy, S. W. (2004). *Altering American consciousness.* Amherst: University of Massachusetts Press.

ACS. (2007). *Cancer facts and figures.* Atlanta: American Cancer Society.

Anderson, N., and Vail, R. (1998). *The backseat flyer.* New York: Safe Goods.

Brown, S., and Lewis, V. (1999). *The alcoholic family in recovery.* New York: Guilford Press.

CDC. (2007). *Obesity trends 1985–2005.* Atlanta: National Center for Chronic Disease Prevention and Health Promotion.

Chen, J., Campbell, T. C., Li, J., and Peto, R. (1990). *Diet, lifestyle and mortality in China: A study of the characteristics of 65 counties.* Ithaca, NY: Cornell University Press.

DeHaro, L., and Panda, S. (2006). Systems biology of circadian rhythms. *Journal of Biological Rhythms, 21,* 507–18.

de la Sierra, A. (2003). Vascular abnormalities in salt-sensitive hypertension. *Current Hypertension Reports, 5,* 93–94.

Dooley, E. E. (2005). Noise pollution clearinghouse. *Environmental Helath Perspectives, 113,* no. 1, 27–32.

Fairechild, D. (2004). *Jet smarter.* Miami: Flyana Rhyme.

Gerstein, D. R., and Lewin, L. S. (1990). Special report: Treating drug problems. *New England Journal of Medicine, 323,* 14–18.

Girdano, D., and Dusek, D. (1988). Smoking cessation. In *Changing health behavior,* 215–38. Scottsdale, AZ: Gorsuch and Scarisbrick.

Harris, D. (1996). *Diet and nutrition sourcebook.* Ft. Lauderdale, FL: Omnigraphics.

Hoffman, J., and Cerbone, F. (2002). Parental substance use disorder and the risk of adolescent drug abuse. *Drug and Alcohol Dependence, 66,* 255–64.

Malone, S. M., et al. (2004). Genetic and environmental influences on antisocial personality disorder and alcohol dependence: From adolescence to adulthood. *Development and Psychopathology,* 16, 943–66.

Meyers, R. J., and Smith, J. E. (1999). *Clinical guide to alcohol treatment.* New York: Guilford Press.

Nadler, S. (2003). Sweet mayhem. *American Scholar,* 72, no. 2, 97–103.

National Institutes of Health (NIH). (2002). *Do you know the health risks of being overweight?* Bethesda, MD: NIH.

Nawrot, P., et al. (2003). Effects of caffeiene on human health. *Food Additives and Contaminants,* 20, 1–30.

NIOSH. (1977). *Occupational diseases: A guide to their recognition.* Washington, DC: U.S. Government Printing Office.

Press, M. R. (2006). Use music in the classroom. *Intervention in School and Clinic,* 41, no. 5, 307–10.

Selye, H. (1976). *The stress of life.* New York: McGraw-Hill.

Shiftwork Alert Editors. (1998). *The practical guide to managing 24-hour operations.* Cambridge, MA: Circadian Information.

Sizer, F., & Whitney, E. (2003). *Nutrition: Concepts and controversies.* Belmont, CA: Wadsworth/Thompson Learning.

Turner, R. J. & Lloyd, D. A. (2003). Cumulative adversity and drug dependence in young adults. *Addiction,* 98, 305–15.

U.S. Department of Agriculture. (2005). *Dietary guidelines for Americans 2005.* Washington, DC: U.S. Government Printing Office.

U.S. Department of Health and Human Services. (2004). *The health consequences of smoking: Nicotine addiction: A report of the Surgeon General.* Atlanta: CDC.

U.S. Department of Labor. (1992). *Hearing conservation.* Washington, DC: Occupational Safety and Health Administration.

Weil, A. (2001). *Eating well for optimum health.* Sanger, CA: Quill.

Willcox, B. J., Willcox, D. C., Suzuki, M., and Weil, A. (2002). *The Okinawa Program.* New York: Three Rivers Press.

Yamaguchi, S., et al. (2003). Synchronization of cellular clocks in the suprachiasmatic nucleus. *Science,* 302, no. 5649, 1408–12.

Zickler, P. (2003). Nicotine's multiple effects on the brain's reward system drive addiction. *NIDA Notes,* 17, no. 6, 1, 4.

Journal Entry 8

Making Choices

Everything you do is preceded by making a choice—whether it's choosing which apple to pick up in the grocery store or which movie to see on TV. You may think that some of the things you do are so unconscious or subconscious that you don't really have control over them, yet at some level you are making a choice.

You choose what to think, what to believe, what to say, how to act, and even how to feel. Many of your choices are governed by the role you are playing at any given time. When you are with your family you may choose one thing, whereas you would obviously choose another if you're hanging out with your friends.

To take ultimate responsibility for your life, your choices must be your own—carefully considered thoughts, words, and actions and their impact on the others around you.

When you defer to others because of indecision, fear, laziness, or ignorance, you give up some of yourself—you give them power over your decisions. That deference costs you something in the long run and appears as stress.

Remember a situation concerning one of the issues in this chapter (for example, food, drink, drugs, alcohol, smoking) where you yielded to the opinions of others. Briefly describe it here:

Write down how you felt in this situation.

Write down what you said to yourself after this experience.

Write down how self-talk affected you and where in your body you felt these thoughts and feelings.

 Sum up your insights into how you make your choices and how you allow others to influence you. Are your choices conscious and well thought-out? Are they out of habit? Do you do your own research? Do you find out the opinions of others around you?

 Write a positive word or short phrase about your choice making (such as "be decisive") that will be useful to you in future situations.

Stress in Relationships

We initiated the discussion on relationships in the very first chapter of this book because we believe that relationships are the proving grounds on which we show how well we have learned to manage stress. The greatest challenge to our serenity is human relationships: intimate partners, friends, children, parents, employers, coworkers, teachers, siblings, even campus cops and store clerks. However, nowhere are emotions so raw and vulnerable as in love relationships. Stress is social.

First, understand the fact that we are social creatures who crave relationship. This is not just a conscious need for attention, it is an inborn characteristic of humans. If we were to second-guess Mother Nature, this need for relationship may be the roots of civilization because newborn humans don't "hit the ground running." They must be tended, fed, and nurtured for many years until they are self-sufficient. So infants must have the neurologic makeup to learn who they can trust, rely on, and feel safe with.

Fortunately, we are wired for social relationship. Unfortunately, we are not wired for automatic, healthy, and fulfilling relationships. Again, we go back to the same trouble we've seen in previous chapters—until we are motivated to learn how to relate in a self-assured, confident, and compassionate way, we are lost in a stress-filled social environment.

Until recently the science of neurology had a fairly static picture of the social brain, but with the advent of functional magnetic resonance imagery (fMRI) instrumentation, the brain at work can now actually be seen. We now know that when you have a social encounter (for example, the person in the seat next to you turns and says, "Hi"), that stimulation goes immediately and directly to your limbic system (which by now we know is the seat of emotions). Your immediate limbic response is to anticipate the movement of that person, mirror their body movement or posture, and also mirror the mood of that person. After the immediate automatic response, your limbic system sends out messages to other brain sites where you might more consciously dwell on the meaning of the interaction and design behavior to go along with it (Insel and Fernald 2004). How well this process is carried from the subconscious to conscious manipulation is the basis for healthy relationships. Why? Because using the conscious mind is how we inhibit the behaviors that do not work for us and encourage the behaviors that do work for us when it comes to interacting with others (Oschner 2006).

All of the issues discussed in the last few chapters such as self-esteem, anxiety, decision making, patterns of behavior, and so on will influence how well you handle the stress inherent in relationships. That stress comes from a combination of perceptions of failure to get your needs met and failure to meet the expectations of others. Intimate relationships test us on such issues as loyalty, values, morals, defending lifestyle choices, competition, rivalry, compatibility, jealousy, and control. Remember that you're in life's school and you're here to learn how to do relationships. We are here to learn consciousness, not perfect it. You can make it easy on yourself, or you can go on crying and screaming at all those who are "making life difficult for you."

Three Layers of Love

In studying stress management, we find that many aspects of it are hierarchical; that is, we deal with basic aspects, then proceed to intermediate and then advanced. For instance, we noted that the brain evolved from physical, to emotional, to mental layers. We move from physical, material energy toward divine energy in our spiritual search. It is no surprise that social relationships also reflect this model with three layers of relating: sexual attraction, attachment, and then nurturing or caretaking. To progress from level to level requires increasing maturity and self-evolvement if we are to have rewarding relationships that are not continually fraught with fear and anxiety. Here are the three levels:

Level 1, as you'd imagine, is *sex/lust*. It is the lowest on this ladder because it the most physically defined aspect. It is driven by androgens, estrogens, and pheromones.

Level 2 is the *attachment* level, where the two people get to know each other and explore the likelihood that the other would be a good caring, loving partner with whom they feel safe and nurtured. This exciting phase is fueled by the neurohormones dopamine and serotonin.

Level 3 is the *nurturing* level, where each seeks to find in each other the nurturing necessary for long-term bonding and parenting. The chemicals that drive this level are oxytocin and vasopressin. You might remember oxytocin from the discussion about women's unique "tend and befriend" response to stress that we spoke of in Chapter 5.

Goleman's book, *Social Intelligence* (2006), is a great source for researching the phenomenon of relationships, and will be cited several times in this chapter. Unless otherwise indicated, when you see "Goleman" herein, go to his book for detailed clarification.

Love/Lust/Being "In Love"

As we described in the chapter about emotions, feelings cannot be described adequately. Only after the emotion centers communicate with other brain sites does the conscious mind try to put things together. And only then can feelings be translated into words and outward behavior. One of humanity's greatest frustrations throughout history has been the inability to define and explain feelings, especially love.

We are drawn into physical, sexual relationships by our very genetics, responding to the drive for survival of the species. Beyond the physical drive for human propagation, sexual closeness also offers meaningful loving contact with a partner, and at the highest tantra yogic practice, an ecstatic state. At this level, we need to begin to talk about love and "falling in love." Many at this stage of a relationship substitute the word "lust" with "love" and that would not be so far off the mark. This is the beginning of the relationship dance—the flirting with eyes, body postures, and clever and/or suggestive phraseology that signals physical attraction to someone.

"Falling in love" occurs at the beginning of an intimate relationship. It is an exhilarating, druglike high, yet, after a period of time, the "in love" stage fades, and either a couple proceeds into the attachment phase of the relationship or they break up. Some people never get into the real attachment phase because they need that druglike high of being in love. They continuously seek new partners without committing to a relationship. They're not able to make the transition to a mature love and thus are robbed of the happiness that comes from building a strong foundation of mutual support. Obviously, for these people relationships are constant sources of stress in their lives (see **Table 9.1**).

Freud described human psychosocial development in terms of six stages of love: narcissistic love in infancy, imitative love in the first few years, Oedipal love between the ages of four and seven, homosexual love in later childhood, idealistic love at puberty, and heterosexual love in early adulthood. Children first learn how and whom to love from those who provide pleasure, security, or relief from pain; later they learn how to voluntarily control and inhibit expressions of love according to personal feelings and social dictates. In essence, this process is one of learning the voluntary control over a basic emotion: love. If you inhibit the expression of love, you may eventually lose the ability to feel the emotion. If you overcontrol it, you may begin to manipulate it. The result is that an involuntary, natural phenomenon becomes a servant of the logical, analytical self; love becomes a servant of the social-psychological self: I will love you if . . . I will

Table 9.1 People in Love

People in Love
According to Branden and Branden (1981), people who are in love exhibit the following traits:
• They express love verbally.
• They are physically affectionate with each other.
• They express their love sexually, making love frequently.
• They express their appreciation and admiration for one another.
• They participate in mutual self-disclosure, sharing more of themselves and their inner lives with each other than with any other person.
• They offer each other an emotional support system, being there for each other in illness, difficulty, hardship, and crisis.
• They express love materially, with big or small gifts, but on more than the routine occasions or with tasks performed to lighten the other's burden.
• They accept demands or put up with shortcomings that would be less acceptable in another person.
• They create time to be alone together.

love you when. . . . In this way love becomes conditional: I will love you if you are pretty . . . thin . . . smart . . . kind . . . obedient . . . I will love you if you love me, or when I need you, or when I am not busy, or when I am not angry with you.

As we learn what and whom to love and when to love, love may become a consciously and subconsciously manipulated commodity—because it has so many conditions attached to it, a scarce commodity. And we may learn to save it for a certain person to show that person that this relationship is indeed special. So we learn voluntary control over the outward expression of love and, to a large degree, the inner feelings of love as well.

The sex drive is a basic and unconscious urge. Testosterone drives the male (and female, to some extent) to mate. We know that if this urge is not controlled by conscious inhibition, all kinds of irrational behavior could result from "thinking below the belt." Luckily, humans have prefrontal cortex "brakes" to apply that prevent rash sexual behavior. However, alcohol and other drugs often interfere with those brakes.

The Need for Attachment

When a couple seems compatible at all three levels (sex, attachment, and nurturing), we see a full-blown romantic relationship. When one or two are missing, romance falters.

You know what the beginning attachment phase of a relationship looks like. The couple cuddles and talks, they walk hand-in-hand, slow-dance, gaze into each other's eyes, write love letters (or text messages), maybe even baby-talk with each other, give little gifts. They are excited to be with each other and think of the other person virtually all the time when they're apart; they can't wait to be back together. Just thinking of the other, or gazing at their picture, gives them a "zing." The hormones dopamine and serotonin are active here; dopamine to excite them, serotonin to make them feel relaxed and wonderful.

It is in the attachment phase that couples may actually become "addicted" to each other (Goldstein 2002). The brain sites that light up when craving, intoxicated with, and/or binging on drugs are the precise ones that are stimulated when lovers are focusing on their loved one. Addiction-gratification biology mimics the natural pleasure that we feel when connected to someone we dearly love. Goleman notes that brain chemicals cement our family ties and friendships and love relationships.

This is a getting-to-know-you phase that is more than what it seems overtly. On a deeper level, each partner is looking for someone who makes them feel important, special, safe, and nurtured. She is deciding whether this is someone who can take care of her (and her/their children). He is deciding if this is the one who will give him support, nurturance, and mother his/their children.

Gallith and colleagues (2005) have noted three attachment styles, two of which are major stressors in all relationships. These attachment styles are:

Adjusted

Avoidant

Anxious

An infant's attachment system begins early on in order for the child to obtain care and protection. How the infant learns to attach at a very early age carries into later life. How it makes early social connections reflects strongly in its later connections. A secure child will likely become a secure adult; an anxious child will likely become an anxious adult.

As you would guess, the adjusted attachment style doesn't tend to have large relationship problems. Sure, there will be problems, but this person, because he or she *is* adjusted and has a healthy self-concept doesn't let problems shake the foundations of the relationship. Adjusted individuals find it easy to get close to others and feel comfortable trusting them, depending on them. They expect their partner to be caring, be attuned to them, and be there when they need them because that is what they expect from themselves. Their relationships, therefore, tend to be intimate and trusting. They are comfortable talking about emotions and problems, but don't stay preoccupied on them. Problems come up, they deal with them, and the relationship may actually be enhanced by working together to resolve the problem.

The avoidant attachment style is one where the person feels uncomfortable getting close to others. They tend to solve their own problems in their own way, not trusting in or sharing with their partner. They suppress their emotions and would rather not talk about them. They find it hard to trust a partner and feel nervous or anxious when pressured to share their thoughts and feelings. The neuro-social biology behind their emotional distance and uninvolvement with life seems to lie in the fact that they are unable to stop suppressing worry, even when they are asked to (Goleman 2006).

The anxious attachment style is one in which the person is highly dependent on their partner for nurturance and solace. They are obsessed with clinging to their relationship, even though they may feel they are unworthy of their partner. They fear that they will be abandoned. Insatiable neediness often pushes their partner away from them. At the neurological level, these people cannot seem to shut down the emotional memory of relationship anxiety and sadness.

What are the stressors of these three attachment styles? Those of the adjusted style have many of the possible normal stressors that we talk about later in the chapter—money, in-laws, and so on—but these are the folks who can and are willing to resolve their problems.

The anxious and avoidance styles? Imagine this relationship: He has a job where he has had to work late several weeks in a row. She is convinced that he's not coming home for dinner and spending the evenings with her because he doesn't love her anymore (the classic anxious style). When he comes home, she cries and begs him to talk to her, tell her how he feels about her, reassure her. He just wants to go to bed and not deal with her emotional demands (the classic avoider). Perhaps you know this couple. Had either picked someone with an adjusted style, perhaps there would be less strain on the relationship. Stress management techniques that would likely help both of these individuals would include meditation to retrain the brain and cognitive behavioral techniques such as assertiveness training and self-concept enhancement.

Herein is the importance of the attachment phase of a relationship. When you are in search of a new relationship, you throw out a pretty big net, let it be known to everyone around you that you're ready and willing. You get a few hits, the possibilities are there, and you decide on one in particular. You flirt, you draw them in, you begin to attach. **Now is the time!** The attachment phase is the time where it is your job to find out the other person's strengths, weaknesses, philosophy, politics, aspirations, skills, talents, and all the other characteristics that you need in a partner to make your relationship a happy one where both partners get their needs met; where both are loved and cared for; and where there is a strength of union that can withstand crises and hardships. This is the hunting phase. If you are interested in a low-stress relationship, hunt with care.

We are attracted to another person and desire them in our lives because they fill a perceived need. Introverts often are attracted to extroverts. They recognize that they need some extroversion in their lives, so they are attracted to that person. On a subconscious level, they find it easier to couple with the desired trait than to develop it themselves. Often a relationship becomes a substitution for self-development, and because self-development is life's path, you have an eventual confrontation with your self. Some philosophers call this an existential crisis. Letting the other person really know you and still love what they come to know is the ultimate gamble. We are looking for unconditional love, rather like the way your mother loved you, or loves you—only better, but that is a nearly impossible situation in relationships.

The ultimate question to ask regarding a relationship is "What do I want to become in this relationship?" You are the only one who knows that (for help, see **Table 9.2**).

Nurturing

The third "layer" of relationships is of the highest order: what we referred to as compassion and empathy in Chapter 4. Here we have a nurturance, a caretaking that goes beyond a barter for protection. It is the feeling that is turned on when we care deeply for the well-being of someone or something else. It is the "warm fuzzies" you feel in your heart when your toddler looks up and smiles at you, or when your golden retriever puppy cuddles in your arms. You demonstrate that ability when you instantly snatch up the child that has fallen or envelop the partner who is in pain. Again, body chemicals

Table 9.2 Finding Mr./Ms. Right: Being Mr./Ms. Right

The work of finding the right partner starts with some realistic and honest soul searching. When a few great dates turn into an almost constant togetherness, you should come up for air long enough to assess the situation. Logically, how does this relationship stack up?

- How do you feel about yourself when you are with this person?
- Does he or she bring out the best in you, or do you feel inhibited, put down, or confined? Does this person energize you or drain your energy when you are together and after you have been together?
- How does your partner feel about him or herself?
- How do you feel about yourself?
- How well does your partner express feelings and emotions?
- How well does this person let his or her needs and wants be known?
- Does this person give you positive feedback frequently?
- Is he or she able to express appreciation, affection, and caring by word, deed, and touch?
- How does this person handle anger, conflict, and differences? Is he or she placating, explosive, and sulking?
- Are this person's goals, values, and viewpoints on life generally similar to yours? More specifically, what are his or her attitudes toward money, sex, fidelity, roles, and children? Have you ever discussed these topics?
- What changes would you like to see this person make?
- What changes would this person like to see you make?

are at work, helping to produce a feeling of love that is very different from sexual arousal or the love addiction during the attachment phase of relationship.

During the nurturing phase, you become the nurturer. If the attachment phase has been successful, you know that are loved, you are important, touched, listened to, and taken care of. Safe and secure. Now it is your turn to do the nurturing.

It seems that this stage is delayed until grandparenting for many adults. Parenting is so new and hectic, especially if there are a number of children in the family, that nurturing may be put on a back burner. But when grandchildren come along, there is more time and opportunity for caretaking. To picture nurturance, think of the doting grandmother.

On the opposite side of the nurturance coin, too many times we see a relationship mode that demonstrates a serious lack of empathy: **narcissism.** As you may recall from mythology, Narcissus was in love with himself. In modern terms, the Narcissist thinks only of himself, his desires, his goals; he has an exploitative attitude and is vainly self-centered. Other people are only support cast in his life. A love partner is objectified to the point of using her for his own gratification. Bushman (2003) reports that 20 percent of U.S. women claim to have been forced into unwanted sex despite resistance—and this was most often perpetrated by a spouse or partner with whom they were currently in love. Indeed, ten times as many women are forced to have sex by someone they love as by a stranger. The Narcissist feels entitled to sex if his partner has encouraged and aroused him, even when she clearly demands that he stop.

Which brings us to the discussion of date and spousal abuse and rape. Domestic violence is recognized as a serious public health problem, but abuse problems among unmarried, dating teens are understudied and underreported (Ko 2007). Recognizing abuse is the first step for young people. Abuse may occur as emotional abuse (for example, a partner calls you fat and ugly, shouts, curses, screams at you); psychological abuse (for example, destroys your property, intentionally spites you, keeps you from seeing friends or family); sexual abuse (for example, talks you into kissing or touching when you don't want to, gets you to drink or do drugs so you will have sex, forces you into unprotected sex); physical abuse (for example, pushes, bites, or grabs you; twists your arm; pulls your hair; threatens you with a deadly weapon); economic abuse (for example constantly calls at work, won't allow you to go to work, uses credit card/money unauthorized). When any of these kinds of abuse occur, not only must they be reported, they must be stopped. From long-term, in-depth domestic violence research, we know that violence between couples escalates.

Making a Relationship Work

No one really knows the exact ingredients for a successful relationship between any two people, but one thing is known: whether as a result of a conscious effort by the couple or a natural way of relating, most successful relationships seem to possess the qualities of love, independence, self-authenticity, openness and honesty, room for personal growth, and personal freedom.

Obviously you cannot have a love relationship without love. After a relationship stales due to "incompatibility," there is a tendency to try to save it by appealing to logic, to stay with a person with whom we should be able to make a go of it. No matter how intelligent, handsome, or beautiful the other person is, no matter how mutual the interests, without love there can be no real love relationship. Although you can have a relationship without love, you cannot have a love relationship without love, and there is no way to fool your emotions. Stress is the inevitable consequence of living with this deception.

Every relationship must have some independence. To reduce the chance of relationship failure, couples often seek "togetherness insurance" by trying to be everything to each other. Most couples are convinced that relationships fail because of a lack of togetherness, when just the opposite, too much togetherness, may be at the root of the problem. Nothing is as stressful as being smothered and forced to buy into your partner's expectations. Both partners must be able to keep their own friends, male and female, and must be free to interact with them on a regular basis. Each partner must feel free to participate in the activities they enjoy, regardless of whether the other person is involved.

Both partners must remain authentic, true to their own selfhood and true to their values. They each should live a lifestyle based on their own values and not sacrifice their own needs for their partner's needs. They should always move toward being their own person. Stress has often been defined as the distance between who you really think you are and how you act. Stress will tell you through physical symptoms or behavioral manifestations exactly how big the difference is.

The opposing life forces of individuality and togetherness must somehow be balanced. It takes a differentiation of the separate "self " superimposed on the together "self " in the relationship. Beware of the partner who leans too far in either direction (Gilbert 2002). However, be careful. When couples go their own way in activities that are most engaging and save the mundane things for togetherness, the relationship can become associated with boredom and tedium. This often happens when one of the members travels a lot for work and has no energy and interest in going places and doing things on the weekends or when time together is just maintenance, cleaning house, doing laundry, and resting for the hard workweek ahead (Carlson 2001).

Each partner should strive to remain open, honest, and assertive and not be held back by fear of hurting, fear of being rejected, or guilt. Both need to feel free to verbalize their wants and not expect their partner to somehow "know" what they want. Each needs to be able to talk about everything openly and honestly, and most of all to express hurts, anger, and disappointments as they occur and not allow resentments to build up.

There should be room for personal growth (that is, room to change and room to be independent). Expectations should be kept to a minimum, or resentments will follow. A healthier love relationship is just that, the love relationship. Each should realize that the other is not a business partner, playmate, housekeeper, or errand runner.

Each partner needs to be allowed to do those things they enjoy and not be expected to give them up just because the other person may be able to do them more efficiently. Interest should be more important than expertise or cultural bias (usually sexist) in the choice of activities.

Obligation—out of guilt, prior commitment, or security needs—should not rule the relationship. Binding commitments and lifetime security are a myth and usually work to increase complacency.

Brown describes a healthy family unit as being nonmeshed, meaning a healthy mix of interdependence with independence in which each person is encouraged to be sharing, cooperative, and interested in each other's lives but also be independent and pursue independent goals. The primary goal in any relationship is for each to become the best possible person. This allows individuals to bring freshness and happiness to the relationship that by its very nature promotes too much togetherness and dependence (Brown 2002).

Partners, to the best of their ability, should strive to keep themselves healthy, physically active, fresh, interesting, playful, and growing. Neither partner should change or postpone change in order to stay in place with his or her partner. Mutual support is essential, but becoming a crutch or excessively leaning on a partner usually spells disaster for a relationship. And as the relationship goes, so go your stress level, your health, and your happiness.

There's nothing new or profound in any of these statements, but by recognizing them and reminding yourself of them, you might keep a relationship with real promise from dying of neglect. If you are a free, loving, honest, and interesting person who is working to become the best possible you and who is acting to foster your partner's growth, and if you love each other and have a fair number of mutual interests, then the relationship will be fulfilling. If not, it will become old, boring, dependent, and stifling, and you'll be better off finding someone else and starting over.

It seems as though the philosophers, marriage counselors, and other professionals in this field are saying that success for a relationship adds up to experiencing mature love, maintaining independence and self-sufficiency, and being in touch with personal need fulfillment. When two people can respect where they are and work to develop their own identities, it is impossible for them to become clinging, jealous, and dependent—the three factors that most often undermine a relationship. The experts also seem to agree that although love may just seem to happen, good relationships do not. A strong, lasting relationship is not a matter of luck; it is a matter of two mature, healthy personalities being realistic in working to make it work (Bartels and Semir 2000; Feeney 2004; Fisher 2004).

Living Together

If you are lucky enough to have a good loving relationship going for you, then life together should be a stress-free walk in the park. Well, perhaps not. No matter how healthy and happy you are, trying to fit two lives together on a day-to-day basis is not stress-free. After you have attached and feel comfortable with a mate, the next step is usually living together or marriage. This cohabitation puts all of your positive psychological traits to the test. After the other person hangs their toothbrush next to yours, you may find that the candlelight dinners with wine and soft music have turned into pizza and beer in front of a TV, and that leisurely discussions of love and life become play-by-play accounts of the NCAA basketball finals.

Dating, no matter how frequent or fantastic, does not prepare a couple for living together. After months of dinners out, breakfast in, studying together, vacationing together, and so on, you may feel you know everything there is to know about this person. But life is made of many more routine things than dating is. Meals need to be fixed, floors and furniture dusted, dishes and laundry done, and bills paid. People also need time to be alone. Everyone has his or her own living habits. Men sometimes leave the bathroom sink full of whiskers, guzzle orange juice from the bottle, and expect to have their dinners cooked, not to mention leaving the lid up! Women often leave their makeup all over the bathroom sink, want the garbage to be taken out, and expect their cars to be in running order and filled with gas. Little annoyances, perhaps, but they often precipitate arguments and make you wonder why you ever gave up the romance for the routine. There are more serious difficulties when the "strong silent type" is in reality sulking, withdrawn, and continually depressed; when the forceful, take-charge type turns out to be extremely pushy; when knowing just what is wanted turns into unforgiving perfectionism with high expectations of the right way to do everything; when the seemingly insatiable appetite for sex starts to take a backseat to other needs, pressures, and activities; and when the cozy little apartment that made a great little love nest affords little space for privacy and time alone.

While you were dating you had time to spend alone, wind down from the day's work or school, and rejuvenate yourself before going out. Now you both come home needing that time, but there you are together with new, constant demands. You expect to see the same warm, witty, wonderful person alive with enthusiasm—the one you used to date. Unfulfilled expectations can engender excess stress that can eat away at a relationship, so the time to learn exactly what to expect is before you make the big move.

Although toleration of those little idiosyncrasies does grow, some major problems must be worked out if the relationship is to survive. Some problem areas in a relationship are handling money, basic communication, and jealousy. Of these, basic communication compatibility is probably the most important factor in keeping you and the relationship healthy.

Communication

Good communication is mandatory. It means being open and honest with your feelings; it means being assertive enough to get your needs met; it means not being so afraid of losing your partner that you always give in; and it means knowing how to fight fairly and constructively. As we discussed in Chapter 6, one essential to honest communication is learning assertiveness.

Assertiveness Assertiveness promotes the best communication in a relationship; people who are assertive are able to state their likes and dislikes without demeaning the other person. Aggressive people, on the other hand, make demands and state their likes and dislikes in a way that damages the other person's self-esteem. Passive placaters do not have the skill to ask for what they want; instead, they manipulate others by means of guilt and blame into getting what they want. Being assertive makes for happier communication in all facets of life, including sexuality. You can determine your verbal impact on others by watching the effect your words have. If you think that the words you use will intimidate or give the other person a feeling of low self-worth, you're probably being aggressive. However, if you tell the other person what you like or dislike without degrading them, then you're probably being assertive. Being assertive does not always guarantee that the other person will not choose to be hurt. For example, you may have had an instance in which a very good friend of yours wanted your friendship to become sexually intimate, but you did not want that kind of relationship. If you were assertive, you told the person that you regarded their friendship very highly and that you really liked having them as a friend but preferred to keep your relationship on a best-friend basis rather than let sex enter into it. At that point, the friend could choose to be hurt or to continue to be one of your best friends. You asserted your rights in a caring way, and the response is up to the other person. If they choose to be hurt, it was not because you said something degrading.

Feeling assertive is incompatible with stressful feelings and anxiety. The more you feel one, the less you feel the other. Assertiveness is sometimes called "feel-good communication." If you feel good after a conversation or confrontation, you have communicated effectively and positively. When people choose to respond in nonassertive, passive ways, they do so for some payoff. Some reasons for not being assertive are fear of retaliation, fear of losing affection or esteem, being rewarded for not rocking the boat, and being unaware that it is all right to be assertive. Recall a situation in which you did not say how you felt, did not stand up for your rights, or did not express your opinion. What kept you from being assertive?

Aggression also carries payoffs. Among them may be the feeling of power, of being right, or of getting others' attention. When was the last time you were aggressive? What was the payoff? There may indeed be a short-term period of feeling good or righteous or smug after having been nonassertive or aggressive, but there's a long-term effect of feeling good that goes with assertiveness. We always have these three elements: the monster, the mouse, and the assertive me. The goal of assertiveness is responding less and less as a monster or a mouse and more and more as the assertive me.

Being passive never has payoffs. Lack of assertiveness has continually been identified as one of the root causes of anger. In a survey of African American women who had difficulty managing stress, it was found that when women allow people to, as they put it, "walk all over them" without saying anything, there was an inevitable complete loss of control (Childs 2002).

Suggestions for assertive communication were given in Chapter 6. With regard to relationships, a good way to start being assertive is to tell others when they're doing something right—it will make both of you feel good. The next step might be to work on saying outloud what you like and what you dislike without expressing a judgment of the other person's personality. A good follow-up to this step is to also suggest outloud a positive alternative for the thing you dislike. Remember that the most powerful block to communication in a relationship is being negative. Use positive words and give positive suggestions instead of filling your sentences with "don't," "shouldn't," or "can't."

Many people have the most trouble being assertive in sexual situations. This is probably due to society's lingering attitude that sex is something that we should not discuss. Being able to talk about sex with a sex partner in an assertive way greatly enhances the sexual relationship and makes for a more mature relationship. In the sexual silence of the bedroom, neither partner knows what the other one wants or enjoys, but knowing how to ask and then asking for what you want enhances your chance of getting that need met.

Perhaps the most important sexual assertive communication is letting your partner know whether you wish to engage in sexual activity. It is important to say what you feel instead of giving vague signals. No matter how you ask for your needs to be met, you always risk being rejected, but having been asked to join a partner in sex, there are assertive ways of making rejection less painful. It is well to remember that, although you are not being assertive or not being entirely truthful verbally, your body/subconscious will communicate your true feelings somehow. This stressful behavioral communication will in the long run be much more damaging to the relationship and your health than just saying honestly how you feel. If you're feeling anxiety or resentment about saying "yes," you may carry that bad feeling about the same experience to the future. A caring, assertive "no" frees you from that anxiety.

Fighting Fair

Quarrels between daters are usually less frequent and less intense than those between couples who are living together. Couples who are just dating spend much of their time pleasing each other; they do not like to waste time arguing. When a couple is living together, there is no escape; the disagreement usually concerns the entire lifestyle, and each partner is more apt to want his or her own way. Also, the preliminary period of trying to continually please each other and impress each other ended when they began to live together.

No two people want to live exactly the same way, so disagreements are bound to arise. The "we never fight" couple usually spends a lot of energy burying the problem, and resentment builds up over time. If these resentments are triggered, a major battle that can undermine the relationship is apt to occur. The "we always fight" couple is usually a pair of unhappy individuals who are dissatisfied with themselves and the relationship and are venting a lot of emotion without really discussing the issues. Fighting too much is a sign of real problems in a relationship, problems that are never really resolved. Fights that resolve problems can strengthen a relationship, whereas those that do not are merely emotional outbursts that destroy the relationship. Most couples, furthermore, do not know how to fight fairly. The major obstacles to fighting fairly are the following:

1. The concept that there must be a winner and a loser. Actually, no one ever wins a fight. Each time one wins a point, the other feels resentment. The point is to resolve your differences and continue living with and loving each other. The basis for diplomatic negotiations applies—that is, give a little, receive a little. The outcome should be a win/win situation rather than a lose/lose or a win/lose one.

2. Charged emotions and hurt feelings. Attacking with the use of statements such as "I don't like the way you . . ." elicits defensiveness, and the real issues become sidetracked as the attacked tries to protect his or her feelings.

3. Trying to change the behavior of a partner by nagging, sulking, or withholding. This is manipulation, and true feelings never get expressed.

4. Killing effective communication with verbal and nonverbal turnoffs. These techniques signal that you do not wish to discuss the issue. Another technique is punishment—making your partner pay for weeks for bringing up the issue. This usually takes the form of recurrent sarcastic remarks, sulking, and withholding.

Akin to assertive communication described earlier is Rosenberg's system of Nonviolent Communication (2005), which provides an effective outline for effectively communicating what you want.

Nonviolence means letting your positive aspects emerge—the aspects we recognize as respect, compassion, empathy, love. In a world of TV violence and global terrorism, it is easy to fall into that kind of communication, a relating that is filled with self-centeredness, greed, hatefulness, prejudice, suspicion, and aggression.

In a capsule, Rosenberg's model of nonviolent communication (2005) teaches us how to both express ourselves and to listen or receive openly and empathetically what the other person is trying to communicate.

First, about expressing yourself:

1. Honestly express *yourself* without blaming or criticizing:
   a. what I observe that contributes (or not) to my well-being
   b. how I feel in relation to what I observe
   c. what I need or value that causes the feelings I've expressed

   Then:
   a. request clearly what would enrich my life *without demanding*
   b. request specific and concrete actions I would like taken

Second, about receiving others' *communication:*

2. Openly and empathetically *receive* how the *other person* is without blame or criticism
   a. what *you* observe that contributes or not to *your* well-being
   b. how *you* feel in relation to what *you* observe
   c. What you need or value that causes your feelings

   Then
   a. receiving with empathy that which would enrich *your* life without hearing it as a demand
   b. receiving openly the concrete actions *you* would like taken

Once communication is under way, you may experience an emotional overload before the issue is resolved, so feel free to say that you need a break or time to think things over. Stress builds up over time. Too much stress in a short time and too much emotion inhibits communication. You are wise to know your limits and realize that more will be accomplished by coming back to this at a later time when you are less stressed and tired. The key is to make it known that the issue is not resolved and that you would like to resume the discussion later. In the meantime, try not to withhold affection. Do something fun together—it signifies that things are basically all right and that you just have to work out a few details. Many couples live by the rule that they will never go to bed angry. Fatigue may cause you to bury the problem for a while, but unresolved problems do not go away; they will reemerge later, usually dragging along a train of resentment. Try to maintain a normal existence while resolving the problem. Do not allow problems to get buried under a "return to normal." Renew the discussion the next day simply by saying that you do not feel the issue has been resolved. By then there is usually less emotion, and elapsed time has helped each to absorb the other's position. Always resist the temptation to play "shrink," which gives the impression that anyone holding those views has serious psychological problems. Use the model of labor and management, and enter into good-faith negotiations. With labor and management, both parties come in wanting everything and settle for less. Changes can be made only if parties consent, and that occurs only if both parties give some.

It is well to remember that most conflict begins with you. It's usually more about one's general stress, disillusionment, and disappointments than what the other person has done or not done. If you're often in "a bad mood," then arguments will eventually follow. If you are, on the whole, at peace you will find you engage in far fewer arguments (Simmons 2002).

Avoiding the Stress of Arguments   To the ego-centered person, feeling good is synonymous with being right. Being right means appearing to be knowledgeable or smart enough to buy the right car, go to the right school, belong to the right religion, eat the right foods, and to prevail in decisions or disputes at home, school, and work. To be wrong is to lose face and feel bad. As a result, you spend much of your time defending your point of view. Most of the time other people are doing the same thing, so in reality, defending is fruitless because the other person is not listening. Trying to be right is responsible for most of the arguments between people.

When you choose not to defend your point of view, there will be no argument. In addition, there will be no hurt feelings, no anger, no withholding, no put-downs, no passive-aggressive getting even, and no winning or losing.

When you remain open to all points of view, not attached to one, and stay flexible, there is less friction and less resistance; thus life flows effortlessly. If you do need to justify yourself, simply declare your intent to yourself and do what you want. As an application of these principles try the following exercise:

Think of a recent experience where an argument could have been prevented. Describe it.

How could you have done what you wanted without the argument?

What is your plan for acting differently next time?

Common Areas of Stressful Conflict in Relationships

It is no secret that unhappy couples fight more than happy couples. Many times the problems are due more to style than to the issues, and those unhappy couples have problems with their quality of interaction. Unhappy couples often use aversive problem-solving styles, show less appreciation for the other person, and have more difficulty initiating interesting conversation and expressing emotions clearly. The actual issues and fights do not really differ that much between happy and unhappy couples. The major issues most couples fight over involve sexual relations, money, personal habits, jealousy, and in-laws. When these problems become overwhelming or go on for a long time, the couple may have reached the "burned-out" stage.

Sexual Relations   One standard problem area is sexual relations. An inability to be close and get sexual needs met eventually leads to frustration. Partners become irritable over this issue, and they begin to haggle over other areas. Sexual problems are related more to intensity of feelings than to skill deficiencies. Frequency of sex is usually a matter of need and satisfaction. Even though many couples complain about infrequent sex, the fact is they're not enjoying sex and therefore do not engage in it as often. Time limitations are often mentioned as one of the major limiting factors in decreased frequency of sex; however, studies show that a large proportion of young adults who work sixty hours a week have sex more than eighty times a year, far out distancing the average of fifty-eight times per year for most couples (Welch 1995).

Because it is difficult to have sex with someone you're not happy with, sexual problems usually grow out of other hostilities, and mutual resentments are often carried over into the sexual arena. Sexual problems are also bound up with communication problems. The inability to solve long-standing problems invariably has repercussions in the bedroom. Likewise the fatigue of a stressful lifestyle usually catches up with a person by making him or her self-absorbed and a less considerate romantic partner.

Sex is sex—not a manipulation. You can't trade sex for getting the trash taken out. Even if sexual ploys garner the desired attention or win some other battle for its perpetrator, the real problems go unsolved. Feelings of disappointment, anger, and frustration begin to take over. Sex, which should be enjoyable on a physical, emotional, and spiritual level, is degraded. When you use sex as a tool of power, it interferes with the pleasure and togetherness it could bring to the relationship and the beauty of the sexual experience is impeded.

In some cases, couples have a healthy relationship, but only outside the bedroom. This can be a problem in the long-term monogamous relationship, especially for couples busy with careers. Fatigue and pressure can leave them vulnerable. They may see their declining sex life as a symbol of a decline in their relationship. Sex sometimes becomes just something you do because you're supposed to—a habit. The greatest challenge confronting monogamous relationships today is maintaining the sexual passion. A couple needs to set aside time to make their partner and sex life a priority (Barbach 1997).

No one can instinctively know what his or her partner enjoys. A frequent obstacle to complete sexual fulfillment is a lack of communication on the part of one or both partners. Whether due to fear, embarrassment, or a general reluctance to discuss sex, an honest and open dialogue will help you to have sex the way you want it—in the manner that will bring you the most enjoyment possible.

Recall Exercise   Recall a time in your life when you felt you had a very special sexual or romantic experience. Who was your partner? Where were you? What was the setting? What made that particular experience so enjoyable? It may help to close your eyes, relax, and let the images come to you.

Describe the experience in the following terms.

1. When was it? _____

2. Who were you with? _____

3. Look around; describe what you see; describe your feelings and sensations:

Next recall a time in your life when you felt you had a not-so-pleasurable sexual or romantic experience. Who was your partner? Where were you? What was the setting? What made that particular experience less enjoyable?

Describe the experience in the following terms.

1. When was it? _____

2. Who were you with? _____

3. Look around; describe what you see; describe your feelings and sensations:

Now compare your favorite experiences with your not-so-good ones. Make a list of the significant factors that made the sexual experience good for you. Was it the location, the person, or other circumstances?

Now rewrite the list, placing the most meaningful items at the top and the least important on the bottom. This revised list will identify the conditions you associate with more enjoyable experiences, as well as those that are less satisfying.

Finally, analyze the items that appear high on your list. Are they reasonable? Which apply to your current partner? Can you work with your current partner to achieve more of the "optimal" conditions and to eliminate the ones that are less fulfilling?

Take this a step further into the realm of fantasy. See yourself in the best possible sexual or romantic experience. Make a list of the significant factors that made this fantasy special. How does this list compare with the other two? This is what you really want. What keeps you from getting it? What can you do to make it happen for you? Can you communicate this to your current partner?

It is impossible to have a good sexual relationship without clear communication. But an amazing number of people find it difficult to talk honestly and openly about their sexual desires. The best time to broach the subject with your partner is when you are both feeling warm and intimate. The worst time to try to communicate your needs is when you or your partner feels angry, frustrated, or resentful. If you choose the time and the words carefully, you run little risk of offending or intimidating your partner. If you speak out of anger, you risk offending your partner. Remember that sexual criticism cuts deep and is not easily forgotten, and your attempts at reducing stress will only cause more stress instead.

Money   Money, how is it made, and the style of spending it are other major areas of conflict in most households. More than married couples, cohabitating couples often feel that "what is mine is mine," not "ours." How the money is spent is often a bone of contention. If spending and savings styles and values are incompatible, major negotiations are usually necessary to save the relationship. If couples cannot agree on this issue, then separating money is essential. Passivity in this area always results in resentment, long-term low-level stress, and an attitude of "getting even." Most financial counselors such as Suze Orman (2007) recommend that each partner have their own money and each put into a joint account enough money to pay joint obligations. This way each can buy what they want without begging or "convincing" or laying guilt trips on the other. What often happens is "competitive buying." He wants a new bike, so she feels that to be fair she will get some goods or services of equal value. And before you know it the credit cards are maxed. Special situations require creativity. If, for example, a woman is out for a while on maternity leave then the man could share his income equally so the woman still has her own money. Adults cannot be put into a position of asking for money as if they were a child who is asking "mommy or daddy." They will resent the situation and hard feelings will result. It is well to remember that we don't romance parent figures. Reduce a lover to a child and you can forget the lover part. Each adult must manage his or her own money or there is trouble in paradise.

Personal Habits   Poor personal habits, or (perhaps better stated) incompatible personal habits, are often the source of conflict in a relationship. The list here is endless, and often the items seem trivial. Things such as bad temper, jealousy, discourtesy, poor driving habits, moodiness, chronic lateness, household neglect, unhelpfulness, drinking too much, overemphasizing cleanliness, nagging, and infidelity may signal that a couple is mismatched or cannot communicate well enough to resolve these issues. Either way, if differences exist, they must be resolved or overlooked or the stress will eventually trigger conflict.

Jealousy   Still another area of frequent conflict is jealousy and the way it limits the freedom and independence of partners in a relationship. What makes the problem of jealousy so difficult to solve is that jealousy entails a threat to self-esteem as well as to a valued relationship. It does not really matter if that threat is real, potential, or just a figment of the imagination. In other words, jealous individuals will be jealous even if there is no actual, physical reason for that jealousy. Jealousy, then, is more a personal behavioral trait of persons who may themselves be faithless and have a tendency to stray. Jealous people often have poor self-images and constantly feel that because they're basically not good enough for their partners, their partners will eventually stray. Interestingly enough, even people who are not particularly happy with their partners or the quality of their relationship are nevertheless very often jealous. Thus, it is more the loss of self-esteem than the loss of the relationship that threatens them. Naturally, individuals whose self-esteem is heavily dependent on their partner or who are emotionally overdependent on their partner or the relationship are more often jealous than individuals who are healthily independent (Friday 1997; Pines 1998). As was outlined in Chapter 6, this is a good example of how poor self-perception can be at the root of stress problems.

Often the idealized dating phase does not reveal the true emotional personality of your mate. It is difficult to know if you are in love with an emotional vampire. These are charming, talented, together-looking people who somehow manage to bring you down emotionally. These usually loving mates, who are okay as long as life is going their way, easily slip into negative, even hateful emotions when things are not going their way. They have poor impulse control and are mostly selfish, slyly enticing you to rescue them from their emotions. This is especially dangerous if the other person secretly likes playing the rescuer role (Bernstein 2002).

It is also interesting that the sexes customarily react to jealousy in different ways. Jealous women tend to concentrate on enhancing their attractiveness and strengthening the relationship, whereas men tend to concentrate on saving face by becoming more sexually aggressive with other women and seeking new relationships. In addition, men are more likely than women to end a relationship because of their partner's infidelity. Jealousy always limits freedom in a relationship; it leads to suspicion, insecurity, and resentment, and if not resolved, it usually spells the end of the relationship in one form or another.

In-laws   Even though you may not be married, if your partner has parents, you have "in-laws," and in-laws are often a source of conflict in a relationship. Young adults have usually not been out of their parents' control and influence for very long—not long enough to establish themselves as adults in their parents' eyes. Thus, parents still try to influence their children's decisions and the young-adult children are trying to live up to their parents' expectations. There is a big difference between "you and I" and "we." If a couple is really getting close and starting to think of themselves as "we," then each needs to be more important to the other than to either set of parents. This is a giant step in the development of a relationship. Often young couples get caught between pleasing their partners and pleasing their parents—a good definition of stress if ever there was one. Parents often create difficulties by not accepting partners, thus making it uncomfortable, to say the least, for partners to interact with them. Parents often have a difficult time accepting the living-together arrangement, and consciously do whatever they can to break it up. They make no attempt to get to know their child's live-in partner. The presence of the parent or even a telephone call can be the source of stress or conflict. If the couple cannot stand together as one in the face of such opposition, their relationship will be short-lived.

Although there are many more areas of potential conflict in a relationship, the ones just described are most often mentioned. As discussed earlier, a couple's communication style is usually more important than the substance of their differences. If there are too many differences or if there are too many communication problems, then chances are the relationship is not worth saving. After a prolonged period of damaging interaction, a couple can become "burned out," and the individuals will exhibit the same burned-out symptoms as mentioned in Chapter 7, a state usually associated with work-related overloads.

The Blended Family and the Single-Parent Family   The classic movie *Yours, Mine, and Ours*, with Lucille Ball and Henry Fonda, is still a good watch for the second-time-around couples who come into a new marriage with children from a previous marriage.

Each situation has its own stressful relationship problems: only child with new mom or dad ("You can't tell me what to do, you're not my mom/dad."); one new partner with child(ren) and the other with none; both with one or more children.

The new stepparents are torn between loyalty to their own children, being fair to the stepchildren, quality time with their new partner, disciplinary modes, chores, and just about every aspect of life that is going to be different after the marriage. A major stress management technique for these families is learning the communication skills we've presented in this chapter.

The stress of most single-parent families is apparent: not enough time to spend with the children, usually due to the demands of work. True, there are some financially secure men and women who choose to rear a child by themselves, and the child enjoys a rich home life. Unfortunately that is not the case in most instances. Divorce, death of spouse, unwed motherhood, and abandonment are some of the issues that face many mothers, and they must not only make financial ends meet, but also nurture and protect their children. Every moment that a single mother can snatch for herself, even if it is to do a few deep breaths before going back into the fray, will better enable her to cope.

Separation

Is separation a personal tragedy, a family embarrassment, or a social problem? Or is it a new lease on life, a chance to start over, and a chance to make something positive out of something that has turned negative? It is a matter of perspective, but either way it is the most stressful aspect of relationships. The end of a relationship may be accompanied by an introspective period often filled with self-doubt.

Did I give up too soon, did I not try hard enough, or was it obvious that it was a failure and I was not seeing it for what it was? Did I bail too soon or too late? After a separation, friends will tell you they never thought the two of you were right for each other. Do they say that to make you feel better, or did they see something you were unwilling or unable to see?

What happens when two people do not see the incongruities in their paths? They are unhappy for a long period of time and resent the partner, which allows the low-level stress to fester for long periods of time. When love dies, it is difficult to overlook the partner's faults. It is as though there is a hole opened in the dike. Without love, the wear and tear from the stress and strain of everyday life come rushing in that hole, making it bigger and bigger. Gradually you start to dislike yourself for putting up with things that you feel diminish you. On the surface, at least, you deny your anger, keep it bottled, and don't talk to anyone about it, especially your partner. People often say, "Hindsight is perfect. Looking back now, I realize that I didn't know what was going on. I let our love erode to the point that we were fighting over whose turn it was to take out the trash. I couldn't seem to stop it, or I didn't want to stop it."

However, we are not victims of life circumstances. The stress of overwhelming financial, social, and professional responsibilities is a challenge presenting opportunities for us to join together and find ways to be happy with what we have. Relationships are supposed to add to our feelings of joy and abundance. When they don't, it may be time to move on.

For any one of a thousand reasons, a couple may suddenly see each other as being worlds apart. Usually it is not because the personality for which each was chosen is not there, but because the unrealized, unallowed-for differences are deeper than either bargained for. After months or even years, living with these differences and experiencing the frustration, fights, hurts, and angers, a couple may see that going their separate ways is the only viable alternative. Everyone should be allowed to change their minds, change jobs, move to a new place, or choose a new partner. People move into relationships to prove their sense of commitment and to find security. However, many find that commitment is situational and security is a figment of their imagination. With all couples there is a real possibility that the day may come, no matter how strong the prior commitment, no matter how much love was shared and shown, that the relationship may end. One may find oneself companionless, jobless, childless; and in a matter of a few months, one's entire life can change. Although separation cannot help but be stressful, the length of time one remains in this stressful state is an indicator of how well they manage stress and will be the determining factor in how quickly they return to positive health and happiness.

When children are involved, separation and divorce take on a whole new aspect. No longer can each partner think of him or herself first (unless violence and abuse are involved in the issue). Always do what is best for the children. Making their lives better may or may not lessen the stress, but will elevate their feelings of self-worth.

Loneliness

One of the more stressful aspects of relationships is the absence of relationships. In a society that gives a high rating to togetherness, it is often very stressful to find yourself without a partner. Here again, the relationship arena provides the proving grounds for how well you deal with the stress of boredom and loneliness (Hawkley et al. 2003). There is a difference between being alone and being lonely, and that is most often determined by the spiritual health of the individual. Very often, being single does not mean being alone at all. The singles who seem to enjoy being single tend to be young; most are in college or just out of college. They like themselves and are content with what they are; they have many friends and many interests, are physically active, have fulfilling jobs, are emotionally fit, have a sense of humor, and generally are content with their lives and not overzealous in their search for a mate. A sharply increasing number of young people are choosing to remain single for reasons such as freedom and privacy (Sanders 1998). **Table 9.3** shows pros and cons of being single.

In our society, being alone is seen as a symptom of social pathology; being less worthy, less lovable, something to be pitied. If being coupled is the norm, then everyone who is not part of a couple is abnormal. Few people consider that being alone is an integral part of everyone's journey. It may be even more noticeable in the lives of those people who are working on self-reliance issues. What do you learn from being alone? Many things, especially how to be alone. Only in your aloneness will you find out who you really are. If you are concerned about aloneness, reframe the reason you are alone. There is a large difference between being lonely and unlovable or undesirable and experiencing aloneness as a precondition to philosophical integration. If you need to be alone to

Table 9.3   Being Single

Advantages

- privacy
- no one to clean up after
- money goes a lot further; you can spend your money on whatever you want without answering to anyone or feeling guilty
- not being tied to a schedule; working when you feel like it, not having to prepare meals on time or when someone else is hungry
- generally not being responsible to or for anyone else
- enjoying the feeling of being in control of your life

Disadvantages

- loneliness; not having anyone to talk with, to share with, or to support you when you are down
- lack of emotional intimacy; no one to touch, hug, and share thoughts and moods with
- lack of steady sex
- having to find a date and being stuck with someone undesirable
- lack of opportunity to meet companions; most singles do not like the "meat market" atmosphere of single bars
- fear that being single will become permanent
- an overemphasis on looks and outward appearance in the singles scene; there is little opportunity to really get to know someone
- not being able to have children

gain that experience, you'll find some reason to be alone. And if you need to be alone, you're going to have to practice being alone, or you're not going to be able to pull it off. Even if it's sometimes painful, you're learning how to do it. If you cannot be alone, then you will not be able to be alone, and you will constantly seek the comfort of relationships. As a rule, we fixate our loneliness on other people and thus try to rid ourselves of loneliness by being with other people or being entertained. People are more afraid of what being alone means to them and society than the actual state of being alone (Middleton 1999). Even battered women are reluctant to get out of their relationships, not because they love the creeps but because they are terrified to be alone.

How does one go about being comfortable with being alone? By trying it in varying degrees. One might start out with short sessions of solitary meditation. That is quality alone time. When rewards and insights come from being alone, the time will increase. One may learn that relationships, especially dependency relationships, hinder. And if you are at a point in your path where you need to integrate what you have learned about who you really are, then you will seek aloneness.

When being alone hurts, that is, causes us to feel lonely or incomplete, it is a purely physical or material state. Our physical body is alone, but our spiritual bodies are still joined. When we access our spiritual bodies, we are able to know the soul's will. We are able to be alone in our physical bodies and at the same time be in constant oneness with our divine part, or God part, if you prefer. What we find in our quality alone time is that we are never alone. Each of us is a part of the whole.

There is a difference between "alone" and "lonely." Both are free-will choices, but being lonely carries with it the negative baggage of the ego, that of self-doubt, and lack of self-respect, self-regard, and self-love. We have an agenda for the time we spend alone—it's part of our experience. How can we resent being alone when we have chosen it as our tool? Resentment of being alone is the feeling we are trying to overcome. Loneliness is an emotional choice we can make to know our aloneness. When we integrate that emotion with the sense of free will, we can choose to experience joy in our aloneness.

Experiencing your aloneness as being lonely with its accompanied socially and psychologically promoted pathology is an indication that you have not understood the purpose of the aloneness and that you are not ready to give up either the loneliness or the debilitating fear of it. Fear, as we know, has as its companion, anger, and the antisocial behavior that goes with it.

If you do not know what you need, look at what you have. If you do not know what you want, look at what you have. You create what you need and what you want. What have you created? You could also be ready to create relationships if that's what you think you want. Or you could create a whole new attitude about aloneness.

Relationships! Both the advantages and disadvantages inherent in them have their accompanying stressors. Relationships can, and will, be as stressful as your perception allows them to be. Perhaps more than any other arena, the stress of relationships is largely dependent on one's perception. One's self-perception; patterns of behavior; communications skills; ability to deal with change, frustration, and overload; and ability to manage stress before it gets out of control will greatly affect the stress engendered by relationships or the joy they can bring.

SUMMARY

Most of us will go through life in and out of various relationships. Relationships are consistently one of our most prevalent stressors. It is important for stress management to know which relationship pitfalls to avoid and some techniques to use to reduce these difficult stressful situations. Consider the following points:

- Love occurs in stages and degrees. The euphoric "being in love" stage is usually not highly stressful, but as love changes to the conjugal (living together or marriage) stage, the potential for stress increases.

- A great many people, especially young people, follow a pattern of serial monogamy relationships, one short-lived relationship after another.

- Living together brings in new stressors in the area of intimacy and privacy. Other major stressors include handling money, jealousy, in-laws, sexual relationships, personal habits, and openness in communication.

- The most obvious and immediate stressors are fights and quarrels. They have the capacity to destroy the relationship and evoke stressful emotions such as fear, anger, and hurt.

- A growing number of people by either divorce or personal choice are single. The stress of relationships diminishes but is often replaced by potential stressors of loneliness or diminished feelings of self-worth.

- List the strengths and weaknesses of your relationship and examine ways of reducing the stressful aspects. Alternatively, weigh the pros and cons of not being in any love relationship.

- Successful relationships seem to possess the following qualities: love, independence, self-authenticity, openness and honesty, room for personal growth, and personal freedom.

SOURCES CITED

Barbach, L. (1997). *Fifty ways to please your lover.* New York: E. P. Dutton.

Bartels, A., and Semir, Z. (2000). The neural basis of romantic love, *NeuroReport,* 17, 3829–34.

Bernstein, A. (2002). *Emotional vampires: Dealing with people who drain you dry.* Berkeley, CA: McGraw-Hill.

Branden, N., and Branden, E. D. (1981). *The romantic love: Question and answer book.* Los Angeles: Torcher Publishing Co.

Brown, N. (2002). *Whose life is it anyway?* Oakland, CA: New Harbinger Press.

Bushman, B. J., et al. (2003). Narcissism, sexual refusal, and aggression. *Journal of Personality and Social Psychology,* 48, 1027–40.

Carlson, R. (2001). *Don't sweat guide for couples.* New York: Hyperion Press.

Childs, F. (2002). *Going off: A black woman's guide for dealing with anger and stress.* Torrance, CA: Griffin Trade Paperback.

Feeney, B. (2004). A secure base: Responsive support of goal strivings and exploration in adult intimate relationships. *Journal of Personality and Social Psychology,* 87, no. 5, 631–48.

Fisher, H. (2004). *Why we love.* New York: Henry Holt.

Friday, N. (1997). *Jealousy.* New York: M. Evans.

Gallith, O., et al. (2005). Attachment style differences and ability to suppress negative thoughts. *NeuroImage,* 28, 835–47.

Gilbert, R. M. (2002). *Extraordinary relationships: A new way of thinking about human interactions.* Hoboken, NJ: John Wiley and Sons.

Goldstein, R. Z. (2002). Drug addiction and its underlying neurobiological basis. *American Journal of Psychiatry,* 159, 1642–52.

Goleman, D. (2006). *Social intelligence.* New York: Random House.

Hawkley, L., et al. (2003). Loneliness in everyday life: cardiovascular activity, psychosocial context, and health behaviors. *Journal of Personality and Social Psychology,* 85, 205–20.

Insel, T., and Fernald, R. (2004). How the brain processes social information. *Annual Review of Neuroscience,* 27, 697–722.

Ko, M. (2007). Improving identification of dating abuse using the conflict tactics scale. *American Journal of Health Education,* 38, no. 2, 108–11.

Middleton, D. (1999). *Dealing with feeling left out.* Center City, MN: Hazelden Information Education.

Oschner, K. (2006). How thinking controls feeling. In *Social neuroscience.* P. Winkleman and E. Harman Jones, eds. New York: Oxford University Press.

Orman, S., (2007). *Women & money: Owning the power to control your money.* New York: Random House.

Pines, A. M. (1998). *Romantic jealousy.* New York: Routledge.

Rosenberg, M. B. (2005). *Nonviolent communication.* Encinitas, CA: PuddleDancer Press.

Sanders, J. (1998). *Facing loneliness.* New York: Discovery House.

Simmons, G. (2002). *The I of the storm.* Unity Village, MO: Unity Publishing.

Welch, L. (1995). *Sex facts.* New York: Citadel.

Journal Entry 9

Relationships and Conflict

Relationships can give you pleasure and they can give you misery. When a relationship becomes stressful, you have to examine what it is about that relationship that causes you to be upset. Two common causes of stress in relationships are expectations and power. Given any two people, it is rare that they have the same motivations and that they allow the other to have more or less power in the relationship.

Healthy relationships are based on the premise that both people in the relationship are equal. You cannot work to exert power over others, and you expect the same from them—expect, but don't get attached to outcomes.

Even in physics we know that every act generates a force of energy that cannot be destroyed. What you put out, you get back; no debt ever goes unpaid in the universe, so give what you want in return. What we seek in all of our relationships are things that make us happy: attention, caring, love, appreciation, reward, and the like.

One other aspect to remember is that someone else cannot make you feel a certain way. You have the choice to feel the way you want, to react and respond to the actions of others. You may perceive their actions and motives to be hurtful, and so you feel hurt. Or you can perceive their actions as products of their own experiences that really have little to do with you. In reality, what others think of you is not your business.

EXERCISE LEARNING FROM OTHERS

Name a relationship in your life:

What is the gift in this relationship? What are you learning?

How are you going to be a less stressed person because of what you have learned?

Recall Exercise

This chapter described the twofold method of nonviolent communication (Rosenberg 2005). Think of a time of conflict when you could have used these steps for better communication, and then fill in each step with your observations, feelings, needs, and requests.

Here are the steps to fill in:

First, about expressing yourself:

In the situation you have chosen, write how you could have honestly expressed *yourself* without blaming or criticizing:

a. What did you observe that was contributing or not contributing to your well-being?

b. How were you feeling in relation to what you had been observing?

c. What would you have needed or what did you value that caused the feelings you've expressed?

d. What could you have clearly requested *(without demanding)* that would have enriched your life at that time?

e. How could you have requested specific and concrete actions that you would have liked taken?

Second, about receiving the other person's communication:

In the situation you have chosen, write how you could have empathetically *received* how the other person was at the time, without blame or criticism.

a. Did you ask the other person, "What are you observing?" If yes, what was it? If no, **guess** what the answer would have been.

b. Did you ask, "How do you feel in relation to what you are observing?" If yes, what was it? If no, **guess** what the answer would have been.

c. Did you ask, "What do you need or value that causes you to feel that way?" If yes, what was it? If no, **guess** what the answer would have been.

d. Did you ask and receive with empathy, what would enrich *your* life?" If yes, what was it? If no, **guess** what the answer would have been.

e. Did you ask, "What concrete actions *you* would like taken?" If yes, what was the answer? If no, **guess** what the answer would have been.

 Write down any insights you have had regarding your ability to communicate in an open and caring way.

 Write a positive word or short phrase about conflict within relationships that will be useful to you in future situations.

The Stress of Terrorism and Trauma

In 1992, Walt Disney Studios released an animated movie titled *Aladdin*. It was to become a Disney "classic," entertaining millions. It was the story of a man who had discovered a genie in a bottle, a genie that would grant him three wishes. The promotional tagline for the movie was actually, "Imagine if you had three wishes, three hopes, three dreams and they all could come true."

The Disney movie *Aladdin* was actually based on an Arabian fable translated in the mid-1800s by Sir Richard F. Burton and called *Tales of the Arabian Nights*. But Burton's description of the genie was somewhat different from that created by Disney. Burton described the genie as an ancient and powerful evil force that was inclined to destroy those who released him from the bottle. Only through the calm, strength, and wisdom shown by those who discovered him, was the genie safely returned to his bottle.

At 8:15 on the morning of August 6, 1945, an atomic bomb named "Little Boy" was dropped on Hiroshima, Japan, by a Boeing B-29 bomber, the *Enola Gay*. This detonation over Hiroshima created an atomic holocaust. The devastation was so complete, so profound that many feared that we had unleashed a powerful "atomic genie," a genie that was so powerful it could spell the end of humanity as we know it. In the August 19, 1946, issue of *Life* magazine, Admiral William H. P. Blandy called the atomic bomb "a poison weapon."

Terrorism and the Genie

Terrorism represents a form of "evil genie," an ancient and powerful force capable of remarkable devastation. Indeed, it may be a "poison weapon" as Admiral Blandy remarked. To briefly review, *terrorism* can be defined as the illegal, immoral use or threatened use of force designed to create conditions of fear, helplessness, and demoralization as a coercive or punitive force. More important, terrorism is psychological warfare, the goal of which is to demoralize the target group to the point that it surrenders to the will of the terrorists. From a planning perspective, it is important to see terrorism as a strategic weapon that targets the sources of a nation's military, economic, and political power—the civilian population!

Terrorism targets:

Your sense of safety ("I'm afraid to do what I normally do.")

Your sense of justice and fair play ("That's not right, fair . . .")

Your sense of order, meaning ("It doesn't make sense . . . How could anyone do such a thing?")

Death and destruction are merely means to an end; they are not ends unto themselves. Terrorism seeks to create "psychological casualties," that is, individuals who become impaired as a result of the terrorism. The adverse impact of terrorism may, therefore, be estimated not just in terms of physical destruction, but in terms of psychological "toxicity." Factors that may serve to increase psychological toxicity might include:

1. An unpredictable pattern of attacks

2. Ability to affect large numbers of victims

3. Intent to harm noncombatants, especially targeting women and children

4. Ease of weapon delivery

5. Delay and difficulty in assessing exposure, especially lethality

6. Long latency or incubation period, at least several days

7. Potential for contagion (physical or psychological), especially if it deters emergency response and/or treatment

8. Potential to scar and disable rather than kill

9. Ability to overwhelm public health and other resources, while altering the accepted and preferential way of life

10. Motivation that is immune to rational, measured deterrence; willingness to use self-destruction as a weapon; all-or-nothing strategic thinking

A Brief History of Terrorism

One of the earliest of documented terrorist movements was that of the Zealot-Sicarii, an extremist group in ancient Rome circa 70 CE, which attempted to foster a rebellion against Roman rule. The Zealot-Sicarii would murder Roman sympathizers in broad daylight and in crowded areas as a way of instilling fear and unrest. Ultimately, these murders were done as a way of inciting a rebellion so large that it was thought that it would necessitate the coming of the Messiah.

A medieval (1090–1275 CE) Muslim Shiite group known as the Assassins used terror tactics in an attempt to purify the Muslim community. They promoted what was a form of "murder suicide" (similar to the notion of the modern-day suicide bomber). The Assassin would murder the victim in public then wait to be arrested and executed. The calm resolve shown by the Assassins was based on the belief that they were becoming martyrs who would be rewarded in the afterlife (once again similar to modern-day suicide bombers).

In the late eighteenth century, the French Revolution was marked by Robespierre and his "Reign of Terror." No longer was terrorism exacted in the name of God, but in the name of political expediency.

This theme of terrorism to serve political ends was continued in an influential book titled *Revolutionary Catechism* by Michael Bakunin and Sergey Nechayev. This book, published in Tzarist Russia around 1869, painted an idealistic picture of the terrorist who willingly dies in an effort to destroy social, religious, and economic institutions.

Terrorist movements since these early variations have had similar characteristics:

1. The goal has not been military victory; rather, political, social, or religious goals are sought.

2. Infiltration, deception, and disguise are often used as means of setting the stage for the attack.

3. Suicide/self-sacrifice are seen as viable, if not desirable, means to achieve the end point of a successful attack.

4. The ultimate mechanism by which the terrorist hopes to achieve the desired end is psychological demoralization with a resultant "giving up."

Defining Moments of a Generation

For the generation of "baby boomers," it has been said that the assassination of President John F. Kennedy was the defining moment of their generation. For the generation of individuals who are currently college students, it may be said that the defining moment of their generation was the attacks of September 11, 2001.

On September 11, 2001, at approximately 8:45 A.M., the hijacked American Airlines Flight 11, en route from Boston, crashed into the north tower at the World Trade Center in New York City. Shortly thereafter, at 9:06 A.M., the hijacked United Airlines Flight 175, also en route from Boston, crashed into the remaining south tower. At 10:00 A.M., the south tower collapsed, sending a wave of debris for blocks and trapping hundreds of firefighters and law enforcement officers who had rushed to rescue those working in the tower. At 10:29 A.M., the north tower also collapsed.

Approximately fifty-five minutes after the World Trade Center was attacked, a similar terrorist attack was perpetrated against the Pentagon in Washington, DC. American Airlines Flight 77, en route from the Washington Dulles Airport to Los Angeles, crashed into the Pentagon as an apparent secondary target after possibly intending to crash into the White House.

Although the resultant physical devastation and physical human suffering were beyond anything this nation has ever experienced, the psychological devastation may not be known for years, perhaps even for generations!

To expand this notion of terrorism and its resultant stress, there exist four credible and significant threats to our nation at this time, based on the most recent of current events as described above: (1) the objective threat of incidents of physical destruction and death; (2) the perceived threat of injury/death to individuals, families, and communities; (3) the threat of sociological upheaval; and (4) the threat of economic recession, with the potential for specific industrial sectors to collapse.

Logistically, it seems a low-probability event that groups of terrorists could defeat our nation militarily. However, a higher-probability event would be that the terrorists could cripple our nation to such a degree that they achieve desired political and foreign policy victories. How could such an outcome occur? The answer rests on understanding that three of the four threats described above are actually psychological in nature. Fear, albeit subjective, is an agent of change. It can destroy one's personal health through excessive stress. It can split apart families. It can split apart communities and destroy political unity. It can destroy businesses and cause economic collapse (as evidenced by the technology crash).

The attack on September 11, 2001, was obviously different from the attack on the World Trade Center perpetrated eight years earlier. The amount of physical destruction and the loss of life are clearly incomparable. However, the psychological destruction is incomparable as well. In the wake of the first attack on the World Trade Center, the illusion of safety was largely maintained by the American people. That illusion appears to be eroding as terrorist attacks become more prevalent. Remember, stressors, like beauty, lie in the eye of the beholder!

Virginia Tech Massacre

On April 16, 2007, the deadliest school shooting in modern U.S. history took place at Virginia Polytechnic Institute in Blacksburg, Virginia. A shooter, Seung-Hui Cho, killed thirty two people and wounded fifteen more before committing suicide. He had a history of unsettling incidents at the school, including allegations of stalking and a 2005 declaration of mental illness by a Virginia special justice. The shootings came just four days before the eighth anniversary of the Columbine High School shootings wherein two students killed thirteen people and themselves near Littleton, Colorado. Was this another example of terrorism? The video messages left behind by Cho suggest that the intention was indeed to intentionally punish, and the shootings did indeed induce a reaction of "terror" in survivors, but the missing element was the notion of demoralization with the intention to cause capitulation or "giving up." So from our strict interpretation, the Virginia Polytechnic shootings were not terrorism, per se, but were examples of trauma.

What was your reaction when you first learned of the shootings in Virginia? Was there concern for your own safety?

Psychological Contagion

Considering that a primary goal of terrorism is to create pervasive fear and uncertainty, or in other words large-scale psychological morbidity, among its survivors, and given that other forms of trauma can induce significant distress, the mechanism of contagion warrants exploration. The term "contagion" has typically been associated with medical diseases, emotional and behavioral reactions, and sociological phenomena. Regardless of its context, contagion implies a surge or spread of events. From a medical perspective, mostly in relation to infectious agents, contagion refers to transmission of disease by direct or indirect contact, or "something that serves as a medium to transmit disease"

(*Merriam-Webster's Collegiate Dictionary,* 10th ed.). From a psychological or sociological perspective, the concept of contagion was first introduced by the French sociologist Gustave Le Bon (1903) to account for the emotionally charged "collective mind" of people in a crowd. In the present context, psychological contagion refers to how the effects of terrorism are transmitted to those not directly affected by the initial event. In essence, it represents a surge of events, both behavioral and psychological, that threaten our safety and security (Everly and Castellano 2005).

Considering that a primary goal of terrorism is the proliferation of fear, understanding the potent mechanisms of transmission is particularly critical. For example, do factors such as physical proximity, personally knowing someone directly involved in the event, lack of social support, or perceived personal threat account for the potent terrorist effect?

Bioterrorism and Contagion Theory

Given terrorism's potential to create large-scale psychological morbidity, from a contagion perspective there are no more potentially devastating terrorist weapons than biological, chemical, or nuclear agents. Research has indicated that human-made disasters are more psychologically pathogenic than natural disasters (Baum and Davidson 1985). The implementation of biological agents against a human population, or bioterrorism, is associated with our most fundamental fears of disease and death. Bioterrorist events, due to their possible invisible nature, extreme lethality, long incubation time, and lack of defined perimeter, expose our societal vulnerability.

An intentional bioterrorist attack using agents such inhalation anthrax, botulism, plague, smallpox, tularemia, or sarin, or a combination of these or other agents, will clearly have profound medical effects. Yet the psychological impact in the aftermath of a bioterrorist attack may be equally daunting. In fact, estimates suggest that for every one physical illness produced by a biological agent, between 50 and 100 individuals will experience psychological distress at a level that impairs their daily functioning (DeMartino 2002).

From a larger perspective, terrorist acts, as well as traumatic events that may not be terrorism, may be seen as capable of creating psychological crises. Let's learn more.

The Stress of Terror and Trauma

Have you ever experienced a crisis? Just what constitutes a crisis, from a psychological perspective?

A crisis is a response to some threatening or adverse event wherein three conditions are evident:

1. Your normal state of psychological balance (homeostasis) is disrupted, leading to a state of distress.

2. Your normal coping strategies are not successful.

3. You are unable to perform at your normal level of effectiveness; that is, some level of impaired functioning is evident. (Everly 1999)

Just as a physical crisis threatens your physical health, a psychological crisis threatens your psychological health. The most severe form of crisis is the psychological trauma, and a traumatic event is the most severe form of stressor. Psychological trauma has existed as long as humanity. The earliest accounts of posttraumatic stress reactions come to us from the battlefield. Terms such as battle fatigue, soldier's heart, war neurosis, and shell shock were often used as labels for posttraumatic stress reactions (Chalsma 1998; Parrish 1999). But such reactions are not limited to warfare.

In 1865, Charles Dickens wrote of a railway accident in which he was involved (Trimble 1981). Dickens's diary contained numerous accounts of the accident, and he subsequently described his reactions to the disaster in the following way: "I am curiously weak—weak as if I were recovering from a long illness." The description is intriguing in that Dickens himself was not physically injured but rather was an observer of several hours of "horrifying" sights and sounds during which many people did indeed die.

The year 1666 was the year of the Great Fire of London. Trimble (1981), in his historical account of posttraumatic stress, notes that the fire not only destroyed lives and property but also engendered numerous accounts of posttraumatic stress reactions including phobic reactions, nightmares, flashbacks, and many stress-related physical complaints.

In 1980, the American Psychiatric Association (APA) officially described a mental disorder that may develop in response to psychological or physical trauma. That disorder is now referred to as posttraumatic stress disorder (PTSD). Thus, with PTSD's recognition as an official "legitimate" affliction in 1980, further inquiry and preventive programs became possible. Recent events in the world have further underscored the need to recognize and investigate posttraumatic stress reactions. In 1992, the American Red Cross and the APA cooperated to create a national-disaster mental health network. The purpose of this network was not only to provide disaster mental health services to Red Cross personnel working in disaster venues but also, more important, to provide acute mental health support for primary disaster victims throughout the United States. Shortly after this network was created, the United States saw a virtual plague of disasters including Hurricane Andrew, Hurricane Iniki, the Los Angeles earthquake, the floods in the Midwest, the California firestorms and floods, the first World Trade Center attack, the Oklahoma City terrorist bombings, numerous airline disasters such as TWA 800 and Swiss Air 111, the earthquakes in Turkey, and the "holy war" targeted against Americans called for by Osama bin Laden.

Recognizing the fact that emergency response professionals such as law enforcement, fire suppression, emergency medical personnel, and rescue workers were at high risk for PTSD, another organization was formed that actually predates the network just mentioned. In 1989, the International Critical Incident Stress Foundation was formed to provide support for all emergency services professionals because they are at greatest risk for developing PTSD. Although this foundation predated the national-disaster mental health network of the American Red Cross and the APA, it has a far more selective constituency.

Just how widespread is crisis? Consider the following:

- Recent evidence suggests that more than 60 percent of adults in the United States will be exposed to a traumatic event during their lifetime.

- The rate of trauma exposure for children and adolescents has been estimated at about 40 percent.
- Suicide rates have been seen to increase after natural disasters.
- The lifetime prevalence of criminal victimization was assessed among female HMO patients and was found to be about 57 percent.
- Violence at work costs more than 1.75 million lost workdays.
- Homicide is the third leading cause of death from injury at the worksite (NIOSH) in the United States, but in California and the District of Columbia it is the leading cause of workplace death.
- Each year, approximately 1 million people become victims of violent crime at work.
- The prevalence of PTSD was found to be 13 percent in a sample of suburban law enforcement officers.
- Law enforcement officers are 8.6 times more likely to die from suicide than from homicide and are 3.1 times more likely to die from suicide than from accidental circumstances.
- Clinical health care staff sampled reported that 62 percent of their employees were exposed to a traumatic stressor at work.
- The prevalence of posttraumatic stress disorder ranged from 15 to 31 percent for samples of urban firefighters based on a traumatic exposure prevalence ranging from 85 to 91 percent.
- Symptoms of distress and PTSD are correlated with exposure to traumatic stressors, such that there exists a virtual dose–response relationship; that is, the more crises you are exposed to, the greater your risk of developing PTSD (adapted from Everly and Mitchell 1999).

Posttraumatic Stress Disorder

Widespread research and prevention programs did not develop until PTSD became an official psychiatric phenomenon in 1980. The American Psychiatric Association's diagnostic nosology, *Diagnostic and Statistical Manual of Mental Disorders* (APA 1994), retains the PTSD diagnosis under the heading "Anxiety Disorders." The official diagnostic criteria are as follows:

1. The person has been exposed to a traumatic event in which both of the following were present:
   - The person experienced, witnessed, or was confronted with an event or events that involved actual or threatened death or serious injury or a threat to the physical integrity of self or others.
   - The person's response involved intense fear, helplessness, or horror.
2. The traumatic event is persistently reexperienced in one (or more) of the following ways:
   - recurrent and intrusive distressing recollections of the event

- recurrent distressing dreams of the event
- acting or feeling as if the traumatic event were recurring
- intense psychological distress at exposure to internal or external cues that symbolize or resemble an aspect of the traumatic event
- physiological reactivity on exposure to internal or external cues that symbolize or resemble an aspect of the event

3. The person persistently avoids stimuli associated with the trauma and experiences a numbing of general responsiveness as indicated by three or more of the following:
   - efforts to avoid thoughts, feelings, or conversations associated with the trauma
   - efforts to avoid activities, places, or people that arouse recollections of the trauma
   - inability to recall an important aspect of the trauma
   - markedly diminished interest or participation in significant activities
   - feeling of detachment or estrangement from others
   - restricted range of affect
   - sense of a foreshortened future

4. The person presents persistent symptoms of increased arousal (not present before the trauma), as indicated by two (or more) of the following:
   - difficulty falling or staying asleep
   - irritability or outbursts of anger
   - difficulty concentrating
   - hypervigilance
   - exaggerated startle response

5. Symptom duration is greater than one month.

6. The disturbance causes clinically significant distress or impairment.

The Consequences of PTSD   The consequences of prolonged PTSD are nothing less than profound. There exists evidence that prolonged PTSD represents chronic neurotransmitter and neurohumoral cascades that may result in a wide variety of behavioral and health-related consequences that extend far beyond the diagnostic criteria themselves, for example:

1. irritability and aggressiveness

2. difficulty concentrating

3. difficulty in assimilating new information

4. reclusive, avoidant behavior

5. self-medication

6. symptoms consistent with attention deficit hyperactivity disorder (ADHD) formulations

7. narcoleptic symptoms (inappropriate sleepiness)

8. symptoms consistent with those of complex partial seizures

9. existential crises

10. compulsive eating, buying, and/or sexual behavior

11. an acceleration of physical diseases of degeneration

12. presenile dementia-like symptoms

The Nature of Posttraumatic Stress   The symptoms just listed provide a working definition of a complex psychological condition. As we can see in Criteria 2, 3, and 4 of the preceding list, PTSD exhibits three specific symptom clusters that reveal the pathological nature of the disorder:

1. Reexperiencing the traumatic event

2. Numbing and withdrawal symptoms: persistent avoidance of people, places, and things associated with the trauma, and/or a psychological numbing in which the victim seems to withdraw into a shell

3. Persistent increased stress arousal

PTSD may also be seen as a combination of recalled images and excessive arousal, especially of the sympathetic nervous system (Everly and Lating 1995). The numbing and withdrawal is then understood as a secondary reaction to the intrusive recollections and increased arousal. **Figure 10.1** depicts the postulated relationships.

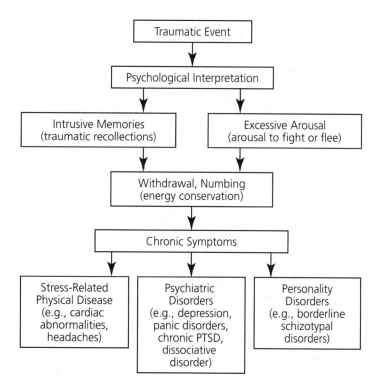

Figure 10.1 A Process Model of PTSD

Source: Adapted from Everly and Lating (1995).

This latter formulation may help us to better understand PTSD and other traumatic stress syndromes. For example, PTSD may represent an extreme variation of survival mechanisms. Remember that PTSD arises from exposure to some event that is life threatening or otherwise capable of overwhelming normal coping mechanisms. The mind's survival response may be to deeply ingrain that event in the memory so that similar situations may be avoided in the future (or so that the person will be better prepared to cope with them). The body's survival response may be to create a chronic state of arousal that keeps one prepared for fight or flight at the slightest provocation or threat. Finally, the numbing, and especially the withdrawal symptoms, may represent an energy-conservation mechanism designed to allow recovery of strength after a traumatic event (Everly 1991).

Figure 10.1 indicates that chronic acute traumatic syndrome has three potential outcomes:

1. Stress-related physical disease

2. Psychiatric syndromes such as depression or chronic PTSD itself

3. Posttraumatic personality disorders such as borderline personality disorder

An analysis of PTSD reveals two underlying factors: a neurological hypersensitivity and a psychological hypersensitivity (Everly 1991). In neurological terms, exposure to a traumatizing event may result in hypersensitivity within the neural networks of the subcortical limbic system (described earlier in Chapter 2). Functionally, such hypersensitivity represents a lowering of the threshold for excessive arousal or excitation. Thus, the slightest irritation or provocation could result in rage, impaired general memory, panic, withdrawal, impulsive reactions, or other forms of extreme stress reactions. The biological foundations for such neurological hypersensitivities and abnormalities may include massive catecholamine release, abnormal cortisol secretions, and endogenous opioid release (Everly and Lating 1995). Mukerjee (1995) has even reviewed evidence that suggests that nerve centers in the hippocampal area of the limbic system of PTSD victims may be so adversely affected by trauma that a 13–26 percent reduction in cellular mass may result. Semple and colleagues (1993) found that persons diagnosed both with PTSD and as substance abusers show abnormal blood flow patterns in the frontal cortex as well as in the subcortical hippocampus.

Psychologically, exposure to a traumatizing event may create hypersensitivity within important mechanisms used by all individuals to maintain psychological homeostasis. More specifically, trauma shatters some important assumptions about the nature of our world. It was Abraham Maslow (1968) who noted that a basic human need, second only to the need for food and shelter, is the need for safety.

To make the unknown aspects of the world somewhat safe, we all create assumptions about life in general. For example, one assumption many people hold is that life is "fair." Another is that you get what you deserve and you deserve what you get—it is a "just" world. Another assumption might be that "good" always conquers "evil." Traumatic events by their very nature violate, challenge, and sometimes destroy these presuppositions about life and the world around us. In so doing, they create a psychological void. This void represents a "psychic puzzle" that yields a hypersensitivity to perceptions of threat, demoralization, and panic.

There appear to be five core belief systems that when violated yield posttraumatic stress syndrome:

1. the belief in a just and fair world

2. the belief that one is not helpless in the world (self-efficacy)

3. the belief that one can trust most people

4. the belief that the world is generally a safe place

5. the belief that there is some order to our lives and the world (Everly and Lating 2003)

When violated, these beliefs become

1. a sense that justice was not served;

2. helplessness, hopelessness, and guilt;

3. betrayal;

4. pervasive insecurity; and

5. chaos, spiritual crises, and existential crises.

PTSD is not the only form that posttraumatic stress can take; however, it is the most severe. In addition to physical illnesses and personality dysfunctions, a posttraumatic reaction may manifest itself in the following ways (Horowitz 1997):

- fear of a recurrence of the trauma
- shame over being a victim
- rage over being a victim
- rage toward the person or thing that caused the trauma
- phobic reactions
- fear of a loss of control
- depression
- mourning
- guilt

Traumatic Events

What sort of events can cause traumatic stress reactions? Initially, psychologists defined a traumatic event as any event outside the usual realm of human experience that would be markedly distressing to virtually anyone who encountered it. That definition has been drastically narrowed to not only embrace particular events but to also include one's appraisal of the event, for example, appraisals of helplessness, fear, or horror. **Table 10.1** contains a list of potentially traumatic events.

Even though all of the factors listed in Table 10.1 can clearly lead to traumatic stress reactions, one's psychological appraisal of the adverse experience can serve to mitigate or augment one's personal traumatic response. This phenomenon not only helps us explain why not every person exposed to a traumatic stressor develops the same level of

Table 10.1   Traumatic Events

Personal Traumas	Community Traumas
robbery	flood
physical assault	earthquake
rape	fire
automobile accident	building collapse
a "life-or-death" struggle	airplane crash
physical abuse	multiple-injury accident
psychological abuse	terrorism
sexual abuse	injury or death of a child
a perceived serious threat to one's well-being	
a perceived serious threat to a family member or close friend	
observing any of the personal or community traumas listed here	

posttraumatic reaction, but it also gives us clues into how we might more effectively treat and even prevent PTSD in high-risk individuals.

Coping with Traumatic Stress   A number of strategies that consider both neurological and psychological hypersensitivity have been used to cope with traumatic events. Neurological hypersensitivity manifests itself in the form of excessive arousal. This arousal is based on either a biological propensity for arousal or a failure of the brain to dampen arousal.

Relaxation training is usually the best generic approach to lower the level of arousal. No one technique appears to be superior to others. One should practice the relaxation technique that seems easiest and most convenient to utilize. However, some individuals will find that during relaxation they tend to recall the traumatic experience. Such recollection can be stressful and therefore counterproductive. It is sometimes recommended that a more active relaxation technique be employed to reduce the intrusive ideation. Biofeedback is one such technology. In some instances, psychotropic medications are used to dampen the excessive arousal that is a natural constituent of PTSD.

Psychological hypersensitivity arises from a violated worldview, or assumption about the world. The strategies often employed to reduce the disequilibrium associated with a violated worldview include (1) reinterpreting the traumatic event, (2) reinterpreting the role that one played in the event, (3) active behavior oriented toward increasing one's sense of control over similar events, (4) behaviors designed to increase one's general sense of control, (5) utilization of social support, and (6) changing one's worldview so as to assimilate the trauma and thus reduce the anxiety associated with disconfirmation. Let us take a closer look at each of these.

One of the most common coping mechanisms for reducing stress and a sense of chaos is to reinterpret the traumatic event, perhaps by trying to find some positive aspect to it. For example, one might say that the trauma allowed one to finally "grow up" and face problems like an adult. Or one might say that the trauma revealed a previously unknown inner strength. In general, these strategies allow the person to find "meaning" in an otherwise meaningless catastrophe. Although it may seem like a pedestrian effort to find the "silver lining" in a cloud of trauma, reinterpretation can prove quite useful as long as it doesn't stifle further growth and development or create new problems of its own.

Another strategy is to reinterpret the role one played in the trauma itself. Survivors of disasters sometimes cope by considering themselves fortunate even to have survived. A similar strategy might be to compare oneself to victims who were more adversely affected. Often, victims of physical harm cope by focusing not on the event but on recovering from it beyond anyone's expectations. If one tends to blame oneself for the traumatic event, it is sometimes helpful to search for other reasonable explanations for the event. If one is truly responsible, however, one should try to accept responsibility and then consider how to assist the recovery process and/or reduce the chances of similar events occurring. Also, when viewing oneself as partially responsible for the traumatic event, one quickly discovers a reason for it. This coping strategy of self-blame is commonly used by victims, even when their role in the trauma was minimal, as a means of restoring order and predictability to the world.

The third common coping mechanism is engaging in some action that reduces the likelihood of a similar event, actively pursuing rehabilitation, or even pursuing punitive action through proper authorities. For example, a burglary victim may place locks on windows and dead-bolt doors or even install an electronic alarm system. These strategies are likely to reduce the probability of a repeat trauma. The victim of an automobile accident may install an air bag in the car. Often, traumatized persons who are physically injured will not only pursue rehabilitation but will also use the opportunity to become more health conscious. Finally, the victim of a crime or of human negligence may pursue punitive action through the court system. Such action may not only reduce the likelihood of further crimes or negligence, but it often also results in a feeling of empowerment for the victim.

A fourth strategy to reduce psychological hypersensitivity after trauma is to engage in any activity that creates a sense of empowerment and control. It is well known that victims of trauma commonly suffer feelings of self-doubt, helplessness, and a general lack of control. Any activity that helps develop a sense of self-control tends to restore order to a worldview whose assumptions have been violated. The activities do not have to be related to the trauma; rather, any activity that increases self-esteem will prove valuable.

Trauma often leaves the victim believing that the world may be a malevolent place. This is in direct contradiction to the more deeply ingrained assumptions that the world is safe and secure. A strategy that helps refute the malevolent-world perspective is social support. We all need some form of social support; humans are social animals. Trauma increases our inherent need for social support. Yet trauma victims often hesitate to seek social support out of a dislike for showing "weakness," a concern over being taken advantage of, and even a reluctance to have others feel sorry for them. Nevertheless, trauma actually increases the need for social support, and thus appropriate social support can have powerful healing effects. Sometimes that support must be obtained from a trained mental health professional such as a psychologist. Failure to obtain social support can needlessly protract psychological suffering. Pennebaker (1995, 1997) argues that translating emotional events into language increases both physical and emotional health. On the other hand, "holding it all inside" can be destructive to both in the long run.

In some cases, the trauma may be so overwhelming, the victim's ability to cope may be so meager, or one's previously held assumptions about the world may have been so ineffective (or blatantly inappropriate) that the only reasonable coping strategy is to change one's worldview rather than try to salvage it.

A brief summary of the various coping strategies follows:

1. Dampen the tendency for overexcitation, overreaction, and excessive arousal.
2. Reinterpret the traumatic event.
3. Reinterpret your role in the trauma.
4. Increase your control over the traumatic situation.
5. Increase your personal sense of control.
6. Obtain social support (perhaps professional support).
7. Verbalize or journal your feelings.
8. Change your assumptions about the world.

The earlier one recognizes the symptoms of psychological trauma and seeks help, the more rapid the recovery is likely to be. The victim of psychological trauma usually requires assistance to recover. Professional help should always be sought in fully developed cases of PTSD. This information is offered not as a way of treating trauma but rather as a way of familiarizing you with this extreme stress response so that formal treatment can be sought more readily when and if trauma strikes.

Violence: A Special Form of Crisis

In the fall of 2002, two snipers randomly killed thirteen victims, most in the Washington, DC, area. Although this series of murders justifiably accrued national news attention, what was not mentioned was that a similar number of people unceremoniously died in the Baltimore-Washington megalopolis from all-too-common street violence at the same time that the sniper killings occurred.

Regarding youth violence, a 1998 Department of Education report covering a sample of 1,200 schools indicated that there were 11,000 fights using weapons, 4,000 rapes and other sexual assaults, and 7,000 robberies (Flannery 1999). Dr. Flannery concludes that there is an epidemic of violence in the United States. He notes that Americans do not feel safe because we are not safe!

In the search for the causes of our violent society, Flannery lists the following contributing factors:

- disrupted familial relationships and domestic violence
- poverty
- discrimination
- inadequate schooling
- media portrayal of violence as acceptable/desirable
- disruption of prosocial values

- drug abuse
- disruption of caring attachments with others

As a solution, Flannery (1998) notes that the remedy to the epidemic of violence resides in the restoration of a sense of community, restoration of the family and caring attachments to others, improvement of the educational system, and restoration of religious values. It is likely that the pursuit of such outcomes will result not only in a less violence society but a less stressful one as well.

SUMMARY

Every day ordinary people around the world undergo extreme fear situations that evoke terror, resulting in extreme psychological and physical stress reactions that may result in a prolonged stress response (known as posttraumatic stress disorder, or PTSD). Consider the following points:

- Evidence suggests that more than 60 percent of adults in the United States will be exposed to a traumatic event in their lifetime.
- During extreme trauma, one's psychological balance (homeostasis) is disrupted, leading to a state of distress.
- Research has indicated that human-made disasters are more psychologically pathogenic than natural disasters.
- Psychological contagion refers to how the effects of terrorism are transmitted to those not directly affected by the initial event. In essence, it represents a surge of events, both behavioral and psychological, that threaten our safety and security.
- Normal coping strategies are not usually successful in extreme trauma cases.
- Terrorism engenders a large-scale psychological response that occurs in others besides the actual victims of the event.
- The purpose of terrorism is not necessarily harm to the victims, but large-scale psychological distress to a generalized population.
- The prolonged consequences of PTSD are profound and clinically recognizable as a set of symptoms.
- PTSD appears to be the result of core belief systems being violated.
- Coping with traumatic stress starts with generic relaxation training.
- Strategies for advanced trauma include professional intervention techniques such as behavior-oriented therapy.
- Prevention of trauma can include environmental manipulation so as to reduce the incidence of physical attack, burglary, and so on.
- Even though current emphasis seems to be on foreign terrorists, our violent society appears to be the number-one cause of terror-related stress.

SOURCES CITED

American Psychiatric Association (1994). *Diagnostic and statistical manual of mental disorders,* 4th ed. Washington, DC: Author.

Chalsma, H. W. (1998). *The chambers of memory: PTSD in the life stories of U.S. Vietnam vets.* London: Jason Aronson.

DeMartino, R. (2002). *Bio-terrorism. Bio-security.* Las Vegas, NV, as reported on AOL News.

Everly, G. S. (1991). Neurophysiological considerations in the treatment of PTSD: A neurocognitive perspective. *In International handbook for traumatic stress syndrome,* eds. J. Wilson and B. Raphael. New York: Plenum, 356.

Everly, G. S. (1999). A primer on critical incident stress management: What's really in a name? *International Journal of Emergency Mental Health,* 1, 77–79.

Everly, G. S., Jr., & Castellano, C. (2005). *Psychological counterterrorism and World War IV.* Ellicott City, MD: Chevron.

Everly, G. S., and Lating, J., eds. (1995). *Psychotraumatology: Key papers and concepts in posttraumatic stress.* New York: Plenum.

Everly, G. S., and Lating, J. (2004). Personality-guided therapy of PTSD. Washington, DC: APA Press.

Everly, G. S., and Mitchell, J. T. (1999). *Critical incident stress management,* 2nd ed. Ellicott City, MD: Chevron.

Flannery, R. B., Jr. (1998). *Violence in America.* New York: Continuum.

Flannery, R. B., Jr. (1999). *Preventing youth violence.* New York: Continuum.

Horowitz, M. J. (1997). *Stress response syndromes: PTSD, grief, and adjustment disorders.* London: Jason Aronson.

Le Bon, G. (1903). *The crowd.* London: Allen and Unwin.

Maslow, A. (1968). *Toward a psychology of being.* New York: Van Nostrand Reinhold.

Merriam-Webster's collegiate dictionary, 10th ed. (1993). Springfield, MA: Merriam-Webster, Inc.

Mukerjee, M. (1995). Hidden scars: Sexual and other abuse may alter a brain region. *Scientific American,* 273, 14, 20.

NIOSH (2003). *NIOSH intramural research projects addressing occupational injuries for fiscal year 2002.* Washington, DC: NIOSH.

Parrish, I. S. (1999). *Military veterans' PTSD reference manual.* Media, PA: BuyBooksontheweb.com.

Pennebaker, J. W. (1997). *Opening up: The healing power of expressing emotions.* New York: Guilford Press.

Pennebaker, J. W., ed. (1995). *Emotion, disclosure, and health.* Washington, D.C.: American Psychological Association.

Semple, W., Goyer, P., McCormick, R., Morris, E., Comptom, B., Muswick, G., and Nelson, D. (1993). Preliminary report: Brain blood flow using PET in patients with posttraumatic stress disorder and substance-abuse histories. *Biological Psychiatry,* 34, 115–18.

Trimble, M. R. (1981). *Post-traumatic neurosis.* Chichester, UK: Wiley.

Journal Entry 10

Responding to Terror

Terror is defined as "intense fear"; thus the stress reaction is magnified in response to acts of terrorism. Although terrorism is a word common to everyone's vocabulary after the events of September 11, 2001, the word wasn't coined on that day. Each and every day ordinary people around the world undergo extreme fear situations that evoke pure terror in their lives—women are raped, men are tortured, parents see their children killed, men and women in uniform experience the horror of war, firefighters hear the screams of trapped victims. There is an endless litany of terror in the world.

Everyone reacts to terror, and many have prolonged responses to it. These prolonged responses have been named "posttraumatic stress disorder" (PTSD). Chapter 10 describes PTSD, giving the symptoms of this disorder.

As a journaling exercise, you are asked to describe a traumatic experience you have had. Perhaps September 11 produced this kind of shock in your life, or you have had a more personal experience that has shaken you. In the area below, (a) write about your experience and then (b) write about the aftermath of that experience—what recurring feelings/thoughts/behaviors you have had due to the traumatic experience.

a.

b.

Chapter 10 identifies five core belief systems (given below) that, when violated, yield the posttraumatic stress syndrome. Concerning the traumatic event that you journaled earlier, indicate the involvement of each of these beliefs in your trauma in the space provided.

a. the belief that the world is fair

b. the belief that one is not helpless in the world

c. the belief that one can trust most people

d. the belief that the world is generally a safe place

e. the belief that there is some order to our lives and the world

What insights have you had from this exercise regarding the stress of terror and trauma?

Write a positive word or short phrase that may empower you when you think of this trauma.

CHAPTER 11

Stress in the Workplace

The social anthropologist Studs Terkel suggested in his book, *Working* (1990), "Work is about a search for daily meaning as well as daily bread, for recognition as well as cash, for astonishment rather than torpor, in short, for a sort of life rather than a Monday to Friday sort of dying" (5). Work has a qualitative as well as a quantitative aspect, and both can produce stress. It will come as no surprise that work and the relationships among coworkers, superiors, and subordinates are always listed as high on the scale of stressors in just about every survey.

As you might have noticed, this book is in its eighth edition, spanning three decades. This chapter has been written in economic good times, and in recessions. In good times, workers are in demand and get treated somewhat better, which to a large degree ameliorates some of their job-related stress. In a poor economy, workers tend to suffer, and naturally, job-related stress goes up as does the staggering cost of workers' compensation. Stress-related conditions have increased 500 percent in the last decade and represent the greatest threat to productivity, costing companies and society hundreds of billions of dollars and robbing millions of their quality of life (Partridge 2007). Stress, which is the second-highest work-related disease in the United States, accounts for 20–25 percent of all occupational health claims (Cooper 2000). These statistics are mainly mental conditions and do not reflect the stress contribution to physical diseases, which makes the stress-related figure even more staggering (see **Figure 11.1**).

As optimists, we hope that world economy will be robust and as such that alone will play a role in decreasing the stress load on workers. Even if it does, however, there are many stressful factors inherent in the work situation to keep work at the top of the stressor list; further, there are some fundamental changes that have occurred in the workplace over the last few years that will impact workers for years to come. These exist in the areas of employer–employee relationships and worker overload. As the saying goes there is a new sheriff in town. It goes by the name of multinational corporations or globalization. On the positive side, the world is now more than ever seen as new markets with new customers who are buying goods. On the negative side, the entire world is now part of the labor pool and most of the additional workers have a much lower standard of living and are willing to

Figure 11.1 Stressors, Psychological Discord, and Illness

work for much lower wages. Outsourcing to lower-wage countries is an ever-increasing problem for American workers (Karoly and Constantijn 2004).

The United States is shifting from a production economy to one of service and information. Workers in the service sector, comprised of those making around $10,000 per year, usually do not have much trouble finding work, but the flood of illegal immigrant workers ensures that their wages will not keep up and they are destined to barely survive. Wage earners between them and those making the medium income of about $45,000 per year are part of what crusading talk show host Lou Dobbs (2006) refers to as the vanishing middle class, whose jobs and wages are under constant threat to downsizing and outsourcing. The higher-income portion of the middle class, those making between $50,000 and $150,000, are the professionals, those in high-tech positions, and middle managers who are making a good living while working ever harder and going deeper in debt.

In the United Kingdom and Europe, they describe the current workplace changes as the Americanized scenario, that of downsizing, restructuring, and mergers. Although this has produced leaner, more productive organizations, it has given rise to intrinsic job insecurity and a culture of longer working hours. This change is beginning to have an adverse effect on employee attitudes and behavior.

Another added stressor is information overload. A major source of pressure for people at work is the massive weight of information they have to handle daily, particularly e-mails, memos, and "interruptions."

According to research at the University of California, more data will be created in the next two years than in all of human history. Lewis (1999) says, "Convinced that knowledge is power, many people are working themselves into the ground in an attempt to keep up." The result can be a state of mental and physical exhaustion known as information fatigue syndrome. This creates a productivity paradox in which the quest for ever more information often means a decline in performance, resulting in a loss of productivity rather than the predicted gain.

In general, the work pace has increased over the last decade. Half of today's workers feel they work at an increasingly higher pace, three-fourths see poor possibilities for promotion, and one-third see no fit between their work and their education. Thus stress and anxiety on the job and at school contribute significantly to the total stress level of the average person in our fast-paced society. Therefore, the workplace is the natural extension of our discussion of the causes of stress.

Job Stress

Swedish researchers have helped clarify some of the broadest conceptual aspects of work-related stress. Bertil Gardell (1976) was among the first to demonstrate that work environments that contribute to feelings of powerlessness and alienation are stressful for most workers. Marianne Frankenhaeuser (1986; Frankenhaeuser, Lundberg, and Chesney 1991) focused on the variables of **effort** and **distress**. She defined effort as active coping and a striving to gain and maintain control, and distress as feelings of dissatisfaction, boredom, and unpredictability. In her model of job stress, she shows that high effort creates a condition of elevated catecholamine's (epinephrine and norepinephrine) in the body, while high distress is related to elevated levels of cortisol. (Conversely, low effort and low distress are related to lower levels of catecholamines and cortisol, respectively.) High levels of both effort and distress represent the most stressful environment, one in which the worker attempts to overcome boring, routine, repetitive, or unpredictable constraints. Such environments give rise to extraordinary catecholamine and cortisol secretion, which contributes to cardiovascular disease (Karasek and Theorell 1992). Environmental conditions that engender feelings of loss of control, helplessness, and hopelessness are associated primarily with elevated levels of cortisol, depressive syndromes, and perhaps even tumor formation (Diberardinis 1998). Workers who are motivated and who see productive results enjoy a strong sense of personal control, accompanied by a sense of accomplishment and job commitment. Catecholamines increase moderately under these conditions, and cortisol seems to be suppressed.

Whereas Frankenhaeuser's research focused largely on psychophysiological dynamics of the workplace, Robert Karasek and his colleagues (Karasek et al. 1981; Karasek and Theorell 1992) advanced the study of occupational stress by focusing on the psychological dynamics of the workplace. Karasek's work yielded a model of occupational stress that analyzes job stress by two primary interacting variables: (1) the psychological demand of the job and (2) the degree of control (or decision latitude and flexibility) that the worker possesses with regard to the job function.

The combination of high job demands and low control over the job create an unhealthy, pathogenic environment. **Table 11.1** is an adaptation of Karasek's and Frankenhaeuser's models.

For some, it may be surprising that the condition that yields high job satisfaction is the high demand–high control condition. There are many workers who genuinely enjoy the challenge of their work; they simply wish to have some control over the working conditions. Since the advent of Karasek's model, repeated empirical investigations have not only demonstrated the validity of the model (Radmacher and Sheridan 1995) but have also consistently validated the pathogenic nature of a work environment characterized by high psychological demands and low decision latitude (see Karasek and Theorell 1992). Such work situations appear to put people at greater risk for heart disease, a risk similar to that of smokers or those with elevated serum cholesterol levels.

Table 11.1 Job Stress, Psychological Demands, and Control

| | | Control | |
		High	Low
Psychological Demands	**High**	High job satisfaction	Most pathogenic, high catecholamines, high cortisol
	Low	Least pathogenic	Second most pathogenic

Karasek's research underscores two critical concepts in the study of occupational stress: (1) beware of any job that gives you high levels of responsibility but provides you with low levels of authority, and (2) the essence of most jobs from a psychological health standpoint resides not in the actual job responsibilities, but in the worker's perceptions of the job.

Another situation that imbalances the control element is attachment. There is a fine line between being a passionate, committed employee and being overattached. Overattachment is, of course, a detrimental state as it inevitably leads to expecting too much. Dashed expectations lead to natural disappointment. Overexpectation from overattachment can lead to devastation. America is leading the rest of the world down the path of being obsessed with work. The disturbing trend is to expect work to fill the emptiness in our lives. To many people, work has become the core of their emotional and spiritual lives. There are many great people in our work environment, and it is easy to become friends and form attachments to people, but most big organizations are self-serving with no heart and little conscience. Understanding the limitations of workplace relationships and learning to set emotional boundaries can go a long way toward protecting you from emotional problems (Philipson 2002). Those with an extreme attachment and the intense desire to work are often called workaholics and are seen as negatively addicted like an alcoholic. And like the alcoholic, it is not the taste of alcohol that is craved but the effect of the depression. Workaholics can find great enjoyment in their productivity if they really love the work, but more often it's the side effect of depending too much on the work and work environment that they find addicting, and the imbalance in their lives is the usual stressful result (Johnson and Johnstone 2005).

Pain is inevitable in life and at work. The atmosphere in an organization can become toxic, and if unchecked it can contaminate the health of the organization and its employees. There are abusive managers, unrealistic policies, disruptive coworkers, poorly managed change, and, worst of all, unrealistic expectations. If you do not properly insulate yourself emotionally, this pain can diminish your self-worth and decrease your confidence (Frost 2003).

Occupational Stressors

Smith and his colleagues (Smith, Davy, and Everly 1995; Smith, Everly, and Johns 1992) have attempted to answer the question of just how important one's psychological perception of the workplace is in the process of stress and disease. The results of their investigations demonstrate that the primary work-related stressor is not a direct one; rather, the primary influence of job stressors on stress-related illness is through the psychological discord allowed to be caused by the stressor. Such psychological discord has been previously shown to be highly correlated with biological mechanisms of disease. Thus, it may be that stressors, like beauty, lie in the eye of the beholder.

Having made the case that the worker's perception of the workplace is an essential element in workplace-related stress and disease, there is still great value in understanding what workplace factors seem to be almost universally stressful or at least highly likely to be perceived as stressful. In this section of the chapter, we look at three main categories of job stressors:

1. organizational stressors

2. individual stressors

3. work environment stressors

Before we do, stop and complete Self-Assessment Exercise 11. The results will be discussed in the appropriate sections.

Self-Assessment EXERCISE XI

Choose the response that best answers the question, and place the corresponding letter in the space provided.

Questions 1–7: During the typical course of your job, how often do you . . .

_____ **1.** face important time deadlines that you have difficulty meeting?
   a. once a day or more
   b. more than once a week but less than once a day
   c. once a week
   d. less than once a week

_____ **2.** feel less competent than you think you should?
   a. once a day or more
   b. more than once a week but less than once a day
   c. once a week
   d. less than once a week

_____ **3.** wish your work were less complex?
   a. once a day or more
   b. more than once a week but less than once a day
   c. once a week
   d. less than once a week

_____ **4.** feel overwhelmed by your job?
   a. once a day or more
   b. more than once a week but less than once a day
   c. once a week
   d. less than once a week

_____ **5.** feel that you're in the wrong job?
   a. once a day or more
   b. more than once a week but less than once a day
   c. once a week
   d. less than once a week

_____ **6.** feel frustrated by "red tape"?
   a. once a day or more
   b. more than once a week but less than once a day
   c. once a week
   d. less than once a week

Self-Assessment CONTINUED

_____ **7.** perceive yourself as lost in the bureaucracy?
   a. once a day or more
   b. more than once a week but less than once a day
   c. once a week
   d. less than once a week

Questions 8–10: During the typical course of your job, do you . . .

_____ **8.** feel guilty for taking time off work?
   a. almost always true
   b. usually true
   c. seldom true
   d. never true

_____ **9.** have a tendency to rush into work that needs to be done before knowing the procedure you will use to complete the job?
   a. almost always true
   b. usually true
   c. seldom true
   d. never true

_____ **10.** whenever possible, attempt to complete two or more tasks at once?
   a. almost always true
   b. usually true
   c. seldom true
   d. never true

_____ Total Score

Calculate your total score as follows:

a = 4 points   c = 2 points
b = 3 points   d = 1 points

Write your total score in the space provided, and on the Personal Stressor Profile Summary Sheet located in Table Appendix 1 at the back of the book, and _then_ read the section _in this chapter pertaining to this Self-Assessment Exercise._

Organizational Stressors

Organizational variables greatly influence employee job satisfaction. Very few employees report high job satisfaction in high-stress situations. Organizational factors tend to center on financial rewards and opportunities for individual growth.

Lack of Financial Rewards   It has often been said that pay is important only on payday, when employees are reminded that they are more or less valued. Employees want to be recognized for a job well done. While there are many ways of validating performance and motivating employees, substantial financial rewards are a constant reminder that the work is valued and the employee is probably hard to replace. On days when immediate rewards are absent, a high salary may help to bolster self-esteem and reduce frustration. Low pay may increase stress in exactly the opposite way, fueling the negative self-image and self-talk that destroy concentration and deflate the energy often necessary to fight simple depression and anxiety. Employees who are highly satisfied with most other aspects of their work will often overlook low pay, but low pay and lack of job satisfaction represent a deadly duo that greatly contribute to stress. Some employers feel the double edge of salary in that higher pay does not always motivate, but low salary always makes the employee feel undervalued.

Motivation is a complex concept and pay is only one part of the equation. Different individuals are motivated by different things. For example, Maslow's hierarchy has been used in the motivation scheme by trying to match remunerations to where one is on the Maslow scale; however, this is complex. While theoretically plausible, the devil is in the details, and it is doubtful this could be operational on a large scale. The reality is that most people think money is a motivator and most employees feel that they are worth more than they are actually paid. There is a natural disparity between what people think they should be paid and what organizations spend in compensation. When the difference becomes too great and another opportunity occurs, turnover can result (Phillips and Connell 2003).

People think that money is a motivator and they are right, but it's not the whole picture. There are so many books and articles written on motivation schemes, for example, for sales staff. If it were only a matter of money, then it would be easier just to increase pay. Money does have an effect, but motivation involves far more; it comes from good financial and nonfinancial rewards. It is important the employees understand the salary system and their place in it. They must understand the nature of the other perks and related compensation, such as free time, travel, gifts, and education, to mention but a few.

Nonfinancial rewards can be very important for their long-term effect, and a savvy employee can use these for long-term career development as well. The stress of disatisfication can be lessened if one understands this part of the remuneration package. Stress relief is gained as job satisfaction increases and that can be aided by understanding a few compensation issues. The compensation scheme of an employer should be visible to all, and each employee should try to understand it. Be clear as to the extent of your compensation beyond salary, be honest with yourself about what you are worth, and more important, be honest with yourself about what else that you might be motivated by in addition to money. Many workers feel a need to be of service to their country, their community, and to others in general, and your work may be giving you an opportunity to feel good about yourself. If you feel you are worth more than you are getting, kick in your assertiveness training and seek more.

Lack of Career Guidance   Another potential source of stress from occupational frustration exists in the area of career development. The average college student will in the next five years make a series of life-changing decisions. Choosing a life partner, whether to have a family, where to live, and what occupation to pursue will direct his or her life for decades. It is scary to think about the thin foundation those monumental decisions often are based on. Career guidance is most often lacking in the schools and the decision stress, worry, and doubt is often intense. A consideration that is sometimes overlooked is what really motivates one and what kink of work will really augment overall life satisfaction.

Where that particular kind of profession will take you is another consideration. Are you willing to move to different states or countries? If you want to be in ski area management, you had better like snow and cold, or if in marine biology, you had better like water. Both these examples are probably in high-cost areas. Can you afford to live there? And will that position allow you enough money to live and pay off any college loans that you might have incurred. These days very few lower-, middle-, even upper-middle-class families can just write a check to cover the entire cost of their child's education and most individuals leave college with high debts that may take decades to pay off. As the Life Events Inventory discussed in Chapter 7 showed, debt is always considered a stressor. Will your chosen profession afford you the stress relief of allowing you to get out of debt and live at least modestly; and if you have a significant other, how do their job prospects, debt structure, and aspirations fit with yours?

Interesting to note, better career counseling is often more available in the workplace than at school. Valued employees with potential are often given the opportunity to retrain and will advance because of it. Especially in this technological, computer-driven age, advanced skill training is expected in many jobs. The following aspects of career development are considered important components of the working environment and are useful in contributing to job satisfaction and preventing occupational frustration:

- the opportunity to fully use occupational skills
- the opportunity to develop new, expanded skills
- counseling to facilitate career decisions

Thus, it is important for managers to realize that workers at all levels are demanding intrinsic rewards from their jobs more than ever before. Many large corporations and even branches of the federal government (NASA, for example) have instituted formal career counseling and career development programs. Such programs have taken on increased importance as companies enter the age of downsizing, sometimes called "right-sizing." Spawned by massive corporate mergers and efforts to decrease operating costs, many workers are being retired early or simply fired in order to achieve small, less costly workforces. For some, this situation is devastating; for others, it has an unexpected a silver lining. A lot depends on one's resiliency.

Overspecialization   In this era of highly specialized work, another source of occupational frustration is overspecialization. It has been accepted wisdom in industry that a high specialization—that is, having workers become experts in highly specific job areas—is a way of increasing the efficiency and quality of work. Conceptually, this is a sound procedure. However, because workers are searching for greater intrinsic rewards from their jobs, having them work in an overly fragmented or specialized job area may frustrate them. In our own consulting work with industry and business, we are impressed with the number of employees on all levels and in all professions who express a desire to "see the completed fruits of their labor." Workers do not want to perceive themselves as an insignificant cog in an immense wheel of industry; they want to identify with their companies and products. Far too often, overspecialization robs the worker of this reward. This problem is a serious one on the assembly line, and it may even reach into the professions. In a local hospital famous for its emergency shock-trauma department, we were surprised to find nurses expressing desires to follow patients through recovery rather than seeing them only in the emergency room and never knowing how their treatment progressed.

Work Overload   Job design and technology can contribute to occupational stress. Jobs without freedom produce more stress than autonomous and flexible ones. One of the most damaging situations involving a lack of freedom is excessive deadline pressure, resulting in overload.

Sometimes there is simply too much work to do, or the work is too difficult. When these conditions result in mistakes on the job or contribute to ill health, work overload exists. Overload affects the individual by overstimulating psychological and physiological mechanisms. In effect, overload is a condition in which the individual is bombarded with excessive job demands—excessive in that they cause excessive stress when the worker attempts to meet all the demands.

There are three types of overload: (1) quantitative, (2) qualitative, and (3) a combination of both. Quantitative overload exists when too much work has to be done in a limited time. The individual is capable of completing all of the work, but the time restriction causes the reaction. Qualitative overload exists when the work to be completed exceeds the individual's technical or intellectual capabilities at that time. This form of overload is encountered most often in research and development organizations as well as in many of the professions—health care, law, and so on. Finally, the combination of quantitative and qualitative overload is commonly encountered in administrative-management positions in all industries, in all levels of the sales industry, and in entrepreneurial endeavors.

The occupational conditions that seem to predispose one to overload are the following:

- time pressures, which may develop into quantitative overload
- job complexity, which may develop into qualitative overload
- decision making, which may evolve into a combination of both forms of overload

Time pressure can take two distinct forms: time spent working and time urgency.

Hours Worked.   Even though most CEOs do not recognize it or do want to recognize it, the fact is that everyone in the company is working longer hours. Almost everyone else in their organizations, including directors, indicate they and their subordinates are working significantly longer hours. Surveys (Cooper 2002) report that 45 percent of people always work more than their contracted hours, and a high percentage work evenings and weekends. Eighty-one percent of executives work more than forty-hour weeks, 32 percent over fifty, and 10 percent over sixty, and most report they also work frequently on the weekends. Most indicated that their employer expected them to put in these hours. The health impact of this trend toward a long-hours culture was also assessed. Seventy percent said this was damaging to their health, 70 percent said that it was damaging productivity, and 80 percent said their relationship with their partner and their children was adversely affected (Cooper 2000). Data continues to show this trend in that the average worker in the United States increased the hours worked each year during the last decade, and especially professionals and managers reported that they are asked to work longer hours each year. Seventy-five percent of those earning more than $100,000 a year reported that managing their time was a much bigger problem than managing their money. They used the term *constant time crunch* to describe the "too much to do and not enough time to do it" lives they lead (Milliken and Dunn-Jensen 2005).

Until recently, this has been largely an American phenomenon. American workers work on average 320 hours a year more than either their German or French counterparts. That is almost two months a year. On average, there has been a slow steady increase of nine hours per year in work over a twenty-year period. American productivity has increased in all but five of the last fifty years. Employees produce as much in twenty hours today as they did in forty hours, fifty years ago. One would think that this increased productivity would result in a great deal of leisure time. Not so! The trend is just the opposite. It is interesting and somewhat amusing that in the 1970s, the hot new area of study was leisure counseling. It became popular as Americans geared up to help people deal with the anticipated thirty-hour workweek and the inevitable boredom that would accompany it. Somewhere along the line, obviously, things changed—at least in the United States. Whether it was the fear of boredom or the cranking up of the advertising and public relations effort, the modern age of hyperconsumerism was born. An exciting array of goods and services became available with so much variety that shopping became the national pastime. Americans spend more time shopping than any other people in the world and certainly have been convinced that life is not worth living without these products. Workers worked harder and made a better living, which largely consisted of the accumulation of more goods, which fueled economic growth, and a vicious cycle developed. As with most addictions, tolerance and dependence increased the need for more. Ironically, with all that money being earned, Americans are in more debt now than ever before.

Time overload is a chicken-and-egg phenomenon. Companies demand it, employees need it to keep up, and we go round and round. In its wake lies less free time, less time to sleep and exercise, less time to give to the rearing of children, more stress, and paradoxically more debt.

Time Urgency.   Our society's race against the clock has been proven to be a major source of stress. Virtually every organization exerts some form of time pressure over its employees. It may be in the form of deadlines for work projects, deadlines for reports, sales deadlines, seasonal working limitations, or even unit production quotas (as in assembly line or other factory environments). Time urgency is the most obvious condition that fosters the development of quantitative overload because time limitations create restrictions on the quantity of work that can reasonably be completed. When the employee attempts to complete more work than is reasonable for the time restriction, a case of overarousal will arise—the heart will pump harder and faster as the individual attempts to work beyond his or her normal work rate. In addition, worry about what will happen if the work is not completed will cause the heart to work even harder. A vicious cycle has begun.

In some cases, deadlines will motivate a worker to achieve high levels of performance. However, when the time urgency causes mistakes or contributes to ill health, a condition of quantitative overload exists. At that point, time urgency becomes destructive.

An interesting paradox has developed since the Internet has become a part of daily life. The great time and productivity tool, e-mail, was supposed to save time and energy. Has it? Or has it become one of those "yes, but" tools that on the surface looks like it's saving effort but in reality is costing us more time and effort responding to the deluge of messages that are now so easy to crank out.

An international survey of managers reveals that the average manager deals with 190 messages daily and is interrupted once every ten minutes. The survey also suggests that more than 50 percent of American and 40 percent of British managers believe information overload is set to increase in future years. With this in view and the premise that overload leads to stress, we lose motivation and end up overwhelmed (Lewis 1999).

What gain has all this hurry produced?

Has technology delivered us from excess toil?

Among the impacts of excess time urgency are massive declines in morale, motivation, and perceived job security. Even the threat of impending quantitative overload has an adverse effect on workers. Many employees tend to demonstrate contempt and suspicion for management—they resent management telling them how to do more work in less time. In some instances, the results are work slowdowns and sabotage if time/work output analyses are implemented from an authoritarian point of view.

Time urgency appears to be a way of organizational life. However, in Chapter 7 we discussed ways in which individuals can reduce the harmful effects of time urgency on their minds and bodies while still meeting most organizational demands.

Job Complexity. Many people believe that life is growing more and more complex. The most common factor contributing to qualitative overload is job complexity, or the inherent difficulty of the work that must be done. The higher the complexity, the more stressful the job. The complexity of the work can easily evolve into qualitative overload if the complexity exceeds one's technical or intellectual capabilities at the time. Job complexity is usually increased by the following factors:

- increase in the amount of information to be used
- increase in the sophistication of the information or in skills needed for the job
- expansion or addition of job methods
- introduction of a contingency plan

Although these four strategies will increase the probability of a better product, when excessive they will also increase the individual's stress arousal level to where it actually inhibits his or her performance. Therefore, there is a point at which increasing the complexity of the job no longer proves productive but instead becomes destructive. At this point, the individual's abilities to reason and solve problems have been surpassed and mental fatigue and emotional and physical reactions ensue—all forms of the stress response. Medical research suggests that emotional and mental fatigue, headaches, and gastrointestinal disorders are common outcomes of chronic qualitative overload.

Decision Making Decision making pervades all aspects of life. Yet it has special applicability to the world of work. Decision making represents a unique combination of factors that may eventually lead to the development of simultaneous quantitative and qualitative overload (Smith 1998).

Decision making involves making a choice. Inherent in this process is evaluation—that is, determining the relative merits of one alternative versus another. The stressfulness of decision making is determined largely by the following factors:

- the importance of the decision's consequences
- the complexity of the decision
- the amount of available information
- the locus of responsibility for the decision
- the amount of time allotted for the decision-making process
- the expectation of success

The importance of the consequences of any decision greatly contributes to the stressfulness of decision making. You know, for example, that deciding what kind of car to buy is more stressful than deciding where to eat lunch. There is simply more at risk, more to be lost should your decision be a poor one. The key to successful handling of a complex decision is being able to ascertain what is meaningful and what is superfluous information, and being able to organize and synthesize that information.

Although too much information can make decision making stressful, insufficient information can lead to even greater stress. If you have ever lacked sufficient information to make a decision, you know how frustrating this can be. We have chosen to discuss this topic in terms of overload because of the way most people react to such a condition. If you are faced with insufficient information for making a decision, your first reaction is usually to guess or to extrapolate the needed information. In most cases, this guessing game results in a significant psychological strain as you attempt to foresee all of the possibilities. This strain is overload. Another factor that surely increases the stressfulness of decision making is the locus of responsibility—that is, who will be responsible for the decision? It is more stressful if one person alone has responsibility for a decision than if that responsibility can be shared. It is interesting to observe that many executives insist on single responsibility, for in many systems the individual will receive full recognition for a job well done. Such systems are also very quick to point out consistent incompetence. The fact remains, however, that single decision-making responsibility can be highly stressful and thus may stifle creativity in some individuals; upholding the status quo may be perceived as the safest decision.

Time is another factor in the stressfulness of decision making. With only a few exceptions, we can say that the shorter the amount of time allotted for decision making, the more stressful that decision process will be. One notable exception is the case in which far more time is allowed than is really required. Such conditions seem to breed worry and reconsideration; you might go back and change your mind, a habit that often leads to a less effective decision.

Finally, the expectation of success figures into the stressfulness of decision making. The self-fulfilling prophecy theory suggests that if the decision maker fully expects to make a correct decision, his or her stress level will be lower than if there is doubt (Farmer 1999). Typically, the probability of making a correct decision will be enhanced as well. However, if the decision maker fully expects to fail, his or her stress level may be low also. Such a negative self-fulfilling prophecy may be used to cope with the stress involved in decision making because there will be no disappointment when the individual does indeed fail—after all, it was expected. The only problem with this stress reduction strategy is that it greatly increases the probability of failure and loss of self-esteem. Therefore, it is a destructive coping mechanism.

The amount of stress involved in decision making may be expressed as follows:

$$\text{Decision-Making Stress} = \text{Importance} + \text{Complexity} \\ + \text{Lack of Information} + \text{Responsibility} \\ + \text{Lack of Time} + \text{Lack of Confidence}$$

The multifaceted nature of the decision-making process explains why decision making can result in quantitative and/or qualitative overload. How many of these factors adversely affect your day-to-day decision making?

Organizational policies—not to be confused with human interactions and politics, which will be covered later—contribute to the stressful climate of the workplace. Policies that are rigid and insensitive to employee needs increase employee stress levels and can create an atmosphere in which decision making, the job of most employees and all managers, is fraught with stress.

Individual Stressors in the Workplace

Individual stressors are perhaps the greatest contributors to occupational stress because they include human interaction, the greatest source of stress in general. Another stressor of special concern is occupational frustration, which in turn is influenced by such stressors as job ambiguity and role conflict, stifled communication, discrimination, bureaucracy, inactivity, and boredom.

Frustration   Have you ever thought that your job was holding you back? Have you ever considered yourself lost within the organization? Have you ever wished for more of a chance to use or develop your job skills? These are the types of thoughts that result from being frustrated on your job. Occupational stress from frustration exists when the job inhibits, stifles, or thwarts desired expectations and/or goals. The body reacts adversely to the frustration of psychological desires, resulting in what we know to be the stress response. If we understand occupational frustration as this sense of being inhibited, then several major sources of occupational frustration immediately come to mind.

Job Ambiguity and Role Conflict.   Two of the major contributors to frustration on the job are job ambiguity and role conflict. Job ambiguity refers to the condition in which the job description or the level of job performance is confusing or virtually unknown to the employee. In a case like this, you might find yourself asking questions such as "What should I do now?" or wondering "How did I do on the last assignment?" Job ambiguity may be caused by the following:

- unclear work objectives (goals)
- confusion surrounding responsibility
- unclear working procedures

- confusion about what others expect of you
- lack of feedback, or uncertainty surrounding your job performance

These phenomena result in what is termed the disengaged employee. Actively disengaged employees are physically present but psychologically absent; they are unhappy with their work situation and insist on sharing that unhappiness with their colleagues. Disengaged employees have a low level of commitment or achievement and can be disruptive in the workplace, while engaged employees have consistent levels of high performance and are more likely to stay with the company over time. A lack of clarity around what is expected of employees at work can bring on disengagement (Donaldson 2007).

Job ambiguity and role conflict consistently result in job dissatisfaction and significant stress levels. Role conflict exists when a job function contains roles, duties, or responsibilities that may conflict with one another. This is most commonly found among middle managers who find themselves caught between top-level management and lower-level management. Research has clearly demonstrated the middle-management position to be the most stressful of the three management levels. Role conflict may also be caused by work roles that conflict with personal, familial, or immediate societal values. Individuals in the law enforcement profession are those most frequently caught in this conflict. Once again, the result of such role conflict is job dissatisfaction and stress from frustration.

Stifled Communication   The term **organizational communication** refers to the patterns and networks along which communications flow through an organization. Stifled organizational communication has been found to be the single most prevalent source of frustration in organizations today. Do you find yourself feeling isolated in your job or relying on information that comes too late or not at all? Have you ever had a conversation with someone and walked away asking yourself what that person really said? These are common communication problems. Proper planning and organizing depend on effective communication. Ideally, communications flow upward from subordinates to superiors and horizontally from department to department, as well as in the traditional downward direction from superiors to subordinates. In many cases, organizations frustrate employees by keeping open only the downward channels. Typically, the last channel to be maintained is the upward channel. This is not only frustrating but also a gross waste of human resources. Efficient organizational communication is perceived as so important that organizational communication is becoming a field in itself. University graduate programs are offered in this area. Efficient communication can be a powerful source for stress reduction and increased performance on the job. Unfortunately, it is often overlooked or assumed to be working well.

Discrimination   Discrimination exists when non-work-related factors such as age, attractiveness, disability, race, and sex are used to determine such issues as who will receive promotions, increased job training, mentoring, or who is hired in the first place. Discrimination has long been known to be correlated with intense frustration and anger, and thus is a prime workplace stressor. Employees old and young enter the workplace carrying several individual and group identities. These differences in identities predispose the worker to a subconscious bias that becomes the bases for discrimination.

Individuals who are different form the decision maker, and his or her model of the world (e.g., racial minorities, females, disabled, unattractive, homosexual), experience many more discriminatory practices in the workplace that are unrelated to their actual or predicted job performance. On the surface, it seems like it would take a conscious effort to discriminate, however the opposite may be truer—it takes a conscious effort not to discriminate (Thomas 2005). Discrimination of any type is harmful to the organization and the individual worker because it leads to job dissatisfaction, anger, resentment, and a sense of hopelessness embodied in the "What's the use of trying to do a good job?" attitude (Stone-Romero 2005).

Bureaucracy   Another source of occupational frustration, and perhaps the most insidious source of this form of stress, is bureaucracy. Bureaucracy is a form of organizational planning. The man most responsible in the twentieth century for formalizing and advocating bureaucracy was Max Weber (1864–1920). Weber was concerned with designing an "ideal" organizational structure based on logic and rational thought. According to Weber, there are four major characteristics of a bureaucracy:

1. Specialization and division of labor
2. A set of rules governing all aspects of organizational behavior to ensure uniformity and organizational stability
3. Emotionless management; relationships within the organization should be typified by objectivity and a lack of enthusiasm, hatred, and so forth.
4. A hierarchy of positions; the entire organizational structure must follow the principle of centralized hierarchy—that is, offices built upon offices—so that there exists absolute control over subordinate functions. (Bureaucracy literally means "rule by office.")

It must be understood that Weber's design was intended to be an ideal one. No bureaucracy yet created has lived up to his expectations. The major reason for this failure is probably that the complexity of the human personality is simply not applicable to the bureaucratic structure. In theory, bureaucracy is the most logical and efficient organizational structure possible; in practice, it may be the most counterproductive form of organized work effort.

The most common criticisms of this form of management are the following:

- Frustration or thwarting of personal and professional development
- Fostering mediocrity on the job
- The reinforcement of complex rules (red tape)
- Stifled communication due in part to excessive paperwork (more red tape)
- Impersonality of supervisors and supervisory practices
- Arbitrary rules virtually written in stone
- Stifled creativity

Especially in this age of participation, most new, eager, creative workers find bureaucracies stressful places to work.

Inactivity and Boredom   Have you ever noticed that some people become nervous when they don't have enough to do? Have you ever gone looking for something to work on when you didn't really have to? Inactivity and boredom on the job can cause a stress response. It may manifest itself as nervousness, an inability to sit still, or a noticeable tenseness. Hans Selye categorizes this form of stress as **deprivational stress.**

If you suffer from depravation stress on the job, then your job is failing to provide you with meaningful psychological stimulation. Two occupational settings are noted for this form of stress: the assembly line and the large bureaucracy.

Perhaps the best place to begin to look at boredom is on the assembly line. Here the employee is asked to perform some highly repetitive task. After a relatively short orientation period, he or she will be able to perform the required task with minimal challenge. Before long the task will become boring, and stimulation of another kind will be sought—something to occupy the mind in a more meaningful manner. If such stimulation is found and does not distract from task performance, all will be fine. However, in some cases the thing that the employee chooses to occupy his or her mind with detracts from job performance; the worker makes more mistakes or works more slowly. In other cases, the employee may be unable to keep his or her mind occupied; job satisfaction then begins to decline.

The industrial literature from the last half century is full of examples of worker reactions to job boredom. Cases of low production efficiency, alcohol and drug abuse, and even assembly line sabotage have been recorded, not to mention employee turnover. The majority of cases seem to occur under the following conditions: (1) job boredom, (2) repetitive tasks on the job, (3) no opportunity for workers to communicate, and (4) low job satisfaction.

Boredom and inactivity may affect professional workers as well. In our own consulting work with large bureaucracies, we have observed the results of the boredom that overspecialization and job redundancy create. A common complaint from these workers in such organizations is that there is "not enough stimulating work to do." Many federal agencies appear to manifest this problem. To maintain sanity, people find ways of compensating for their low job satisfaction and stifled creativity. The most common compensation device we've seen is employees working at minimally acceptable levels of job performance during the week and then expressing themselves on the weekend through their avocational pursuits. This "living for the weekend" attitude is obviously debilitating to the organization.

Environmental Stressors

Environmental stressors range from the physical environment of the work station and the organization's location in the community to the location of the community itself. More often, the stress in this category is that of adapting to the environment and living with the changes that accompany most work situations. As Dilbert working in his cubical has made famous, unfavorable environments and changes result in more severe stress; however, even positive changes require adaptation and can be stressful. As with most stressors, the severity level of environmental stressors forms a continuum. The competitive environment, for example, might range from boring and nonexistent to cutthroat.

Change   Change within an organization is a necessary and vital component of growth and continued productivity, yet it can also be a source of stress for many employees. Change is stressful because it disrupts the psychological and physiological rhythms that accompany all human behavior. Whether the change is good or bad, it requires the expansion of psychological and physiological energies. Hans Selye summarizes this point by stating that the expenditure of adaptive energy is what makes change stressful. Change becomes harmful at the point at which adaptive energy is depleted.

There are numerous sources of **adaptive stress** (stress due to change) within the organizational world. To most people, technology is a very positive force in the working world; still, it requires role changes for those whom it affects. Such changes require adaptation. As mentioned earlier, sometimes it seems like work is an endless reeducation and more time is taken learning how to use new technology than working.

Another common source of adaptive stress is relocation, both vocational and residential. When you are forced to relocate, a great deal of stress generally follows. Even if the relocation is in conjunction with a raise and promotion, you will still have to cope with a new environment. The following factors intensify stress from relocation:

- the complexities of moving possessions from one location to another
- the severing of interpersonal relationships
- the formation of new interpersonal relationships
- the necessity of adjusting to new cultural and/or socioeconomic conditions

All of these factors are compounded if you must relocate your residence and work setting simultaneously.

For many individuals, change is exhilarating. Even so, change, whether good or bad, requires the expenditure of adaptive energy and can be stressful. So even positive changes should be carefully considered during periods of high stress unless of course the change removes you from the stressors.

Promotion.   The stressfulness of being promoted is considered by most to be a small price to pay for the rewards of the promotion. Take a moment to consider the impact of the following factors that generally accompany a promotion, in addition to the obvious rewards:

- significant changes in job function
- increased responsibility for people, production, and money
- changes in social role (some promotions come with certain social obligations that cause intense social and even financial stress)

These factors involve considerable adaptation for most individuals. Even if they are all positive, they take some getting used to.

Reorganization and Downsizing.   Departmental or organizational restructuring often happens when a new administration takes over. Such major reorganizations are occurring with greater frequency, and can be a major source of adaptive stress. Feelings of insecurity, anticipation, and apprehension usually dominate the minds of those affected by reorganization. If you are ever involved such reorganization, the first thing on your mind will probably be job security. Your next question will typically be, "How do I fit into this new arrangement?" During such uncertain periods, your work will probably fall off, or you may stress yourself through overload in an attempt to demonstrate your worth to the new management. In either case, it behooves you as well as the new management to quickly resolve questions of job security following reorganization.

A generation ago, a worker would typically work for one or two employers throughout his or her career. It is estimated that the average worker now will work for numerous employers throughout his or her working life. As workers progress through their working lives, change will likely be no longer an exception but the rule, the way of the new working world. One big change is the trend toward outsourcing employees, which makes more use of the part-time and contract worker. The outsourcing mentality has led to more part-time or short-term contracts, fewer full-time contracts, and the creation of a "flexible workforce." These combined elements have served to break the psychological contract between employers and employees (Cooper 2000). From the vantage point of the employee, the "flexible worker" is a "disposable worker" with no job security.

Some logical questions are being asked. Can organizations continue to demand commitment from employees they don't commit to? And what will this long-hours culture do to the two-earner family, which is now the majority family structure? The levels of job insecurity and dissatisfaction are high and growing. Developing and maintaining a "feel good" atmosphere at work is not just about bottom-line factors such as profitability. In a civilized society, it should be about quality-of-life issues as well, such hours of work, family time, manageable workloads, control over one's career, and some sense of job security (Cooper 2000).

Deterioration in job conditions can lead to an increase in anger and depression and a decrease in job satisfaction. Aiken et al. (2001), in their report of 43,000 nurses from more than 700 hospitals in five countries, provided an example. They state that, as a result of a shortage of hospital nurses, job dissatisfaction is at high levels in most of the countries surveyed. Inadequate nursing staffing and a decrease in the quality of services provided by the hospital were seen as a result of hospital downsizing. Nurses felt devalued and unable to deliver the high-quality care they were trained to provide. As has been mentioned several times in this chapter, perception of the quality of work experience impacted their job satisfaction (Greenglass et al. 2002).

The workers of this decade need to prepare themselves for the inevitability of occupational change and learn how to use it to their advantage. The first step in that process is learning to cope personally with adaptive stress.

Violence in the Workplace   Other than motor vehicle accidents, violence in the workplace is the leading cause of worker death and injury on the job. Workplace violence not only includes homicides of workers but also encompasses injuries sustained from battery, assaults, sexual assaults, verbal abuse, threats, and mental anguish caused from actual or threatened violence.

Preincident training, anger management programs, and stress reduction programs can be useful deterrents to workplace violence. Also, employee counseling programs, especially in response to downsizing, can be effective in reducing employee anger, frustration, and violence.

Biological Factors in the Workplace

Time Change.   If you must rotate work shifts, you don't need this book to tell you that this is stressful and requires significant adaptation. Even changes in time zones during travel are stressful. Two common occupational examples of how stress affects the body when the natural biological rhythms have been disturbed are jet lag and shift work fatigue.

Jet Lag.   Jet lag commonly affects transcontinental and transoceanic travelers. This problem can prove costly for those who must conduct high-level business affairs. Jet lag has also been found to be a major problem for pilots and airline crews who frequently make long flights (See Chapter 8).

Shift Work Fatigue.   Workers who must alternate shifts report many of the same symptoms found in jet lag. The most severe symptoms occur when changing to or from the 11 P.M.–7 A.M. shift. Some workers can adapt to the time change in about a week, others require three weeks, and some never properly adjust. It is important to note that the increased stress associated with shift work is not directly related to the shift work per se but to one's efforts to adjust to an unnatural pattern of sleeping (Moore-Ede 1999).

Workers who are subjected to shift work over long periods of time appear to have a higher risk for cardiovascular disease, neurotic disorders, and dysfunctional alterations in appetite, diarrhea, constipation, and possibly depression (see Chapter 8).

Noise.   Chapter 8 contains a more in-depth discussion on noise in general. As it specifically relates to work, noise is an ever-present stressor both as a psychological irritant and as a pure stimulant causing physical damage.

The physical characteristics of noise (intensity and frequency) are the points most often mentioned in discussions of noise as a stressor. Sound levels above 35 to 40 decibels will typically awaken a sleeping person, and sound levels in excess of 55 decibels are sufficient to make normal conversation difficult. Of greater biological significance are noise levels in excess of 65 to 70 decibels. Evidence suggests that at this level there is increased sympathetic-nervous-system arousal characteristic of a stress response. The major component of this response is increased adrenal functions. As decibel levels increase, the body reacts with greater cardiovascular responses characteristic of stress (Schaefer 1998). Reactions such as increased heart rate or increased blood pressure become evident.

As chronic noise levels approach 85 decibels, the potential for permanent hearing loss increases significantly. Perhaps the most insidious aspect of this process is that chronic noise exposure is typically selective in its attack on auditory acuity. The usual case of hearing loss occurs only on specific frequency levels, depending on the amount of the exposure. Therefore, it may be very difficult for a worker to notice a hearing loss until it becomes severe.

The federal government has mandated that workers exposed to an average eight-hour total of 90 decibels must wear protective ear equipment. In addition to the harmful effects caused by the intensity of noise, frequency can also be a factor. Frequencies in excess of 20,000 cycles per second are most often implicated in the harmful effects of noise. However, it has been shown that frequencies in the 15-to-20-cycles-per-second range appear especially stressful because of their extremely low vibration levels. Such levels appear to harm the internal organs of many humans. In some cases, frequencies between these levels may actually reduce the stressful effects of noise.

Computers and Carpal Tunnel Syndrome.   Carpal tunnel syndrome (CTS) appears to be another computer-related condition, and it may occur in any occupation where forceful and repetitive hand and finger movements are necessary. Before the pneumatic nail gun revolutionized the building industry, many "nail-pounders" nursed this condition. CTS occur when the median nerve is compressed in the carpal tunnel between the transverse carpal ligament and the bones of the wrist and hand. In addition to nerve compression, many people with CTS also have associated problems such as tendonitis, arthralgia (joint pain), and muscle strain. When there is a strong suspicion that activity at work is a contributing factor to CTS, a work site analysis should be done. Its purpose is to identify and minimize contributing risk factors such as positioning and repetitive activity.

Physical Posture.   Cramped muscles and inactivity plague anyone who is deskbound for a period of time, especially at the computer. Muscle tension in the head, neck, and shoulders is the most prevalent example of what can happen from laboring over the computer or piles of paper every day. Leg cramps and even some lower-back problems can result from chronic sitting. Computer workers know all too well the aching forearms, wrists, and fingers that can result from hours of typing at a keyboard. Neck problems, carpal tunnel syndrome, and eye strain are now the leading occupational conditions caused, of course, by logging excessive time on the computer. In addition to these specific problems are the effects of sedentary work on the cardiovascular system. Exercise is a necessity for a healthy mind and body; thus, many office workers participate in some kind of exercise regimen. A good relief for the upper back is to lie on the floor for about 10 minutes with a rolled-up towel between the shoulder blades. This gives the muscles that have been tightened by rolling the shoulder in and hunching forward over the computer a chance to stretch out and relax.

Compassion Fatigue: The Stress of Caring Too Much   We are told that it is important to care about our jobs, to care about our "customers." But can we care too much? Earlier in this volume, we discussed the notion of "burnout" and described its three stages. Burnout is sometimes seen as a result of stress on the job. Charles Figley (1995) has described a special form of burnout that he refers to as "compassion fatigue." Compassion fatigue may be thought of as the stress of helping individuals during or after traumatic, or otherwise serious, life events. Examples could be working with people who experience a terminal diagnosis, a disfiguring injury, sexual assault, a near-death traumatic accident, a mass disaster, or other traumatic incidents.

Compassion fatigue may be thought of as a beleaguering degree of sympathy for others who have experienced extreme suffering. Therapists, nurses, physicians, emergency response workers, and hospice workers are prime candidates for compassion fatigue. Symptoms may arise in two seemingly opposite forms: (1) symptoms of overidentification and enmeshment with the primary "victims," or (2) symptoms of anger, resentment, and even disgust directed toward the primary victims. An example of the first type would be the paramedic who felt so sorry for the victims of an automobile accident (an eighteen-year-old unmarried mother and her nine-month-old boy) that she took them both home with her and allowed them to live with her for three years. An example of the second type of compassion fatigue would be the emergency room physician who became extremely angry at the suicide victim who died while the physician was trying to save his life.

It is clear that compassion fatigue is a very real occupational hazard for some unique professions, namely the helping professions. Although contrary to the professional images conveyed by firefighters and law enforcement officers, they too may be victims of compassion fatigue.

Recent advances in occupational psychology have led to the development of training programs designed to "immunize" professionals who may be prone to compassion fatigue (Flannery 1999; Sheehan 1999).

SUMMARY

In this chapter, we have reviewed core concepts related to the understanding of occupational stress and occupational stressors. The integrative work of a number of researchers points us to this important conclusion: the worker's perception of the work environment and job itself plays a critical deterministic role in the creation of excessive occupational stress. The majority of occupational stressors reviewed in this chapter do not exert a direct stress-to-disease link. Rather, these stressors create a condition of psychological discord, which then leads to stress-related illness. Consider these following points:

- Adverse health consequences in the workplace may be mitigated by (1) creating a more healthy workplace and (2) reducing psychological discord by implementing personal stress management programs.

- Job functions should be designed to provide the worker with a sufficient amount of control so as to mitigate overload and frustration. Authority must follow responsibility.

- The work environment should provide sufficient social support for workers, including adequate leadership. Cohesive work teams and participative management should be encouraged to further workers' involvement.

- Workers should receive adequate clarification of work-related roles and policies.

- Schedules should be flexible.

- It is important to recognize that not all stress can be eliminated from work. Work is a place where people interact, and some stress is inherent in human interactions. Work is also very often done in an impersonal and hurried environment with little social support, because the purpose of work is productivity.

- Reduction of debilitating stress is the primary objective of occupational stress management. A secondary focus is aligning personality, skill level, and task to decrease stress and increase productivity.

- Turnover or functional transfers can reduce organizational strain caused by mismatches of skill and task.

- A more efficient approach to reducing organizational stress is to find and reduce the stress situations before inefficiency, decreased productivity, and ill health occur.

- If stress management programs are effective, we may soon see corporate savings sufficient enough to be passed on to consumers, thereby creating a lever to be used in the marketplace by competition-minded corporations.

SOURCES CITED

Aiken, L. H., Clarke, S. P., Sloane, D.M., Sochalski, J. A., Busse, R., Clarke, H., et al. (2001, May/June). Nurses' report on hospital care in five countries. *Nurses Reports, Health Affairs,* 20, 43–53.

Burnbach, J. (1998). *Job discrimination: How to fight and win.* Ojai, CA: Voir Dire Press.

Phillips, J. J., and Connell, A. O. (2003). *Managing employee retention.* Alexandria VA: Society for Human Resourses Press.

Cooper, G. (2000). The psychological implications of the Americanization of work in the UK. *Stress News,* April, 12 (2).

Diberardinis, Louis, ed. (1998). *Handbook of occupational safety and health.* New York: John Wiley and Sons.

Donaldson, C., 2007 Actively disengaged. *Human Resources 2007,* April 11, 2007

Dobbs, Lou., (2006) War on the middle class. New York: Viking, 13–18.

Farmer, R. E. A. (1999). *Macroeconomics of self-fulfilling prophecies.* Cambridge: MIT Press.

Figley, C. R. (1995). Compassion fatigue. In *Secondary traumatic stress,* ed. B. Hudnall Stamm. Lutherville, MD: Sidran, 3–28.

Frankenhaeuser, M. (1986). A psychobiological framework for research on human stress and coping. In *Dynamics of stress,* eds. M. Appley and R. Trumbell. New York: Plenum, 101–16.

Frankenhaeuser, M., Lundberg, U., and Chesney, M., eds. (1991). *Women, work, and health.* New York: Plenum.

Frost, P. J. (2003). *Emotions at work.* Cambridge, MA: Harvard Business School Press.

Gardell, B. (1976). Reactions at work and their influence on non-work activities. *Human Relations,* 29, 885–904.

Greenglass, E. R., Burke, R. J., and Fiksenbaum, L. (2002). Impact of restructuring, insecurity and job satisfaction in hospital nurses. *Stress News,* 14 (1).

Johnson L.U., and Johnstone, A. (2005). The relationship between organizational climate, occupational type and workaholism. *New Zealand Journal of Psychology,* 34, no. 3, 181+.

Karasek, R., Baker, D., Marxer, F., Ahlbom, A., and Theorell, T. (1981). Job decision, job demands, and cardiovascular disease. *American Journal of Public Health,* 71, 694–705.

Karasek, R., and Theorell, T. (1992). *Healthy work.* New York: Basic Books.

Karoly L. A., and Constantijn W. A. (2004). *The 21st century at work: Forces shaping the future workforce and workplace in the United States.* Santa Monica, CA: Rand, 127.

Lewis, D. (1999). *Information overload: Practical strategies for surviving in today's workplace.* London: Penguin Books.

Milliken, F. J., and Dunn-Jensen, L. M. (2005). The changing time demands of managerial and professional work: Implications for managing the work-life boundary. *In Work and life integration: Organizational, cultural, and individual perspectives,* eds. E. E. Kossek and S. J. Lambert. Mahwah, NJ: Lawrence Erlbaum Associates, 43.

Moore-Ede, M. (1999). *The twenty-four hour society: Understanding human limits in a world that never stops.* Cambridge: Circadian Technologies.

Philipson, I. (2002). *Married to the job.* New York: Free Press.

Radmacher, S. A., and Sheridan, C. L. (1995). An investigation of the demand-control model of job strain. In *Organizational risk factors for job stress,* eds. S. Sauter and L. Murphy. Washington, DC: American Psychological Association, 127–38.

Sheehan, D. C. (1999). Stress management in the FBI. *International Journal of Emergency Mental Health,* 1, 39–42.

Smith, C. L. (1998). *Computer-supported decision making: Meeting the decision demands of modern organizations.* Norwood, NJ: Ablex.

Smith, K. J., Davy, J., and Everly, G. S. (1995). An examination of the antecedents of job dissatisfaction and turnover intentions among CPAs in public accounting. *Accounting Inquiries,* 5, 99–142.

Smith, K. J., Everly, G. S., and Johns, T. (1992). *A structural modeling analysis of the mediating role of cognitive-affective arousal in the relationship between stressors and illness among accountants.* Paper presented to the 2nd APA/NIOSH Conference on Occupational Stress, December, Washington, DC.

Stone-Romero, E. F. (2005). Personality-based stigmas and unfair discrimination in work organizations. In *Discrimination at work: The psychological and organizational bases,* ed. R. L. Dipboye. Mahwah, NJ: Lawrence Erlbaum Associates, 255.

Terkel, S. (1990). *Working.* New York: Ballantine Publishing.

Thomas, K. M. (2005). Group-level explanations of workplace discrimination. In *Discrimination at work: The psychological and organizational bases,* ed. R. L. Dipboye. Mahwah, NJ: Lawrence Erlbaum Associates, 63.

U.S. Department of Labor. (1995). *Labor statistics report.* Washington, DC: U.S. Government Printing Office.

Westfall-Lake, M., and McBride, G. (1997). *Shiftwork safety and performance.* New York: Lewis Publishers.

Right Livelihood

According to Deepak Chopra, "What's in it for me?" is the internal dialogue of the ego, whereas asking, "How can I help?" is the internal dialogue of the spirit. A primary factor in choosing right work is doing something that you feel serves humanity. Other important considerations are finding your unique talents, matching those talents to the needs of others, and finding work that serves to develop your higher spiritual self (an important reason that we are on this trip in the first place).

EXERCISE

If you had plenty of money, would you work?

If so, at what?

If not work, then how would spend your time?

What is it about this work or activity that attracts you?

What are your unique talents? Look back at the trail you have left behind (e.g., education, hobbies, volunteer work, and what you loved to do as a child). Describe these talents:

List and describe your best work or school experiences. List at least three of them:

What are the common elements in these experiences?

Could these elements be incorporated into a future job or profession? Which one(s)?

How would this be of service to humanity?

 Looking at your talents and experience, what do you feel would be your "right livelihood"? How might these insights be related to stress management?

 Write a positive word or short phrase about "right livelihood" that will be useful to you in future situations.

CHAPTER 12

Breathing and Relaxation

Breathing and Stress Management

Up to this point in the book, the stress management techniques presented have been about, as we described in Chapter 1, quieting the external environment to reduce stimulation of the individual intended to produce the following effects:

- a cognitive awareness of life events and lifestyle
- a cognitive restructuring of the environment, one's emotional responses, one's thought patterns, and one's behavior designed to change how you think and interact with the people and events in your life

The remainder of the book will focus on relaxation techniques, which are mind-body techniques designed to quiet the internal environment in order to reduce sensory stimulation of the central nervous system and intended to produce the following effects:

- decreased stimulation
- a calming or relaxation response
- reduced mind chatter; fewer arousing memories and anticipations
- increase thoughts that produce peace and tranquility
- increase philosophical awareness

In addition, physical exercise utilizes the stress by-products to:

- decrease arousal
- promote a sense of well-being and a feeling of imperturbability

The relaxation techniques presented here are but a sampling of the thousands that are available. The variety is an attempt to offer a selection wide enough that each reader will be able to find a few that seem to be effective. While they are fun to learn and our stress management toolbox should contain several, the goal is to find a best fit. Besides variety, they all have depth, which means you can benefit from being a beginner or a master. One might view depth as a continuum of the five components of relaxation as seen in **Figure 12.1**.

Without too much effort, all of these activities will give you a sense of *relaxation* and, by using them when you fell stressed, you will be able to physically feel the difference. After a little more practice, a sense of quiet is felt—especially a *quieting* of the endless so-called "chatter" of the mind. In that quiet, one frequently becomes aware of thoughts and physical sensations, often referred to as receiving messages from the subconscious mind and body. Making the connection from physical sensations to feelings, emotions, thoughts, and behavior patterns in light of our history (the past) and dreams (the future) often can produce *insights* into our chosen lifestyle, our illnesses, and our happiness or lack thereof. *Enlightenment* has many deep philosophical interpretations and meanings. Used here it represents the mindful choice of thoughts and behaviors toward the fulfillment of one's dreams and purpose in such a way that is noncontradictory. Put simply, it is behavior in pursuit of goals that do not cause harm, by things such as long-term distress, illness, and disease.

These representative techniques are effective because they are natural to the body and are tried and true, being as old as time. I would imagine that prehistoric humans stretched out their tight muscles and quieted themselves with mind centering breaths. We know that early humans during the axial age occasionally sat quietly in contemplatation

Figure 12.1 The Relaxation Depth Continuum

and meditation, examining the origin, validity, and usefulness of the voices they heard in their heads in ways that are thought to be the beginnings of consciousness and spirituality (Armstrong 2001).

Later these activities were organized into various disciplines and the ancient practice of yoga developed. As humans have always done, some found different and "better" ways of performing and using the techniques and so split off from their teachers. New disciplines were born, and today there are many ways of doing the basic relaxation techniques. Again, some are thousands of years old whereas others are relatively new, such as neuromuscular relaxation created in the early 1900s and biofeedback perfected in the late 1970s. Each represents a slight refinement of the basics to reach a specific audience or to deal with a specific symptom or just to make it simpler.

Breathing is a great example. As taught here, it is a simple, easy, and effective relaxation tool. To the accomplished Yoga master, Pranayama breathing can be a life-long and life-changing pursuit.

Breathing Correctly

Breathing is the most natural thing we do, but over time we often unlearn the natural breathing process and replace it with a less efficient form of breathing. Breathing is a natural and automatic body function, which suggests that we have no control over it. However, any body process can be altered and, if the practice is prolonged, conditioned. For reasons too numerous and involved to discuss here, most of us have developed and conditioned inefficient and improper breathing techniques. And what could be more important than bringing in fresh air and revitalizing the body tissues? Ancient yoga philosophy states that the mind is the master of the senses, breath is the master of the mind, and breathing is the elixir of life.

Actually, the exchange of air is only one aspect of breathing that is important to the relaxation process. Breathing is an involuntary, automatic function that reflects our general state of stress arousal. But breathing is also voluntary and can be manipulated. If we so desire, we can breathe fast or slow; our inhalations can be deep or shallow; our expirations can be partial or complete; and in some cases, we can even "choose" difficult or pathological breathing patterns. By learning to breathe correctly, air is taken in more efficiently, the pulmonary system is strengthened and conditioned, the function of the cardiovascular system is enhanced, greater oxygenation is promoted, the nerves are calmed, and restfulness occurs. The breathing centers in the brain have a facilitating relationship with the arousal centers; therefore, constant, steady, restful breathing promotes relaxation. It is almost impossible to be tense and have slow, relaxed, deep breaths. Thus, control breathing and you control tension. Condition breathing and you condition your system to be more tranquil. The power of deep, steady breathing is instinctual. When you want to control your energy—when lifting a heavy object, for example—you instinctively hold your breath. When you want to center yourself—when pulling the string of a bow or the trigger of a gun, for instance—you instinctively breathe deeply and hold. It is the most natural for you to center yourself or to concentrate. Breath control is essential for control of the mind (Iyengar 1995).

Breathing is used in almost every relaxation technique that has stood the test of time and been evaluated as effective. Scientists have mapped the location of the neuropeptides associated with the relaxation response, and they can be found in the floor of the fourth ventricle, which is where breathing is controlled. Peptides are released into the ventricular fluid and affect how fast the breaths are, how shallow, and how deep. Breathing goes on automatically, but you can instantly take control of it without any training. You can make your will change your breathing, your peptides, and your emotional state (Pert 1995).

Most of our shifts in attention at the body level are subconscious. Although neuropeptides are actually directing our attention by their activities, we are not consciously involved in deciding what gets processed, remembered, and learned. But we do have the possibility of bringing some of these decisions into consciousness, particularly with the help of various types of intentional training techniques such as insight meditation (described in Chapter 16). In some instances, the unconscious can be harnessed for healing or change without the conscious mind being involved. Hypnosis, breathing, and many of the energy-based therapies utilizing body work, massage, and therapeutic touch are all examples of techniques that you can use to effect change at a level beneath consciousness (Pert 1999).

Breathing is often labored and inefficient, and everyone can benefit from proper breathing techniques. At rest, we normally use only one-third of our lung capacity. Through breathing exercises, you will be able to vitalize these functions, regulate breathing patterns, build up respiratory reserve, and increase oxygenation capacity. If you are a singer, you already know the vital part that proper breathing technique plays and how much time is spent improving breath control. Good public speakers also quickly learn that not only does deep breathing slow you down and relax you during that inevitable rush of the jitters, but it also helps in word timing, emphasis, and enunciation.

Practicing breathing techniques not only facilitates relaxation; it also plays a vital role in the prevention of respiratory ailments. Individuals with respiratory disorders such as asthma and emphysema can benefit not only from increased oxygenation but also from learning correct, efficient, and less-stressful breathing patterns.

The biggest breathing muscle in the human body is the diaphragm, the lowering of which can take place only when the jaw and the throat are relaxed, the belly is free, and the hip joints allow free leg movement and flexibility in the lower back. When these conditions are not met, the body compensates by lifting the shoulders, pulling up the chest bone, and contracting the sphincter muscles in the throat, movements that weaken the muscles that assist the breathing process (Buchholz 1994).

In correct breathing, the floating ribs (lower five pairs) are moved by the intercostal muscles between the ribs and the diaphragm as it descends toward the abdomen. This movement allows for expansion of the lower lobes of the lungs, creating a vacuum, and the air rushes in. If you keep the abdominal muscles tight during the breathing movement, your diaphragm cannot descend and the lower lobes cannot fill, so a deep breath is possible only by a hyperexpansion of the top lobes, a method that expends much more energy. Many people have developed the habit of shallow breathing because it is thought to represent better posture—stomach in, chest out. This is not to say that one should not have strong, taut stomach muscles; on the contrary, contraction-relaxation movements will further strengthen stomach muscles without a chronic shortening developing. It is also important not to neglect exhalation. You must exhale deeply to get the stale, used air out or there is less room for fresh air to enter. Generally, exhalation lasts longer than inhalation. Correct breathing, once mastered, becomes a chronic exercise that expands and contracts the lung tissue, building strength and endurance.

Learning more efficient breathing patterns can be facilitated by the ability to perform and differentiate between the following exercises.

Upper Costal Breathing

Use your hands to sense the action of the respiratory movements. Place your hands on the upper third of the chest wall, preferably crossing the hands with the fingertips resting comfortably over the collarbones. You can easily sense the expansion of the upper lobes of the lungs with your fingertips in the open space between the collarbone and the trapeziums muscle, which runs behind that bone. Keeping your abdominal wall relaxed, inhale through your nose, expanding the upper ends of your lungs as fully as possible. Hold your breath for three seconds, then let go, exhaling slowly, letting the air gently flow from the mouth. Repeat the exercise five times, resting for five normal breaths between each one. The pause in between is important because you want to avoid hyperventilation and allow yourself time to center your thoughts on the activity and reflect on what you sensed or felt.

Middle Costal Breathing

Again, let your fingers be your sensors. Place your fingers on the middle third of the chest wall below the nipples (sixth rib). Keeping your abdominal and upper costal area relaxed, inhale through your nose, expanding the mid chest region as fully as possible. Hold for three seconds and gently exhale through the mouth. Repeat this five times and then relax quietly. Remember to pause between each repetition.

Diaphragmatic Breathing

Breathing with the diaphragm is performed by taking a deep inhalation while the belly is pushed down and out by the movement of the diaphragm, thus allowing the lower lobes of the lungs to inflate fully. Your hands are placed on the lower ribs, where they should easily sense the breathing motion. With the upper chest relaxed, inhale deeply. The abdominal wall is pushed up and out. Hold for three seconds and exhale, feeling the abdominal wall descend toward the spine. Repeat this exercise five times. Diaphragmatic breathing stretches the lower lobes of the lungs, allowing more fresh air to enter. It also acts to correct shallow breathing habits, allowing increasing depth of inhalation.

Very Deep Breathing

Start by exhaling every bit of air from your lungs. Force the air out and feel the space between your belly and spine shrink. When all the air is out, inhale slowly, using the diaphragmatic technique. Picture your lungs as a glass being filled with water—bottom, middle, then top. Hold your breath for three seconds and then exhale gently through your nose or mouth. This may sound like an exaggerated, strenuous action, but it is not. Breathe from your diaphragm naturally and effortlessly. Concentrate on the air traveling through the air passageways. With each exhalation, feel yourself relaxing and letting go. Begin to feel the looseness in your body, an uncoiling feeling as you settle down and pull your mind and body together. Repeat this exercise five times, resting between each repetition.

Now that you know how to breathe correctly, go on to the following breathing exercises. You may want to periodically repeat these learning-to-breathe exercises until you feel that you have fully mastered them. Once you do, start with the following exercises on breathing.

Breathing Exercises

Now that you understand the nature of proper breathing and have spent a few minutes practicing, use the technique in some practical exercises that are designed to use breathing as a focus point to enable achieving deeper relaxation.

Complete Breath

During the course of an average day, many of us find ourselves in anxiety-producing situations. Our heart rates increase, our stomachs may become upset, and our thoughts may race uncontrollably. In such moments, we tend to make poor decisions or overreact. During such episodes, we require fast-acting relief from our stressful reactions so that we can attempt to calmly solve the crisis or problem at hand. The following exercise has been found effective for quickly calming one down in stressful situations.

The basic mechanism for stress reduction in this exercise involves deep breathing. The procedure is as follows:

Step 1: Assume a comfortable position. Rest your left hand (palm down) on top of your abdomen. More specifically, place your left hand over your navel. Now place your right hand so that it comfortably rests on your left. Your eyes should remain open (see **Figure 12.2**).

Step 2: Imagine a hollow bottle or pouch lying internally beneath the point at which your hands are resting. Begin to inhale. As you inhale, imagine that the air is entering through your nose and descending to fill that internal pouch. Your hands will rise as you fill the pouch with air. As you continue to inhale, imagine the pouch being filled to the top. Your rib cage and upper chest will continue the wavelike rise that began at your navel. The total length of your inhalation should be three seconds for the first week or so, then lengthening to four or five seconds as you progress in skill development. Remember to concentrate on "seeing" the air move as you inhale and exhale.

Step 3: Hold your breath. Keep the air inside the pouch. Repeat to yourself, "My body is calm."

Figure 12.2 Complete Breath

Step 4: Slowly begin to exhale—to empty the pouch. As you do, repeat the phrase, "My body is quiet." As you exhale, you will feel your raised abdomen and chest recede. Repeat this exercise four or five times in succession. Should you begin to feel lightheaded, stop at that point. If lightheadedness remains a problem, consider shortening the length of the inhalation and/or decreasing the total number of repetitions of the four-step exercise.

Practice this exercise five to ten times a day. Make it a ritual in the morning, afternoon, and evening as well as during stressful situations. After a week or two of practice, omit Step 1. This was only for teaching the technique. Because this form of relaxation is a skill, it is important to practice at least five to ten times a day. At first you may not notice any immediate relaxation. However, after a week or two of regular practice, you will increase your ability to relax on the spot. Remember: You must practice regularly if you are to master this skill. Regular, consistent practice of these daily exercises will lead to a calmer and more relaxed attitude—a sort of antistress attitude—and when you do have stressful moments, they will be far less severe.

Controlled Tempo Breathing

This exercise develops powers of concentration, facilitates centering, and helps breath control. You may sit or lie down. Keep your eyes closed. The breathing will be diaphragmatic—quiet, natural, and effortless. Concentrate on your breathing. Become part of it. With one hand, find your pulse in the wrist of the other arm. Count your pulse for one minute. While still counting your pulse, bring part of your attention back to your breathing. Count the number of pulses during normal exhalation. Do this several times until you have a rhythm. The average will be somewhere between five and ten. As an example, say the number is five. Still monitoring your pulse, breathe in with five beats of your pulse, hold for five, exhale for five, and remain quiet for five. Continue this for three minutes; then sit quietly and prepare for the Breath Counting Exercise. At first you may tend to lose count, but as your powers of concentration increase, you will make it all the way. You can then increase the time spent doing this exercise.

Breath Counting

This is another exercise to promote relaxation and increase powers of concentration. You may do this sitting or lying down. As in the Controlled Tempo Breathing Exercise, you will use quiet, normal, diaphragmatic breathing. Concentrate on your breathing. As you breathe in, think "in." Let the air out and think "out." Think ". . . in . . . out . . . in . . . out." Now each time you breathe out, count the breaths. Count ten consecutive breaths without missing a count. If you happen to miss one, start over. When you get to ten, start at one again. Do this ten times, and then sit quietly. Concentrate, anticipate the breath, and block all other thoughts from your mind.

Controlling breathing is the simplest and most basic activity in the stress management arsenal because breathing is the simplest and most basic physiological, life-sustaining activity.

Advanced Techniques

In one sense, the practice of breathing is short and simple, but yoga masters have spent lifetimes perfecting the subtle techniques of increasing awareness, generating energy, and reaching deep meditative states using advanced breathing techniques.

Pranayama—The Awareness of Breath

Keep the mind alert.

Focus attention on the breath.

Feel the breath enter and leave the body.

Hear the breath enter and leave the body.

Exhale the chaotic stressful energy.

Inhale peaceful centering energy.

The yoga believes that when we follow the breath we achieve quietness. Our mind does not change with each breath; it is a long-term process that follows the conditioning of the brain and body when we allow positive energy to take over our thoughts. It is not only the exchange of stale air from our body for fresh air, it the exchange of negative, chaotic energy for positive, calming energy. Breathing out is the mechanism for creating mental clarity. How does one know it is happening? We believe it to be so, we feel it, and we see it change our behavior.

The yoga has taught this for 5,000 years; the physiologist has verified that a negative state of mind negatively impacts our breathing and that proper breathing can quiet the mind. What happens in that quiet, the yoga teaches, is an exchange of energy, a harnessing of power, a balance of the body directing in to the chakra system.

Chakra Breathing

Chakra breathing not only promotes general relaxation, it gets one in touch with the subtle flow of energy through the body. While being more advanced than the simple techniques you have already mastered, it is not at all difficult. Try it.

According to yoga theory, there are a number of energy centers in the spine, and these centers (chakras) correspond with endocrine glands. The first chakra (see **Figure 12.3**) is at the base of the spine, the coccyx, and has the connotation of security. Moving up the spine to the level of the ovaries is the second chakra, which denotes sensuality and sexuality. The third chakra is at the "hara" or power center at the center of the body near the naval. Next is the heart chakra, denoting love. The fifth chakra is at the throat, denoting expression. The sixth chakra is at the "third eye" or the middle of the forehead and has the connotation of intuitive, intellectual, and psychic powers. The highest chakra, at the anterior fontanel on the top of the head (a baby's "soft spot"), is the spiritual chakra.

The concentrative practice using the chakras is to focus on each of the chakras, beginning at the coccyx, as you breathe through them. Imagine that you are pulling in energy

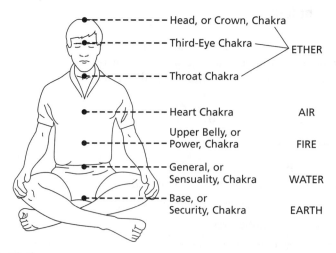

Figure 12.3 Chakras

Writing Exercise

After experiencing this exercise, write about it.

1. Did you locate the energy centers inside you?

2. Did you experience movement?

3. What other insights did you have?

through the first chakra, activating that energy center. You may imagine that it is a wheel that you spin, a glass ball that you are clearing, or any other imagery that helps you feel the energy of that center clearing. Take as many breaths at that level as needed.

Then breathe through the first chakra, taking the energy up to the second chakra, clearing it out. Again, take as many breaths as you need to clear it. As you breathe out, let the energy flow out the first chakra, as though you were continually clearing the pathway up and down the spine between the two chakras. Follow this procedure up the spine to the third, fourth, fifth, sixth, and finally the seventh chakras. Concentrate on the clearing process as you breathe energy in and out of each center.

When completing this process, go into a ten-minute neutral period of meditation. Let thoughts come in and out; touch them and let them go.

Aromatherapy

Aromatherapy is one of those rare forms of treatment that can improve your quality of life regardless of whether it has any other benefits. That's just as well, because little scientific research has been conducted on its significant effects on health. We know that olfaction is a powerful sense that has direct connection to breathing and emotion centers in the brain. Even if it's only short-acting, there may be stress management benefits from emotional response to aromatherapy's pleasing nature. Used as a comforting ritual to reduce stress, enhance relaxation, and relieve anxiety, aromatherapy may indeed relieve stress symptoms and alleviate some emotionally related disorders (Holmes 1995). For some people, it has provided a respite from insomnia. Others have found it an effective remedy for impotence. A few people even report that it eases the pain of arthritis and relieves postpartum discomfort. However, medical science is still searching to document the physical reason for these effects.

Fragrant oils have been used for thousand of years to lubricate the skin, purify infectious air, and repel insects. However, aromatherapy as we know it today dates from the late 1930s. It increased in popularity in the 1980s, when there was an upsurge in the use of "natural," nontoxic healing methods that cost less than conventional medications and produced fewer side effects.

Advocates of aromatherapy propose a variety of mechanisms for its reported effects. The most widely accepted theory suggests that fragrances do their work via the brain. When aromatic molecules enter the nasal cavity and stimulate the odor-sensing nerves, the resulting impulses are sent to the limbic system—the part of the brain that's believed to be the seat of memory and emotion (Cassileth 1999). Depending on the scent, emotional responses then kick in to exert a calming or energizing effect on the body.

Alternatively, some proponents suggest that certain aromas may work by stimulating the glands, prompting the adrenal glands, for example, to produce steroidlike hormones that fight pain and inflammation. Others believe that the essential oils, whether inhaled or rubbed into the skin, react with hormones and enzymes in the bloodstream to produce positive results (Holmes 1995).

Aromatherapists assign specific properties to each essence. According to Price (1991), here are typical claims for some of the more common essential oils:

Lavender: Heals burns and cuts; destroys bacteria; relieves depression, inflammation, spasms, headaches, respiratory allergies, muscle aches, nausea, and menstrual cramps; soothes bug bites; lowers blood pressure.

Peppermint: Alleviates digestive problems; cleans wounds; decongests the chest; relieves headache, neuralgia, and muscle pain; useful for motion sickness.

Eucalyptus: Lowers fever; clears sinuses; has antibacterial and antiviral properties; relieves coughs; useful for boils and pimples.

Tea tree: Fights fungal, yeast, and bacterial infections; useful for skin conditions such as acne, insect bites, and burns; helps clear vaginitis, bladder infections, and thrush.

Rosemary: Increases circulation; decongests the chest; relieves pain, indigestion, gas, and liver problems; lessens swelling; fights infection; helps alleviate depression.

Chamomile: Reduces swelling; treats allergic symptoms; relieves stress, insomnia, and depression; useful in treating digestive problems.

k*Thyme:* Lessens laryngitis and coughs; fights bladder and skin infections; relieves digestive problems and pain in the joints.

Tarragon: Stimulates digestion; calms neural and digestive tracts; relieves menstrual symptoms and stress.

Everlasting: Heals scars; reduces swelling after injuries; relieves sunburn; fights infections such as bronchitis and flu; treats pain from arthritis, muscle injuries, sprains, strains, and tendonitis.

Although many gift boutiques have taken to marketing scented candles, pomanders, and potpourri as "aromatherapy," genuine treatments rely on the use of highly concentrated essential oils extracted from various healing herbs. In most cases, these oils are produced by steam distillation or cold pressing from a plant's flowers, leaves, branches, bark, rind, or roots. The volatile, flammable oils are then mixed with a "carrier"—usually a vegetable oil such as soy, evening primrose, or almond—or diluted in alcohol before being applied to the skin, sprayed in the air, or inhaled.

Rubbing aromatic oil into the skin may be either calming or stimulating, depending on the type of oil used. Some people use it as a remedy for muscle sprains and soreness. Most preparations contain five drops of essential oil blended with light base oil. A higher concentration could irritate the skin. Bathing in aromatic oil is another popular practice for relaxation. No more than eight drops should be used in a tubful of water. Ten to fifteen drops might be added to a Jacuzzi or hot tub, four to five drops to a foot bath, or three to four drops to a hand bath (for chapped skin). During showering, a wet sponge or cloth may be dipped into an oil-water mixture and applied to the skin while the water sprays the body. This technique should not be used if a person has skin allergies.

Warning: Never take aromatherapy oils internally. They are extremely potent, and many can be poisonous. Many essential oils can trigger bronchial spasms. Asthmatics should not use any form of aromatherapy without first consulting their doctor. Also, a person who has skin allergies should not use essential oils in their bath. To check for allergy to oil, place one drop on the inside of the elbow and after twenty-four hours see whether it produces a reaction. As with any medication, it's best to avoid aromatherapy during pregnancy. Be especially wary of sage, rosemary, and juniper oils. These herbs have been known to cause uterine contractions when taken in excessive amounts. Infants and young children are especially sensitive to potent essential oils. Keep the oils away from their faces. Do not use peppermint oil on children under the age of thirty months. Because essential oils are highly concentrated, taking them internally can easily lead to a toxic overdose. Not even the tiniest amount should be ingested without a doctor's approval. Do not use highly concentrated, undiluted oils on the skin, and be careful to keep the oils away from the eyes. Many essential oils will cause skin irritation if used too frequently. They can also increase one's sensitivity to sunlight, making it easier to burn. Excessive inhalation of fragrant vapors can cause headache and fatigue. Remember, too, that certain oils, such as peppermint, can cause insomnia rather than relieve it. If a person develops an allergy to any of the products, stop the treatment immediately and seek another form of therapy (Fisher-Rizzi, 1991).

SUMMARY

Sometimes good things do come in small packages. This is the shortest chapter in the book and is perhaps the most important. Breath control, the simplest technique in the stress management arsenal, may be the most effective. It certainly is the easiest to learn and perform. Consider the following points:

- The simple act of breathing can calm you down.

- Take the time to stop, concentrate on your breathing, and breathe as you learned in this chapter—deep, diaphragmatic breaths.

- Feel yourself slow down as you slowly breathe in and out, repeating to yourself, "I am calm," and in a minute you will be.

- When you get time, practice the breathing techniques and you will gradually condition your autonomic nervous system.

- You will be less tense, more relaxed, and more in control of your stress and tension.

SOURCES CITED

Armstrong, K. (2001). *Buddha.* New York: Penguin.

Buchholz, I. (1994). Breathing, voice, and movement therapy: Applications to breathing disorders. *Biofeedback and Self-Regulation,* 19, no. 2, 141.

Fisher-Rizzi, S. (1991). *The complete aromatherapy handbook: Essential oils for radiant health.* New York: Sterling Press.

Holmes, p. (1995). Aromatherapy: Applications for clinical practice. *Alternative and Complementary Therapies,* 1, no. 3, 117–82.

Iyengar, B. K. S. (1995). *Light on Pranayama.* New York: Crossroad.

Pert, C. (1995). Neuropeptides, AIDS, and the science of healing. *Alternative Therapies,* 1, no. 3, 70–76.

Pert, C. (1999). *Molecules of emotion.* New York: Simon & Schuster.

Price, S. (1991). *Aromatherapy for common ailments.* New York: Simon & Schuster.

Journal Entry 12

Breathing and Awareness

In addition to all of the general health benefits of exchanging stale air for fresh air, breathing has a direct and immediate relationship to stress. In this exercise, you are asked to simply quiet yourself and become aware of the feelings in your mind and body as you concentrate on quiet breathing.

Read through these directions, then put the book aside for ten minutes and practice. Using any of the breathing techniques learned in the chapter, concentrate on proper techniques then stop thinking about it. Let the focus on technique fade. Spend about ten minutes quietly being aware of the feelings in your body and the thoughts or absence of thoughts.

After you have spent some quiet time, think back to how you felt and answer the following questions:

1. Were you able to quiet your body and mind?

2. What techniques or thoughts did you use?

3. What sensations did you feel; what changed from your normal awake state?

4. Could you sense the quietness in your breathing?

5. How would you describe your awareness?

 Write a positive word or short phrase about how quiet breathing may be useful to you in future situations.

CHAPTER 13

Muscle Relaxation

Take a moment and shift your attention from this book to your body. First note your overall position. Are you sitting comfortably? Is your body supported by the chair, or are your back muscles being strained? Are your arms supported, or are you holding the book in the air? Are your fists clenched? Think back to times when you were writing something. Did you ever notice that you were holding the pencil or pen so tightly that it was leaving an indentation in your fingers? Think of another activity, such as driving a car. Have you ever found yourself with a death grip on the steering wheel, producing tension up your arms to your shoulders, neck, back, and even to your head and facial muscles?

These are examples of tension exhibited through the muscles. More specifically, it is excess and needless muscle tension because it is far more than what is needed to accomplish the task. This excess muscle tension is both a response to stress and a cause of stress. The often-mentioned fight-or-flight syndrome is muscular expression, as are speech, facial expression, and eye movements.

Most movements are readily observable; that is, you can see your fingers move a pencil as you write, but it takes a second look to notice whether there is excess pressure. Excess exertion has nothing to do with the writing movement. It is an outward expression of emotional distress over what you are writing and/or it represents the general state of tension constantly with you. It is no mystery that people experienced at observing stress can quickly pick out stressed people by analyzing certain characteristics of their penmanship.

Much of the harmful, stress-producing muscle tension is extremely subtle and almost impossible to detect. If you are thinking defensive thoughts, you start to assume a defensive posture. It is practically impossible to think of an action and not have your muscles prepare for that action. To illustrate this phenomenon, take a pendant on a chain, or tie a key to a string, and hold it out in front of you. Close your eyes and, without moving your hand, imagine the object swinging toward and away from you. After a minute, open your eyes, and chances are it will be moving. Move it side to side, or imagine it circling. Even though your hand did not actually move, the thought was translated to your fingers, and tension developed in a rhythmical pattern with enough force to cause the object to move. This shows that we have the ability to anticipate, and this ability is necessary for preparation. Unfortunately, we often spend so much time in unproductive imagined preparation that our bodies adapt by increasing general muscle tension. At several points in this book we mentioned Selye's concept of the disease of adaptation. Muscle tension represents a good example. The individual who is defensive and is constantly imagining actions creates a situation in which the body learns to adapt by maintaining a chronic state of muscle tension. If such a condition is permitted to exist for an extended period, a wide variety of physical disorders may be produced or exaggerated (Everly and Lating 2007).

The connection between inordinate muscle tension and disease was made hundreds of years ago, but it was not until the end of the nineteenth century that systematic relaxation programs were formulated. The names Schultz, Sweigard, Maja Schade, and Jacobson became synonymous with relaxation training because their pioneering work formed the basis of most of the relaxation programs in existence today. There are literally hundreds of techniques now, but all have the same basic objective of teaching the individual to relax the muscles at will by first developing a cognitive awareness of what it feels like to be tense and then what it feels like to be relaxed. If one is able to distinguish between tension and relaxation, control over tension follows almost effortlessly (Jacobson 1977).

Muscle relaxation techniques can also help the individual learn to remain calm throughout the day by differentially relaxing unneeded skeletal muscles during everyday activities. There are great variations in the actual techniques of muscle relaxation; some are true to the original Jacobson Progressive Muscle Relaxation, and others either are a shorter version or are used in combination with hypnotic suggestion and emphasize the perception of relaxation rather than actual muscle relaxation (Bernstein and Carlson 1993).

The newer combination and shorter-version techniques have been widely used in recent years because they are thought to be more easily learned but produce good results nevertheless. Abbreviated progressive muscle relaxation training seems to be most effective when accompanied by training tapes and when offered to one individual at a time (rather than to groups). In addition, longer sessions offered more times have produced better results (Carlson and Hoyle 1993).

Neuromuscular Relaxation Exercises

Neuromuscular relaxation trains not only the muscles but also the nervous system components that control muscle activity. The benefits are, of course, the reduction of tension in the muscles, and because the muscles make up such a large portion of the body's mass, this represents a significant reduction in total body tension.

The types of stress and medical problems that have been shown to be positively affected by muscle relaxation run the gamut from tension or muscle-contraction headaches, chronic neck and back pain, and essential hypertension to coping with general stress as an adjunct to cancer chemotherapy. It was also found very helpful in post-surgical recovery (Good 1995). In addition, this training helps develop a sense of tension awareness. If you use muscles as a biofeedback device, you can develop an inherent autosensory awareness to the point that a little internal alarm goes off when tension starts to rise.

Another benefit of this training is mental discipline, often mentioned throughout this book. To accomplish any of these techniques, one must learn to center on the task or problem and control the mind's tendency to wander aimlessly in daydreams. Neuromuscular relaxation requires concentration, specifically passive concentration. As you perfect your ability, you can practice relaxation anywhere, even in short spurts, for example, while stopped for a red light, waiting for an appointment, or watching television. Just think of how much time you spend each day just sitting around waiting for things to happen; you might view this "wasted time" as an opportunity to practice relaxation. Two things will happen: first, you will easily get in thirty to sixty minutes of practice a day, and second, you will lose the concept of wasted time—a very important philosophical development necessary for reducing stress.

The Learning Phase

What follows is a detailed set of instructions on how to practice muscular relaxation. The learning phase, of course, necessitates more structured time involvement, more concentration, and more commitment than will be necessary once you master the technique. Once you have perfected it, you will be able to choose the particular exercise sequence that is most beneficial to you and that meets your immediate needs. It is very important, however, that in the learning phase you follow the instructions to the letter. It is also important to note that individuals with heart conditions, high blood pressure, or any condition that results in sore, weak, or otherwise compromised muscular systems should consult their physician for medical clearance before attempting muscle relaxation training.

The exercises presented in this chapter have been used for years in our clinical practice and have been proven to be quite effective and easily learned. Even though they are theoretically based on the concepts of the many relaxation techniques that have preceded them, significant differences exist. We follow a natural pattern to provide a constellation of exercises that we have found more effective and more easily learned than other current relaxation techniques. First you practice the gross muscle actions that you initially developed during the prenatal as well as the neonatal stage. These movements are innate to human locomotion and can be easily identified and controlled. Because these movements provide an excellent basis for cortical learning, you can gain awareness and conscious control over these motor actions. Then you can progress to higher levels of skilled muscle activity. Another important consideration taken into account when these exercises were developed was that they include group-muscle action rather than single-muscle activity. The brain knows nothing about muscles, only about movements involving many muscles working together. Trying to relax one muscle is difficult and retards learning. Finally, the exercises start from distal muscle groups (feet and legs) and proceed to proximal groups of muscles closer to the head and trunk.

Preparation　In order for the learning experience to be as effective as possible, you should do whatever you can to create an environment that enhances concentration. A few minutes spent preparing the environment and the body is a good investment.

Figure 13.1 Preparatory position for relaxation exercises

First, concentrate on the environment. Do whatever you can to reduce external noise. Find a room away from traffic, with no telephone and with indirect or dim lighting. You may want to use earplugs or earphones or play soft instrumental music or environmental sounds. As you become more proficient at these exercises, you will not have to make such elaborate preparations, but anything that might enhance initial learning will reduce learning time.

Next, work on preparing your body. A reclined or semireclined position with proper support under the legs is best (see **Figure 13.1**). Lie down on a mat; place your arms at your sides, elbows flexed at about sixty degrees so that the hands and wrists rest on the abdomen. Your hips will naturally flex to about twenty-five degrees, so don't attempt to hold your legs together. Your legs will naturally rotate outward; don't force them straight. In other words, allow the body to assume a position that does not require muscle action to maintain it. If you wish, you may support your neck with a small, soft pillow. If it is difficult for you to maintain a lying position without pain in the lower back due to unusual pull on the lumbar spine, place a pillow under your knees. This helps flatten the back against its support and relieves strain on the lower back. Also, if you have a history of low-back pain, lumbar-disc disease, or any other musculoskeletal disorder or postural condition including round shoulders, overdeveloped muscle mass, or cervical lordosis, you should take individual precautions and adopt the most restful and comfortable position to promote maximum concentration and learning. Any tight clothing, jewelry, belts, and the like should be loosened or removed. In preparing for relaxation, if you experience tingling or numbness in a body area, change your posture to relieve the pressure on that area. Above all, if pain or cramps develop during relaxation, rest the muscle until they diminish, and then proceed with less intensity.

Lower Extremities

The Ankle. The first exercise involves the ankle joints (see **Figure 13.2**). No other joints should be involved here. You should be lying in the preparatory position shown in Figure 13.1 and should have proceeded through one of the breathing exercises you learned in Chapter 12. It is a good idea to begin every muscle relaxation exercise with

Figure 13.2 Ankle Exercises

one of the deep-breathing exercises. Now pull your feet toward the front of your legs (the movement involved in taking your foot off the gas pedal of a car). The contraction should be felt only in the muscles on the front and outside of the lower leg, not in the calf muscles, which will feel stretched.

Your toes should be pulled forward toward your legs as hard as possible until you feel uncomfortable (short of pain—if pain develops, rest for a moment and proceed less vigorously). Center your thoughts in the muscles experiencing the tension. Try to visualize the tension. Form an image in your mind about this tightness. Hold for a few seconds and let go. Repeat the exercise, this time being sure to synchronize your breathing. Breathe in; pulling the feet up, hold your breath, hold the contraction—then let the air out, relaxing the muscles. Lie quietly for one minute and then repeat.

After you have done this several times and feel comfortable with the activity and the breathing pattern, turn your awareness more toward the relaxation than to the contraction. As you breathe out and relax, allow the muscles to go limp. As you pass over the peak of the contraction, begin to unwind. Try to form a visual image of this relaxed state, and hold it in your mind. Repeat this exercise until you have gained confidence in your ability to relax those muscles.

Next, move on to another group of muscles called the plantar flexor group, or calf muscles. They are the exact opposite of the first group. Thus, tightness will be felt in the calf area, and the stretching sensation will be felt in the muscle group in the front of the lower leg. Start by taking a deep breath, then push your toes down (as in pushing down on the gas pedal) and away from the body as far as possible. Keep the heels down. When you reach the peak of your breath, hold the breath for five seconds, keeping your toes pointed. Now, slowly exhale while allowing the feet to come back to a resting position.

Repeat this exercise three to five times, attempting to synchronize your breathing with the contraction and relaxation phases. As you exhale and let go of the contraction, form a visual image of the tension in the calf muscle flowing out with the air from your lungs. Imagine an unwinding or letting go. Concentrate on the feelings of tension, the feelings of relaxation, and the difference between the two states.

Hips and Knees

A good exercise in this group is the extension of the knees and hips, the knees being pushed down into the mat while the legs are kept straight (see **Figure 13.3**). For this exercise, remove the pillow from under your knees if you were using one. The tightness will be felt in front of the thighs and in the buttocks area. You will not be aware of any apprecia-

Figure 13.3 Hip and knee exercise

Table 13.1   Summary of Lower-Extremity Exercises

Dorsiflexion of Ankle Joints	Bend up the feet . . . Pull hard . . . Harder! And let go.
Plantar Flexion of Ankle Joints	Push the feet down as far as you can . . . Push harder! And let go.
	And slacken off the muscles completely . . .
Extension of Knee and Hip	Straighten the knees as much as possible . . .
	Now press the legs down into the mat . . .
	Hard . . . Harder! Now relax and feel the muscles of the lower legs relax.

ble stretching force because these muscles are long and serve more than one joint. As always, begin with a deep breath, pushing your hips and knees down into the mat. Hold at the peak of your breath, then exhale and allow the muscles to rest. Again, form an image of the tension; feel the letting go.

Table 13.1 summarizes these lower-extremity exercises. Put these together in three successive movements. Allow about thirty seconds between each exercise.

Trunk

The first of these two exercises utilizes the extensor muscles of the lower back. This exercise is particularly good for you if you have lower-back discomfort not related to deformity or injury. Because a large proportion of our population suffers from tension-related low-back pain, remember the earlier warning: If this or any of these exercises produces pain or spasms, stop the exercise and rest. Then continue with only a moderate amount of contraction, gradually increasing the strength of contraction over several weeks. If pain persists, discontinue this type of relaxation training. In this exercise, you hollow or arch your back, as shown in **Figure 13.4**. Move your chest slightly toward your chin. The buttocks are fixed on the mat. You will feel the tension in the lower-back area. Synchronize the exercise with your breathing, concentrating on the feelings of tension and relaxation. Repeat five times.

The second exercise is pulling in the abdominal muscles. Keep the legs, pelvis, and shoulders in contact with the mat. Breathe in, contract the stomach muscles, and flatten the lower back against the mat. Hold for five seconds, exhale, and relax.

The trunk exercises are summarized in **Table 13.2**. Try them both, one after the other, with three-second rest intervals between them. At this point, go back and repeat one time each of the exercises you have learned thus far. Concentrate on the feelings of tension and relaxation. The visual imagery is just as important as the performance of the muscular exercise.

Figure 13.4 Trunk extension

Table 13.2   Summary of Trunk Exercises

Extensor Muscles of the Spine	Push the chest forward until you have hollowed the back strongly . . . Lift a little more! And let go . . .
	Now relax and feel these muscles relax.
Abdominal Muscles	Pull in the abdominal muscles until they are quite flat . . .
	Pull a bit more! And let go . . . And rest . . .
	Now relax and feel these muscles relax.

Upper Extremities

This group of exercises is for the muscles in the upper limbs—around the shoulders, elbows, wrists, and fingers. Remember to start each exercise with deep breathing, and follow all the progressive steps (as discussed in Chapter 12).

The first exercise in this group is the extension of the wrist and fingers (see **Figure 13.5**). Exercise both your left and right extremities at the same time. Pull your hands and fingers simultaneously back toward your forearms, keeping your fingers straight. You should feel the tension in the backs of your hands and the backs of your forearms below the elbows. A little pain might be felt near the wrist—this is ligament stretch, so don't strain. Hold the tension for five seconds, and then relax. Make sure you give yourself a proper rest period so you can focus on the relaxation. Repeat this exercise five times.

The next exercise (see **Figure 13.6**) reverses the previous one. Turn your wrists in (stretching the back of your hand), and clench your fists very tightly. Hold the tension five seconds; then relax. Repeat five times.

Next, straighten your arms against your sides, keeping your fingers straight (see **Figure 13.7**). Press both arms tightly against your sides. Hold the tension for five seconds; then relax. Repeat this exercise five times.

Finally, do the following exercise for your shoulders. Shrug your shoulders up as high as you can—try to touch your shoulders to your earlobes (see **Figure 13.8**). Hold the tension for five seconds; then relax. Repeat five times. This exercise is excellent for stiff necks and shoulders caused by excessive desk work.

Figure 13.5 Wrist and Finger Extension

Figure 13.6 Wrist and Finger Contraction

Figure 13.7 Arms Straight against Sides

Figure 13.8 Shoulder Shrug

For a summary of upper-extremity exercises, see **Table 13.3**.

Head, Neck, and Face

The primary exercise in this group is rotation of the head. The muscles in this region become overworked because we tend to hold a steady partial tension for hours at a time, especially while doing desk work or driving. If you have chronic neck problems, use extreme care. To do this exercise (shown in **Figure 13.9**), first close your eyes. Touch your chin to your breastbone. Return, rest for a breath, and move the head backward toward

Table 13.3 Summary of Upper-Extremity Exercises

Finger and Wrist Extension	Straighten the fingers and pull back the wrists . . . Pull hard. Let go Now relax and feel these muscles relax.
Flexion of the Fingers and Wrists	Clench your fists and curl your wrists inward. Pull a bit more! And let go . . . And rest . . . Now relax and feel these muscles relax.
Adduction of Shoulder Joints	Straighten the arms against your sides . . . Press tightly. Pull a bit more! And let go . . . And rest . . . Now relax and feel these muscles relax.
Shoulder Shrug	Shrug your shoulders high . . . Higher . . . Touch your ears. Pull a bit more! And let go . . . And rest . . . Now relax and feel these muscles relax.

Figure 13.9 Head rotation

Figure 13.10 Facial Exercise

the spine. Return, rest, and then rotate the head so as to look over the right shoulder. Return, rest for a breath, and then look over the left shoulder. Consider these four moves as one exercise, and complete them in succession, but do not hurry. Synchronize each movement with your breathing; contract, relax for a few breaths, and continue with the next movement.

Another group of overworked muscles is the facial muscles, especially those involved in talking and chewing. To exercise these, clench your teeth together and draw your facial muscles up tightly (see **Figure 13.10**). Always remember the correct emphasis on breathing. Repeat five times and then relax.

Table 13.4 contains a summary of head, neck, and facial exercises.

The learning phase will take time and concentrated effort, but as learning progresses, it will take less time to complete the exercises. In the beginning, you may tend to fall asleep during practice or feel lethargic afterward. If this occurs often, it is probably a symptom of sleep debt, which often occurs with college students and, for that matter, is a common occurrence in our overloaded society. If the only time you relax is when you are too tired to do anything else, you may feel this way. However, these are precision exercises requiring concentration (albeit passive), and as you become more proficient you will feel rested, relaxed but alert, and full of vigor, strength, and enthusiasm for your daily activities. These exercises are more than relaxation promoting; they are a learning process that provides awareness of states of mind and body in relation to everyday life. Slowly you will begin to notice your posture, how your hand grips objects, your neck

Table 13.4   Summary of Head, Neck, and Face Exercises

Rotation	Shut the eyes . . . Now roll the head slowly forward, then slowly back . . . Roll the head to the right, then slowly to the left . . . It's heavy . . . and it's rolling easily—front to back, side to side . . . Now stop, with the face turned forward, and rest . . .
Facial Exercise	Clench the teeth together. Now draw up the facial muscles very tightly . . . Tighter! Pull a bit more! And let go . . . And rest . . . Now relax and feel these muscles relax.

position, and your facial expression. Being aware of such neuromuscular states is the first step in the change process, and finally you will be well on your way to not only combating tension but also preventing it.

Other Muscle Relaxation Techniques

Sometime it is better to relax the mind and let the body follow suit. However if muscles are tense, it is usually more efficient to learn to relax the muscles and stop them from bombarding the central nervous system with stimulating impulses. There are a variety of techniques that seek to break the feedback loop between the muscles and the brain. Unlike the Neuromuscular Exercises, all of the techniques listed below require special equipment or a specially trained therapist.

Biofeedback

When you become frightened, anxious, angry, or generally stressed, numerous changes occur in your body—most of them negative. If the stress is moderate to severe, you will have no trouble recognizing the outward signs. For example, your heart rate speeds up, and often you can feel the palpitations in your chest. The palms of your hands become moist with increased sweating, your skin may flush or become excessively pale, the pupils of your eyes may change size, your mouth may become very dry or in some instances salivation may become excessive, your muscles may tense to the point of pain or feel so limp that your legs threaten to give way, your stomach "turns over" and you may feel nauseated, your breathing rate may increase, and you may have a difficult time swallowing.

The body is constantly telling us about its activities. We have learned to key into some feelings, sounds, and outward signs of mind-body function. Stomach contractions are interpreted as hunger, diarrhea and constipation are indicators of gastrointestinal problems, and redness and swelling are signs of possible infection. We have also learned to use physiological parameters such as heart rate and blood pressure to assess the body's functioning. When an increase in blood pressure is detected, the individual has some information about the cardiovascular system, and during treatment subsequent blood pressure readings are a constant measure of the success of treatment.

Biofeedback is to some extent a refinement of that feedback system. Instead of diarrhea, which is a rather gross measure of intestinal action, one could measure the minute muscle contraction of various intestinal segments. Thermal measurement of skin can indicate blood flow to a particular region of the body. Measuring contraction of skeletal muscles can detect muscle action before it reaches the stage of producing pain and discomfort.

Any system in the body that emits energy can be used in the biofeedback process. Because of anatomical and physiological considerations, some systems are more difficult to use than others, and the muscular system is by far the most accessible and useful, especially to stress management.

There are two distinctly different applications of biofeedback to the muscular system:

1. muscle tension and relaxation

2. neuromuscular rehabilitation

Both of these utilize the electromyograph (EMG), an instrument that measures the activity of a muscle. More specifically, the EMG measures the electrical energy emitted by the flow of electrically charged particles in and out of a muscle cell just before contraction. The strength of the muscle contraction depends on the quantity of these particles; thus the EMG can give an instantaneous and continuous evaluation of muscle contraction.

A muscle is a mass of millions of cells with the ability to contract, or shorten, thus producing movement. As we learn how to perform activities, patterns of muscle movements are ingrained in our memory and become automatic functions. You do not have to think about how to pick up a pencil, but rather just think of the act and the muscles respond. Other muscle-action patterns are learned as well, such as fighting back, running away, and bracing for anticipated harm, to mention a few. When a threatening situation occurs, each muscle does not have to be commanded to act; one just thinks of the action "run," and the legs move.

Sit back in your chair, close your eyes, and try to focus your thoughts on your muscles. Bend your arm up so that your hand touches your shoulder. The muscle tension is obvious as movement occurs. Next, just think of the same movement. You may notice a tendency for the arm to move. Feel the muscles contract ever so slightly. Try the same activity with your forehead. Frown; feel the muscles contract. Then just think of an activity that is unpleasant to you, and try to feel the tension that may develop in that area. You are, of course, getting feedback of subtle muscle activity that does not produce movement only because you have not willed the movement.

But just as the gross movement can be controlled, so can the more subtle muscle tension if its existence is known. Unfortunately, most people possess limited ability to sense muscle tension. It is here that the EMG biofeedback instrument can be helpful. If sensing electrodes are placed on the skin over the muscle, subtle contractions can be measured. The signal is specially processed and converted to a light or sound signal and is fed back to the individual, who can use that information to direct the muscle to relax. In most tension reduction or general relaxation programs, muscles of the face and/or neck are used. Tension in these areas generally reflects moods and emotions.

As mentioned earlier in this chapter, Edmund Jacobson, an expert on muscle tension and relaxation, popularized the concept of mind-muscle interrelationship. He indicated that anxiety and muscle relaxation are incompatible and formulated the idea that one effective way of reducing anxiety was to reduce muscle tension. This concept formed the basis for the most common biofeedback program, which uses EMG biofeedback as a technique to develop self-awareness and an awareness of the relationship between emotion and tension. EMG biofeedback has also been used to promote general relaxation, reduce anxiety, treat phobias, and relieve a myriad of other conditions such as tension headache, migraine headache, premenstrual distress, and insomnia commonly associated with muscle tension (Lehrer 1994; Lehrer and Woolfolk 1999).

Massage and Bodywork

There is a substantial body of knowledge and research that indicates that we store emotional energy in all parts of the body, especially the muscles (Pert 1998). The Gestalt bodywork literature describes pain pockets as "depots" in which emotional energy is stored in the muscle and other organs. Manipulation of these pockets by a trained bodywork therapist can release this stored energy. Massaging pain pockets not only alleviates pain of the muscle cramp but can also release the energy of the original emotional experience. Even though not all massage techniques are based on the bodywork principle, it is common knowledge that there is a close relationship between tight muscles and stress arousal. Therefore, it follows that massage can be an effective relaxation and stress management tool. If nothing else, the time-out, self-indulgence, and quiet relaxing environment offer a respite from one's busy day. Although one may realize some results from gently massaging their own body parts or having a friend do the massage, best results can be achieved from visiting a trained professional. The following description of the most popularly available types of massage and bodywork can be viewed as a kind of consumer's guide that may be beneficial for stress management.

Massage   The massage most readily available to us is based on traditional concepts of anatomy, physiology, and soft-tissue manipulation. It includes soft-tissue manipulation tracing the outer contours of the body, usually toward the heart. A very popular technique in the United States was imported from Sweden and is called **Swedish massage.** It uses a system of long gliding strokes, kneading, and friction techniques on the more superficial layers of muscles. It usually goes in the direction of blood flow toward the heart because it emphasizes stimulation of the blood circulation through the body's soft tissues. Swedish massage can be relatively vigorous with a great deal of joint movement included. Oil is usually used to facilitate the stroking and kneading of the body, thereby stimulating metabolism and circulation. Its active and passive movements of the joints promote general relaxation, improve circulation and range of motion, and can relieve muscle tension. Swedish massage is often given as a complete, full-body technique, though sometimes only a part of the body is worked.

More vigorous massage techniques based on the Swedish concept are also popular and generally available. These techniques include neuromuscular massage, deep-tissue massage, sports massage, and manual lymph drainage. The focus is also on relieving muscle tension and increasing circulation, but it has the potential for creating deeper states of relaxation, beneficial states of consciousness, and general well-being.

Neuromuscular massage.   Neuromuscular massage is a form of deep massage that applies concentrated finger pressure specifically to individual muscles. This is a very detailed approach, used to increase blood flow and to release trigger points, intense knots of muscle tension that refer pain to other parts of the body (they become trigger points when they seem to trigger a pain pattern). This form of massage helps to break the cycle of spasm and pain and is often used in pain control. Trigger-point massage and myotherapy are varieties of neuromuscular massage.

Deep-tissue massage.   Moving toward a deeper, more clinical practice, the next level is deep-tissue massage. This approach is used to release chronic patterns of muscular tension using slow strokes, direct pressure, or friction. Often the movements are directed across the grain of the muscles (cross-fiber) using the fingers, thumbs, or elbows. This is applied with greater pressure and at deeper layers of the muscle than Swedish massage.

Sports massage.   A type of deep-muscle massage known as sports massage is a deep-tissue massage more specifically adapted to deal with the needs of athletes and the effects of athletic performance on the body. Sports massage is used before or after events, as part of an athlete's training regimen, and to promote healing from injuries.

Structural/Functional/Movement Integration   These approaches organize and integrate the body in relationship to gravity through manipulating the soft tissues and/or through correcting inappropriate patterns of movement. These are methods that bring about more balanced use of the body and nervous system, creating greater integration and more ease of movement. This category of approaches is interesting in that some do not even involve the practitioner touching the client. There is no clear line of demarcation between where the bodywork therapies end and the movement therapies begin. Furthermore, many practitioners use multiple techniques that integrate massage, deeper-tissue work, and movement, all in the same session with a client.

There are numerous techniques that work on the body structure and how it moves. Remember that chronically stressed muscles can alter their shape, structure, and function. At this point, the very act of moving creates pain and heightened stress-response feedback. Relief must include a restructuring, often called a reorganization of the tissue. The most common approaches include Rolfing, Hellerwork, the Rosen method, the Trager approach, the Feldenkrais method, the Alexander technique, and Ortho-Bionomy.

Rolfing.   Rolfing is perhaps the mostly widely known of these deep-tissue approaches. It is used for reordering the body to bring its major segments—head, shoulder, thorax, pelvis, and legs—into a finer vertical alignment. The technique loosens or releases adhesions in the fascia, the flexible tissue that envelops our muscles and muscle groups. The fascia is supposed to move easily and allow easy articulation, or movement of muscles or muscle groups past each other. However, trauma such as injury or chronic stress can cause stuck points, or adhesions, in which the fascia is in a sense frozen, not allowing full freedom of movement.

The Rolfer works to restore this freedom of movement, resulting in a more balanced, vertical alignment of the body and often a lengthening or expansion of the body's trunk. Rolfing usually takes place over a series of ten organized sessions dealing with different areas of the body.

Feldenkrais.   Another well-known technique is the Feldenkrais method. This approach was developed by Moshe Feldenkrais and uses physical movement to focus learning on the juncture of thought and action. It is known for its ability to improve posture and flexibility and to alleviate muscular tension and pain. It works with the nervous system's capacity for change and learning new patterns for moving, feeling, and thinking. The method involves two applications: awareness through movement and functional integration. These consist of verbally directed, pleasurable, and effortless exercise lessons involving highly sophisticated movement sequences, the use of specific skilled touch, and passive movement. It is known for its ability to address serious muscular and neurological problems and improve human functioning.

Chi.   Even in the Western world, the Asian methods are quite popular. These are based on the principles of Chinese medicine and the flow of energy, or chi, through the meridians. The geography of the acupuncture meridians is relied on to determine points of applying the techniques, and the ultimate goal is restoration of harmony or balance in the flow of chi. These forms may also be used in concert with herbs and acupuncture.

Pressure is applied by fingertips or thumb tips to predetermined points rather than by the sweeping broad strokes of Western-style massage. Strong pressure or very light pressure may be applied. There are over a dozen varieties of Oriental massage and body-work therapy, but the most common forms in this country are acupressure, shiatsu, jin shin jyutsu, and jin shin do.

Acupressure/Shiatsu. Acupressure and shiatsu are similar varieties of finger-pressure massage. They are both based on applying pressure to a pattern of specific points that correspond with the acupuncture points. Pressure is applied with the thumb, finger, and palm rather than with needles. The goal is the efficient and balanced flow of chi through the meridians. It is believed that where tension is being held in the musculature, the flow of chi is impaired through those areas, which can lead to chronic problems not only in the musculature but also in the associated organs. Stretching and movement are also sometimes used.

Acupressure is the more generic term used for this approach, and shiatsu is the Japanese version. Jin shin jyutsu comes from an ancient Japanese healing tradition that uses touch to restore the internal flow of energy through the body by releasing energetic blockages. A session lasts about an hour, and the client is fully clothed, lying on a table. The practitioner uses pulse diagnosis to identify energy blocks and then gently holds or touches a specific combination of two of twenty-six acupuncture points to allow release of the blockage. As practiced in the United States, the holding uses less pressure than other forms of acupressure or shiatsu, and there is no application of massagelike movements to specific points. Rather, the touch is very light and works to balance the flow of energy.

The Asian methods just described are also energetic methods in that they are working with energy according to principles of Chinese medicine and view the human being as an energy system. However, there are other energetic methods that are not based on Chinese principles. The most prominent of these are therapeutic touch, polarity therapy, and reiki.

Therapeutic touch. Therapeutic touch is unique in that it was born and reached its maturation within the context of conventional Western medicine. It was developed in the 1970s by Dolores Krieger (Ph.D., R.N., and a professor at New York University) and Dora Kunz, a natural healer. A contemporary interpretation of several ancient healing traditions, it is based on the principle that the human energy field extends beyond the skin, and the practitioner can use the hands as sensors to locate problems in it that correspond with problems in the physical body. Disease is seen as a condition of energy imbalance or blocked energy flow. Assessment is done by passing the hands over the body from head to toe about two to four inches above the surface.

The practitioner then serves as a conduit for universal energy, consciously and actively transferring energy into the recipient. The hands are used to direct and focus the energy, sometimes in rhythmical, sweeping motions. The method is initially taught "off body," meaning the practitioner's hands do not touch the physical body, though later with experience some physical touch may take place. Because it is not necessary to touch the physical body, this method can be applied in situations in which the client may not be able to tolerate contact. Sessions last up to thirty minutes and can be done sitting or lying down fully clothed. Therapeutic touch is currently taught in more than eighty universities and thirty countries and is practiced by 20,000–30,000 health care professionals.

Polarity therapy. Polarity therapy is a form of energy work that was developed by Randolph Stone, a chiropractor, osteopath, and naturopath in the mid–1920s. The practitioner uses subtle touch or holding of specific points to harmonize the flow of energy through the body and also to enhance the body's structural balance. It is based on the principle that every cell has both negative and positive poles, and the body is gently manipulated to enhance the energy flow. Emotional tension and physical pain are released as the flow of energy becomes more properly balanced. Polarity therapy is often given in a series of four sessions and may be accompanied by guidelines for diet and exercise.

Reiki. Reiki is the Japanese word for "universal life force energy." It is an ancient approach in which the practitioner is a kind of healer in the sense that he or she serves as a conduit for healing energy coming from the universe. The Reiki energy enters the practitioner through the top of the head and exits through the hands, where it is directed into the recipient's body or energy field. Reiki is another very subtle form of healing and may be done through clothing and without any physical contact between practitioner and client.

There are other approaches and combinations of approaches that do not fit neatly into categories. Many massage therapists and bodyworkers use combinations of approaches that could be called integrative massage or integrative bodywork.

Reflexology. Reflexology involves the manual stimulation of reflex points on the ears, hands, and feet. Similar methods resembling shiatsu and acupressure have also been practiced in China for thousands of years. Thumb pressure is applied to specific points that correspond somatotopically to specific areas or organs of the body. Reflexology was introduced to this country by William Fitzgerald, who termed it "zone therapy," in the early 1900s. One of the contemporary explanations for how it works is that compression by specific touch techniques affects a system of points and areas that are thought to "reflex" through neurological pathways to distant parts of the body. The pressure on these reflex points (also called "cutaneo-organ reflex points") is used to relieve stress and tension, to improve blood supply, to promote the unblocking of nerve impulses, and to help restore homeostasis or balance in the body.

Zero balancing. Zero balancing is a painless, hands-on method of aligning body energy with body structure. It is done through clothes and involves the practitioner using gentle pressure at key areas of the skeleton in order to balance the energy body with the structural body. The theory holds that each of us has an unseen energy body that exists like a glove surrounding the physical body. When injury or trauma occurs, healing of these two bodies does not necessarily occur simultaneously. "Balancing" refers to balancing the relationship between energy and structure. Zero balancing seeks to bridge the gap between those methods that work with structure and those that work with energy.

SUMMARY

The following points summarize the concepts covered in this chapter, which discuss the reduction of excess muscle tension through the learning of muscle relaxation techniques. The muscle response to stress covered in Chapter 3 discussed that muscles are our only means of expression. We cannot move toward pleasure or away from danger without muscle movements. Speech, facial expression, and eye movements—indeed, every mode of expression, feeling, and resolution of an emotion—are achieved through muscle movement. The muscles are under the command of the will, but many of the orders are given subconsciously, are counterproductive, and contribute significantly to stress and tension. Consider the following points:

- The stress response is intentional and tries to solve the problem of eliminating the stressor. This usually involves some muscle action.
- Muscle tension is one of the most prevalent stress responses.
- Muscle tension is self-perpetuating and creates a feedback loop; muscle tension exacerbates anxiety, which in turn exacerbates muscle tension.
- You cannot relax the mind if the muscles are tense; thus, muscle relaxation is essential for stress reduction.
- Neuromuscular relaxation is an effective method for reduction of excess muscle tension.
- Neuromuscular relaxation involves learning to feel the difference between tension and relaxation.
- Neuromuscular relaxation involves a voluntary manipulation of muscle tension, alternatively tensing and relaxing each muscle group so as to feel the difference and eventually producing the relaxed state at will.
- Breathing exercises and visual imagery aid in the muscle relaxation process.
- Biofeedback, numerous types of massage, and a variety of complementary and alternative therapies can be used to promote muscle relaxation. Most of these, although effective, involve the use of therapists and thus are passive in nature, so they do not promote the active learning that is essential in developing one's own stress management expertise.

SOURCES CITED

Bernstein, D. A., and Carlson, C. R. (1993). Progressive relaxation: Abbreviated methods. In *Principles and practices of stress management*, eds. P. M. Lehrer and R. L. Woolfolk. New York: Guilford Press, 43–69.

Carlson, C. R., and Hoyle, R. H. (1993). Efficacy of abbreviated progressive muscle relaxation training: A quantitative review of behavioral medicine research. *Journal of Consulting and Clinical Psychology,* 61, no. 6, 1059.

Cassileth, B.R. (1999). *The alternative medicine handbook.* New York: W. W. Norton.

Everly, G. S., Jr., and Lating, J. M. (2007). *A clinical guide to the treatment of the human stress response,* 3rd ed. New York: Plenum

Good, M. (1995). Relaxation techniques for surgical patients. *American Journal of Nursing,* 95, no. 5, 38.

Jacobson, E. (1977). The origins and development of progressive relaxation. *Journal of Behavioral Therapy and Experimental Psychiatry,* 8.

Lehrer, P. M., Carr, R., Sargunaraj, D., and Woolfolk, R. (1994). Stress management techniques: Are they all equivalent, or do they have specific effects? *Biofeedback and Self-Regulation,* 19, no. 4, 353–96.

Lehrer, P. M., and Woolfolk, R. L., eds. (1999). *Principles and practices of stress management.* New York: Guilford Press.

Pert, C. (1998). *Molecules of emotion.* New York: Simon & Schuster.

Journal Entry 13

Muscle Relaxation—A Seven-Day Plan

One of the most prevalent stress responses is muscle tension. Stress exists to accomplish a purpose. Muscle tension as a stress response occurs as an attempt to alleviate stress.

Excess muscle tension heightens anxiety and is responsible for many physical symptoms. Reducing excess muscle tension not only directly reduces total body tension and anxiety, but also indirectly helps eliminate the psychological forerunner of the muscle tension. You cannot relax the mind or fully concentrate if the brain is being bombarded by muscle tension impulses.

The basic technique for muscle relaxation is:

- Separately tense each muscle group.
- As you apply tension, take a deep breath.
- Hold the tension for about five seconds.
- Release the tension slowly as you breathe out while saying silently, "Relax and let go."
- Relax for thirty seconds and silently repeat to yourself, "Relax and let go."

Practice the above sequence with each muscle group listed below. Don't rush it; learn it. Do only one a day. Do each activity several times, spending fifteen to twenty minutes or however long it feels relaxing. Record your thoughts and feeling as to what you did that seemed to work and journal about it after the experience.

A. Head—Day 1

1. Wrinkle your forehead.
2. Squint your eyes tightly.
3. Open your mouth wide.
4. Push your tongue against the roof of your mouth.
5. Clench your jaw tightly.
6. Repeat Steps 1–5 in fairly rapid succession.
7. Relax for five minutes and periodically say, "Relax and let go."

Do you have any tension spots in this area? Because muscle tension has a purpose, what might the tension in this area be indicating to you? Could you feel the tension? What about the relaxation from that tension?

B. Neck—Day 2

1. Push your head back into a pillow.

2. Bring your head forward to touch your chest.

3. Roll your head sideways to your right shoulder.

4. Roll your head sideways to your left shoulder.

5. Repeat Steps 1–4.

6. Relax for five minutes and periodically say, "Relax and let go."

 Do you have any tension spots in this area? Because muscle tension has a purpose, what might the tension in this area be indicating to you? Could you feel the tension? What about the relaxation from that tension?

C. Shoulders—Day 3

1. Shrug your shoulders up as if to touch your ears with them.

2. Shrug your right shoulder up as if to touch your ear.

3. Shrug your left shoulder up as if to touch your ear.

4. Repeat Steps 1–3 in fairly rapid succession.

5. Relax for five minutes and periodically say, "Relax and let go."

 Do you have any tension spots in this area? What might the tension in this area be indicating to you? Could you feel the tension? What about the relaxation from that tension?

D. Arms and Hands—Day 4

1. Hold your arms out and clench both fists.

2. One side at a time: Push your hands down onto a surface.

3. One side at a time: Make a fist, bend your arm at the elbow, and then tighten up your arm, holding the fist.

4. Repeat Steps 1–3 in fairly rapid succession.

5. Relax for five minutes and periodically say, "Relax and let go."

Do you have any tension spots in this area? What might the tension in this area be indicating to you? Could you feel the tension? What about the relaxation from that tension?

E. Chest, Lungs, and Back—Day 5

1. Take a deep breath.
2. Tighten your chest muscles.
3. Arch your back.
4. Repeat Steps 1–3 in fairly rapid succession.
5. Relax for five minutes and periodically say, "Relax and let go."

Do you have any tension spots in this area? Because muscle tension has a purpose, what might the tension in this area be indicating to you? Could you feel the tension? What about the relaxation from that tension?

F. Stomach—Day 6

1. Tighten your stomach area.
2. Push your stomach area out.
3. Pull your stomach area in.
4. Repeat Steps 1–3 in fairly rapid succession.
5. Relax for five minutes and periodically say, "Relax and let go."

Do you have any tension spots in this area? Because muscle tension has a purpose, what might the tension in this area be indicating to you? Could you feel the tension? What about the relaxation from it?

G. Hips, Legs, and Feet—Day 7

1. Tighten your hips.
2. Lying down, push the heels of your feet into the floor.

3. Tighten your leg muscles below the knee.

4. Curl your toes under as if to touch the bottom of your feet.

5. Repeat Steps 1–4 in fairly rapid succession.

6. Relax for five minutes and periodically say, "Relax and let go."

 Do you have any tension spots in this area? What might the tension in this area be indicating to you? Could you feel the tension? What about the relaxation from that tension?

 After you have completed all the areas, what insights do you have about the tension areas in your body? What is the potential for this muscle relaxation technique to alleviate that tension?

 Write a positive word or short phrase about using muscular relaxation that will be useful to you in future situations.

Autogenics and Visual Imagery

Autogenic Relaxation Training

The term **autogenesis** (self-generation) describes almost every form of relaxation exercise; however, the word **autogenic** has become synonymous with a form of relaxation involving self-directed mental images of relaxed states. W. Linden (1999) presents an excellent review of the original technique and its effectiveness.

Although autogenic training has been found highly effective in treating a wide variety of stress-related disorders, most of the research has been done in Europe using what is known as the "full procedure." The abbreviated technique popular in the United States has been found effective as a relaxation and stress management technique but has not been as well researched as a technique to treat specific stress disorders (Linden 1994).

This simple yet advanced technique centers on conditioned patterns of responses that become associated with particular thoughts. Recall those moments when you have allowed your mind to run away and conjure up a tragic event. Recall how thinking of yourself or your loved ones dying or being involved in a serious accident gives you chills or raises the hair on the back of your neck. This represents a conditioned physical response to that particular association. The opposite is just as true and produces an equally dramatic physical response. Imagine sitting on a quiet beach with the sun warming your body, and a relaxation response is triggered. Unfortunately, many of us have become more conditioned to negative thoughts than to positive ones; thus the technique of relaxation recall was developed to help condition relaxation.

Relaxation Recall

Relaxation recall is actually a very advanced form of relaxation training; it is learned more rapidly when the individual already possesses some other relaxation skills. For example, it is difficult to concentrate or control the direction of your thoughts if your mind is being bombarded by arousal impulses from the body. The components of relaxation recall—concentration and relaxation—are facilitated by your ability to vividly imagine a scene or feeling state and by the ability to concentrate without arousal. Let's examine in detail one of the techniques included in the exercise plan.

It is known that one of the physical responses that accompanies relaxation is **vasodilation,** an expansion of the arteries in the skin of the extremities. This produces a warm, heavy sensation as blood flow increases in that area. Generally speaking, relaxed individuals tend to have warmer hands than anxious or stressed individuals. If one can imagine warmth, or on a feeling level can reproduce the heavy sensation, the body has the tendency to "relive" or reproduce that state. A shift in blood flow is impossible without a change in nervous system tone; thus relaxation is facilitated. After a degree of proficiency has been obtained, we will add a more complex imagination process by utilizing personal visual imagery of a time and place that was particularly relaxing to you. If your "feeling memory" is pretty good and if you have developed some fairly good body control and concentration abilities, the memory of the beautiful times in your life can be one of the keys to controlling stress and tension.

We have said that stress arousal is a mind-body response to a particular event. Each situation produces an immediate stress response but also leaves a residual amount of tension in the body. Response to subsequent stressors is augmented by the residual from previous responses. As the day wears on, response overactivity results from the inability to dissipate residual tension. The physical relaxation produced by relaxation exercises is an immediate reaction, but the more the relaxation state is induced, the more the carryover will be to times more removed from the exercise time. Gradually you will experience a decrease of residual tension. Thus each new stressful situation will produce a reaction sufficient to deal only with that particular situation without the added-on effect of previous stress arousal. The longer you practice the relaxation exercises, the more your general state of arousal resembles the relaxed state, and the more the ongoing tensions most detrimental to the body are reduced. After a while, this relaxed state becomes a stable part of your behavior. The overactive, rushed individual can become a slowed, cooler-reacting person having the ability to respond with the intensity demanded of each situation as an isolated incident.

Chronically stressed and anxious people often do not perceive internal states of arousal and do not associate physical states with emotional arousal. As in a positive feedback system, the physical arousal causes anxious feelings, which cause further physical arousal. Relaxation not only diminishes physical arousal but also promotes stress desensitization by allowing individuals to experience previously stressful situations in a relaxed state, gradually diminishing the stressful experience in their lives and reducing anxiety.

One essential ingredient of mental health—happiness—can be thought of as the ability to live each current situation in reality without the effect of adding imaginary consequences of what could or should happen. Perhaps the primary therapeutic benefit of this relaxation program is the development of the ability to concentrate attention on the present, to quiet the imagination, and to distinguish reality from fantasy. You can develop the ability to direct thoughts away from the ego self, the primary source of stress, and direct them to the problem at hand. You can become more problem centered and less ego centered. As you become less stressed, you automatically become more efficient; they go hand in hand. The exercises that are presented in the remainder of this chapter are time-honored, well-practiced examples of the relaxation technique we call relaxation recall. Follow the instructions and practice these for a few days; the effects can be felt immediately, and the long-term benefits can be substantial.

Legs Heavy and Warm   The exercises in this group are quiet concentration activities that can be done either sitting or lying down. The object is to tell yourself to reproduce feelings of heaviness and warmth in the legs. If you are successful, a heavy, warm sensation will occur as blood flow increases in that area. The body will "relive" or reproduce that state, and, as we have said, such a shift is impossible without a change in the nervous system tone. Thus relaxation is facilitated. You must be quiet and undistracted, and you must concentrate.

Start by taking three deep breaths. Repeat the following phrases quietly to yourself. Go slowly; allow time between each phrase to feel these sensations:

I am relaxed.

I am calm.

I am quiet.

My right leg is heavy.

My right leg is heavy and warm.

My right leg is warm and relaxed.

I am calm and quite relaxed.

I am relaxed.

(Pause for a minute or so and feel the relaxation.)

I am relaxed.

I am calm.

I am quiet.

My left leg is heavy.

My left leg is heavy and warm.

My left leg is warm and relaxed.

I am calm and quite relaxed.

I am quiet and at peace.

I am relaxed.

This activity should take about five minutes. When you are done, remain quiet for a few minutes.

Center of Warmth   The exercises in this group are quiet concentration activities that may be done while sitting or lying down. You will need quiet, intense concentration on the trunk area of the body. You are going to try to imagine warmth being emitted from the nerve plexus lying behind the stomach and right above the navel. Focus your attention on what you feel is the exact center of your body. The nerves there form a plexus (or a network) called the *solar plexus*. Softly, slowly, and quietly say to yourself:

I am relaxed.

I am calm.

I am quiet.

My solar plexus is warm.

I can feel the heat radiating throughout my entire body.

My body is warm and relaxed.

I am quiet and at peace.

I am relaxed.

This activity should take about five minutes. When you are finished, remain quiet for a few minutes.

Arms Heavy and Warm   By now you are familiar with the procedure for this exercise. It will include quiet concentration of heaviness and warmth in the arms and hands. If you had any success with the two previous exercises, you will likely do very well here. If you had difficulty with those exercises, this one will likely provide you with a breakthrough because you have better control over your hands and arms than over your legs and trunk, more nerves innervating fewer muscles, and just more practice in using the upper extremities. You may sit or lie down. Start with a few deep breaths. Center yourself. Close your eyes and concentrate on your hands and arms. Your statements are as follows; repeat them to yourself slowly and quietly:

I am relaxed.

I am calm.

I am quiet.

My right arm is heavy.

My right arm is heavy and warm.

My right arm is warm.

My right arm is warm and relaxed.

I am calm and quite relaxed.

I am relaxed.

(Pause for a minute or so and feel the relaxation.)

I am relaxed.

I am calm.

I am quiet.

My left arm is heavy.

My left arm is heavy and warm.

My left arm is warm.

My left arm is warm and relaxed.

I am calm and quite relaxed.

My body is warm and relaxed.

I am quiet and at peace.

I am relaxed.

This activity should take about five minutes. When you are finished, remain quiet for a few minutes.

Freedom Posturing

Another form of autogenic or relaxation recall type of relaxation is what we call freedom posturing. This exercise is designed to change thoughts and behaviors that continually fuel the stress response. The basic premise of freedom posturing lies in the interaction between mind and body—arousing thoughts produce a tense body, and a tense body stimulates central nervous system arousal. The cycle can be broken by changing either the body position or thought process. In addition, this technique seeks to promote self-awareness and reduce stressful behavior, especially as it relates to dealing with the expectations others have of us.

After you learn some of these powerful relaxation techniques, you can then refine your use of them so that you are able to relax at will. Once you have developed the ability to relax at will, you can (1) practice and gradually condition your system to be more tranquil and relaxed, and (2) use your ability to relax for immediate relief when you feel stressed. The catch in Item 2 is that we must be able to recognize stress as it builds and before it pushes us into unproductive emotional states and physical disability.

If you are working with another person, just sit back and have that person read the directions. If you are working by yourself, read the situation, get the idea of what you are being asked to do, then sit back, close your eyes, and work through it. Either way, always close your eyes because it greatly increases your power of concentration.

Situation 1.   Close your eyes, but in your mind's eye see a tense person. It may be someone you know well or just someone you have seen once. What does this person look like when stressed? How is that person sitting? What is he or she doing with his or her legs, arms, and face? Concentrate on the person's breathing. Is it fast or slow, deep or shallow, through the nose or mouth? What sounds is the person making?

Concentrate on the legs. Are they moving or still, crossed or open? Are the feet flat on the floor? Do they seem to be digging into the floor as if to resist movement; or just the opposite, to provide a firm base from which to spring? Are the legs generally taut, ready for action?

Concentrate on the midsection of the person's body. Is this person hunched over from the shoulders? Bent in the abdomen? Is the back arched? Is the back being pushed into the chair?

Concentrate on the hands and arms. Are they moving or still? Are the hands clenched into a fist, or are they open? Are they pushed down onto the arms of the chair? Are they gripping? Are they crossed in front of the body? Are they tensely straight?

Concentrate on the head, neck, and face. Are the eyes wide open or squinted? Is the head pulled down, and are the shoulders up? Is the forehead wrinkled? Are the jaws tightly clenched? Are the neck muscles tightly drawn?

Now assume that position yourself. Tense your muscles as the person you saw in your mind's eye tensed his or her muscles. See yourself in that position. Feel yourself in that position. Where are you? Who are you with? What message (verbal or nonverbal, explicit or implied) is that person giving you? What is he or she expecting from you? Are you feeling pushed to do something you do not want to do? Or are you feeling held back from doing something you want to do? Now leave those thoughts and rest for a moment.

Situation 2.   Close your eyes and switch your mind's eye to a person you see as very relaxed. How is this person sitting? Concentrate on this person's arms, hands, breathing, legs, trunk, and face as you did in the previous exercise. How are they different from those of the tense person? Assume the relaxed position yourself. Where are you? Who are you with? Do you feel free to do what you want to do? In the absence of expectations, this is how your body feels. You can help yourself demand your personal freedom by telling your body to position itself in this fashion. Now slowly open your eyes, and reorient yourself to the world around you. Feel the energy flowing through your system. Vitalize your sense of commitment to your purpose and to yourself. When you feel someone is pushing you or holding you back, assume this freedom posture and be aware of how you are more willing to demand your personal freedom.

Your Special Place

Recall a time in your life when you felt very relaxed, peaceful, and tranquil. It may help to close your eyes, relax, and let the images come to you. Describe the place in the following terms:

1. When was it? _____

2. Who was with you? _____

   Note: Even though you might have traveled with another person, do not list anyone else unless that person's image is vividly associated with the relaxation feeling.

3. Where was it? Look around, describe what you see, and describe your feelings and sensations:

Note: Feelings and sensations are more important than exact topographical descriptions. Here is an example of Item 3, somewhat overdone to drive home the point that the feelings make the scene more vivid.

> See a lonely stretch of beach with the waves forcefully pounding the rocks and teasing the sand. With each wave the sand feels cool, solid, and resisting, then warm and accepting, caressing my feet. The gentle breeze massages my skin, and my hair resembles the grass, bending in response to the wind's gentle persuasion. The sun seductively bathes my skin with warmth, which is then cooled by the breeze. The gulls, precocious and curious, clamor for attention as they proclaim the ecstasy and freedom of flight. My spirit soars with their flight, and as I ride the wind I feel free, open, part of the wind, the sun, the sea, the universe.

Take this a step further into the realm of fantasy. See yourself gently floating on a raft, drifting deeply into relaxation. Your raft may have the ability to float not only on water but also in the air. Feel the wind pick up your raft and gently and safely carry it off the ground as high as you wish it to go, closer to the warmth of the sun. You can fly as high and as far as you wish, looking down on your surroundings, relaxed and calm as you look at the activities of people and events below. Perhaps you wish to visit a special place and view from your gently floating raft the activities of a special event, knowing that you are above it all, relaxed and calm, gently floating on the wind, leaving all your worries on the ground. Continue your travel for a few minutes, and enjoy this special place and experience. As you return from your trip, know that you can return any time you wish just by closing your eyes, taking a deep breath, and seeing yourself floating on your special raft.

Visual Imagery

Aristotle wrote, "The soul never thinks without a picture." It is well documented that the pictures in our minds are closely related to physical arousal and the stress reaction. We now know that what works against us can be turned around to work for us—if we can control the pictures in our mind. The basic premise is that imagery is an experience and can be regarded in many important aspects as equivalent to an actual experience with a concomitant elevation of stress arousal or relaxation response (Roeckelein 2004; Ganim and Fox-Wood 1999).

This exercise is only one type in the broad spectrum of visual imagery that is rapidly becoming perhaps the most widely used and researched area in stress management and healing. A guided imagery or fantasy is one in which an individual, by describing an experience, helps another individual form internal visual images. This differs slightly from what we will use here in that you will be working alone, using a story based on your own experience to elicit internal images that will produce a relaxation response. Construct a guided fantasy illustration to help stimulate your personal imagery that, although based on your personal experience, goes beyond that experience to a relaxation fantasy. Create your own imagined relaxation place and use it in the following exercise:

1. In a quiet room and in a comfortable chair, assume a restful position and a quiet, passive attitude. Take four deep breaths. Make each one deeper than the one before. Hold the first inhalation for four seconds, the second one for five seconds, the third one for six seconds, and the fourth one for seven seconds. Pull the tension from all parts of your body into your lungs, and exhale it with each expiration. Feel more relaxed with each breath.

2. Count backward from ten to zero. Breathe naturally, and with each exhalation count one number and feel more and more relaxed as you approach zero. With each count you descend a relaxation stairway and become more deeply relaxed until you are totally relaxed at zero.

3. Now go to the relaxation place outlined in the previous exercise. Stay there for four minutes. Try to vividly, but passively, recall the feelings of that place and time that were very relaxing.

4. Bring your attention back to yourself. Count from zero to ten. Energize your body. Feel the energy, vitality, and health flow through your system. Feel alert and eager to resume your activities. Open your eyes.

Lusk (1992), Naparstek (1995), and Schwartz (1995) provide imagery scripts for calming, centering, coping, and other aspects of staying well.

SUMMARY

The visual imagery technique involves the use of self-directed mental images of relaxed states. This simple method centers on conditioned patterns of responses that become associated with specific responses. Consider the following points:

- Visual imagery is a method in which you talk to your body and tell it to relax.
- The body physiologically tries to produce the state you direct. States like warmth and heaviness are produced by vasodilatation of blood vessels.
- Vasodilatation is a parasympathetic response associated with the relaxation response.
- With practice the body will become conditioned to the relaxation response, and this will become your "state of being."
- Used as a technique for general relaxation, visual imagery involves the memory recall of relaxing places and/or feelings.
- Chronically stressed people usually worry excessively about the past and/or future.
- Chronically stressed people have become conditioned to negative thoughts and associated feelings.
- Chronically relaxed people tend to live in the now, and think about what is going on in their lives as it is happening.
- Chronically relaxed people have become conditioned to positive thoughts and associated feelings.

SOURCES CITED

Coue, E., and Brooks, C. H. (1974). *Suggestion and autosuggestion.* New York: Samuel Heiser.

Ganim, B., and Fox-Wood, S. (1999). *Visual journaling: Going deeper than words.* New York: Quest Books.

Linden, W. (1994). Autogenic training: A narrative and quantitative review of clinical outcome. *Biofeedback and Self-Regulation, 19,* no. 3, 227.

Linden, W. (1999). The autogenic training method of J. H. Schultz. In *Principles and practice of stress management,* 2nd ed., eds. P. M. Lehrer and R. L. Woolfolk. New York: Guilford Press, 200–15.

Lusk, J. T. (1992). *Relaxation imagery and inner healing.* New York: Whole Person.

Naparstek, B. (1995). *Staying well with guided imagery.* New York: Time Warner.

Roeckelein, J. E. (2004). *Imagery in psychology: A reference guide.* Westport, CT: Praeger

Schwartz, A. E. (1995). *Guided imagery for groups.* New York: Whole Person.

Journal Entry 14

Visual Imagery

Visual imagery is the use of self-directed mental images of relaxed states. This simple technique centers on conditioned patterns of responses that become associated with particular thoughts.

One of the common techniques used in this form of relaxation capitalizes on the body's ability to follow the commands of the conscious centers of the brain. If you can imagine warmth, the body has the tendency to reproduce that sensation. Responding to the conscious demand, blood flow will increase to the desired areas, thereby creating the desired warmth. Such a physiological change would be impossible without a change in the "tone" of your nervous system. Through such a change, relaxation is facilitated and the relaxation response is gradually conditioned.

When you learn that you have voluntary control over normally involuntary bodily processes, you can extrapolate that to controlling thoughts and feelings. Self-control promotes self-concept.

The Power of Suggestion

Read through the following self-commands to familiarize yourself with them. You might even tape them and play them back to yourself or have someone else read the directions to you as you relax.

Keep your eyes closed and place your hands in your lap with the palms facing down and resting comfortably on your lap.

By focusing your thinking, you can make your right hand feel hot. Picture the sun shining on your right hand and let yourself feel that heat. As you think of the sun shining brightly, feel the heat increasing. Feel the sun getting hotter and feel the heat penetrating your skin and going deep into your hand. Think of it getting really hot now, very hot. Feel the heat increasing. Think of the sun getting very, very hot as it penetrates into your hand, making it very hot. Tell yourself that the rays are increasing and the heat is increasing, getting hotter and hotter. Feel the heat penetrating your skin. Feel the heat going deeper in to your skin as you think of the rays of the sun increasing and becoming more and more concentrated, getting hotter and hotter. Feel your hand getting hot from the heat of the sun, a good feeling of warmth as it penetrates deep into your hand; hot, a pleasant hot, penetrating into your hand now. It's a pleasantly hot feeling—pleasantly hot.

Journal this part of the exercise. Could you feel the warmth in your hand? Did it transfer to areas other than the arms and hands? Could you feel relaxation, calm, and quiet?

Center yourself. Take three deep breaths, then repeat the following phrases quietly to yourself:

I am relaxed.

I am calm.

I am quiet.

Then repeat the following passage quietly to yourself:

The sun has great power. The power to warm you, power to heal you. You also have great power, power to do anything that you want. The key to your success is confidence, confidence in yourself, confidence in your ability to do whatever you truly want. Confidence that you can and will accomplish your goals through the power of your own mind, the power of your own thoughts. What you tell yourself has the greatest power over your life. What you tell yourself determines whether you feel cheerful, or gloomy and worried, and the way you feel determines to a great extent the health and well-being of your physical body. When you're unhappy, your body simply cannot function properly. What you tell yourself has an enormous impact on your life. What you tell yourself ultimately determines what you are or are not able to do.

Tell yourself that you will no longer worry unnecessarily about things that happened in the past or about what will happen in the future. Life exists only for each moment. Tell yourself that your mind and body are relaxed and calm, and you are at peace with the universe. And because of your calmness, you have greater energy and your mind will be clearer, sharper, and more focused. Feel the warmth of the sun; feel the power of the heat. Feel the power of the confidence within you.

 Journal this part of the exercise. Could you feel relaxation, calm, and quiet? Did it transfer to other areas?

Did you feel confidence?

How do you feet in relation to how you felt before you started? Write your insights here:

 Write a positive word or short phrase about using visual imagery that will be useful to you in future situations.

CHAPTER 15

Yoga and Stretch-Relaxation

The devastating effects of stress induced by muscle tension have been discussed in numerous places throughout this book. You might recall two important points. First, muscles are our only form of communication and behavior. We cannot speak or move without muscle contraction. And two, muscles tend to remain in a partial contraction responding to the potential for movement, also known as anticipation, whether the movement actually takes place or not. The partial contraction bombards the central nervous system with impulses resulting in muscle tension–generated stress. A positive feedback loop develops where stress or the anticipation of movement generates muscle tension and in turn muscle tension exacerbates the stress. At this point you have two options, reduce the stressful thoughts and emotions (usually anger, fear, or anxiety related) that are generating the tension or reduce the tension that is exacerbating the thoughts. If one wishes to work on the muscle tension directly, which is usually the most direct and efficient approach given the complex nature of our thoughts emotions, beliefs, and behaviors, then this book has presented numerous options. It is so important that we present yet another.

Stretching

Stretching tense muscles is another one on those innate actions that has existed since the beginning of time and is not unique to humans. Notice your pet dog or cat, especially on awakening but at other times during the day also. They usually do not attempt to get up without first stretching. Humans also naturally go through a series of stretches before arising from sleep or after prolonged sitting. When tightness or tension is sensed, stretching is a natural reflex. Just because someone organized it into patterns and sequences does not mean they invented it, although they probably made it easier it learn. The ancient yoga masters who, thousands of years ago perfected the skills and organized its teaching, advanced the practice and took stretching to the next level by combining it with breathing and meditation, incorporating it into a life skill and a lifestyle of awareness, insight, and enlightenment.

Yoga

The word **yoga** is derived from the Sanskrit word meaning "union" or "reunion" and is a method of physical, mental, and spiritual development based on the philosophies of Krishna. Knowledge of these philosophies was passed from enlightened master to student, generation after generation, for centuries before the first written record appeared around 200 B.C. in Patanjali's Sutras. Since then, thousands of books have been written describing the many types of yoga, called "paths," which have developed into many different disciplines, several important to the study of stress management. Pranayama, the yogic awareness of breath, was discussed along with breathing in Chapter 12. Raja yoga, or royal yoga, meaning the path to self-realization and enlightenment, is very similar to the meditative practice described in Chapter 16.

The most popular path in the Western world is hatha yoga, which uses positions and exercises to promote physical and mental harmony. Most yoga practice starts with Hatha yoga because it is thought to provide the body with the health and endurance needed to learn more advanced forms of yoga. Hatha yoga also has been reported to heal the body—strengthen immunity and breath, improve body alignment, open up blocked energy, and aid meditation (Weller 1995).

Hatha yoga can be practiced for its own rewards, which include strength, flexibility, and reduction of muscle tension, and is also used as a technique to quiet the body in preparation for quiet mental states. We have elected to combine some hatha yoga postures with general stretching and present it here; even these few exercises will amaze you in their effectiveness. We guarantee you will feel instant relief from muscle tension and will be anxious to incorporate the activities into your stress management program. We hope you will be motivated to learn more about developing a complete program from the hundreds of books have been written on stretching and Hatha yoga.

Stretch-Relaxation Exercises

The health benefits of stretch-relaxation techniques have been known for centuries; these exercises are an essential part of most exercise programs, and represent an innate pattern of movement. Research shows that flexibility training reduces postworkout soreness, decreases musculoskeletal injury, and increases range of motion. Flexibility is especially important for the aging population. For the professional and recreational athlete, improved flexibility decreases the chance of injury and enhances performance (Grieco 2002). According to stretching guru Bob Anderson (Anderson et al. 2006), in addition to reducing muscle tension the benefits of stretching also include better coordination, increased range of motion, decreased injuries, better circulation, increased body awareness, and a more relaxed state of mind.

Our modern living patterns are directly responsible for a multitude of health problems, many of which are listed in earlier sections of the book. One of the most pervasive is shortened muscles, tendons, and ligaments. Our basic body structure and function have not changed since the days of prehistoric humans, yet our daily activities have changed drastically. Because the body is adaptive, continual sitting during work and leisure will eventually result in shortened muscles, tendons, and ligaments and in restricted movements. It is not unusual for adults in their mid-twenties to be so restricted that touching their fingers to their toes while keeping the knees straight is impossible or at least very painful. The spine will condition itself to the state demanded by chronic sitting and lose its natural erect capabilities; the result will be a sitting-type posture while one is standing or walking. This posture naturally produces pain and tension because body parts are positioned unnaturally. Neck and facial muscles, tendons, and ligaments will pull unnaturally, producing pain in the sensitive tissue around the head and thus causing headache. It is not at all unusual for the posture and tone of the muscles under the skin to resemble those of the very old. Age lines are not a natural process of aging (they occur from constant use) and are surely not natural in the young or even in those in the middle years.

Chronically shortened muscles do not function properly; excess tension and internal viscosity prohibit normal functioning, and a vicious cycle of the tension reflex develops. Gradually, movements become inefficient and labored; more energy than necessary is required, and fatigue causes a chronic tired feeling even after adequate amounts of sleep. It has long been known that a muscle with proper stretch capabilities is stronger, more efficient, and more enduring than one that is chronically shortened. Moreover, such a muscle is more contractible, exhibits less residual tension, and can be relaxed more easily.

Whether you end up becoming a yoga practitioner or just using stretching for the benefits mentioned earlier, it is well to remember that these activities will condition the body as you go starting slowly and then advancing as you condition the muscles. It is difficult for most of us to completely master all of the positions, especially the advanced ones, without daily practice over a period of time. Nevertheless, positive results can be derived especially if the exercises are chosen for specific outcomes in specific muscle groups. For relaxation, we have developed some exercises and postures derived from principles of stretching hatha yoga. These carefully developed exercises have been shown to yield maximal results in the shortest period of time in groups of individuals with no prior experience or special physical conditioning. This program is sequenced to condition natural readiness. There is a fine line between feeling the long-overdue stretch of a chronically shortened muscle and the pain of overstretching. Do not go beyond that point of feeling the stretch and never go beyond your point of pain, or you will tear the tissue and retard your progress. You have spent many years conditioning this state of chronically shortened muscles, and you cannot reverse it overnight. One hard-and-fast rule is to never bounce to achieve greater stretch. The weight and momentum of the body will overstretch the muscle. Instead, use slow and easy movements; take the time to feel the tension relief as you go.

These are powerful exercises with the capability of restoring the natural structure and function to your tissue. Use them as directed until you have reconditioned your body. As was mentioned earlier, if you enjoy these exercises as we are sure you will, and would like a more complete program, there are hundreds of books on the subject. Some are listed in the sources at the end of this chapter.

Specific Positions

Even though muscles will contract during these positions, the emphasis is on stretch of muscles and joints. The large muscles of the legs chronically shortened from sitting are a good place to start.

Toe Raise, Knee Stretch, Toe Touch

The first exercise is a simple toe raise (see **Figure 15.1**). In a standing position with hands on hips or raised in front of you, balance yourself as high on the tips of your toes as possible. Hold for a count of ten and relax. Repeat this exercise five times and relax.

Figure 15.1 Toe Raise

Figure 15.2
Knee Stretch

The second exercise is the knee stretch (see **Figure 15.2**). Sit with your legs folded under you so that your buttocks are resting on your ankles. Your toes should be pointed backward. Place your hands on the floor outside and behind your feet. Straighten your body with your head raised high. Hold for a count of ten; relax and repeat five times.

The third exercise, the toe touch (see **Figure 15.3**), stretches the muscles in the back of the leg in three positions. In a standing position with the heels together, toes angled slightly outward and legs straight, bend forward from the waist and place your hands on your knees. Hold for a count of ten, and return to standing. If this produced no pain, the second repetition should find you reaching for your ankles. If pain was experienced, repeat the position to your knees. Don't force it; your body will tell you when it is ready to go lower. Hold for a count of ten, and return to standing. On the third repetition, place the tips of your fingers on the floor, but assume this position only if no pain was experienced during the last one. Hold for a count of ten and return to standing. The final position, assuming you feel no pain at this point, is to place your palms flat on the floor. Keep your legs straight, bend at the waist, and hold for a count of ten. You will do four repetitions whether you reach the floor or not. Remember, go slowly; your body will tell you when to go on to the next position.

Back Stretch Forward and Reverse, Standing Trunk Bend

Here again, the emphasis is on the stretch of the muscle, the recoil, and the sense of relaxation that follows. Concentrate on the "after feeling" of extreme relaxation. The stretch relieves the partial contraction and allows the muscle to relax fully.

The first exercise is the back stretch forward (see **Figure 15.4**). As its name implies, you will feel the stretch in different parts of your back as the exercise advances. Lie on

Figure 15.3 Toe touch

Figure 15.4 Back Stretch Forward

the floor. Slowly tensing your stomach muscles, raise your trunk through the sitting position to a point where your head is as close to your knees as possible. Once there, place your hands on your knees, thumb on the inside of your leg, and elbow held as high as possible. Hold for ten counts and return to the lying position. Move very slowly. Feel the stomach muscles contract as they raise and lower your upper body. Feel the stretch in the lower back.

On the second repetition, place your hands halfway between your knees and ankles. Try to get your head to your knees; however, go only as far as your flexibility allows. Don't force it—you will likely get there one day soon. Hold for a count of ten, and relax back to the lying position. Feel the stretch and subsequent relaxation in the back slightly higher than in the first repetition.

On the third repetition, try for your ankles. Go slowly; feel the stretch a little higher on the back. It may help at first to use a strap or belt around your feet to extend your reach if you are having difficulties; however if you had success at the first two positions, this should be a success also. Try to get your head on your knees. Hold for a count of ten and relax. For the fourth repetition, try to hold your hands on the bottoms of your feet. Draw the trunk toward your legs. Allow your elbows to rest on the floor. Hold for a count of ten, and slowly return to the lying position. Relax, feeling the tension release.

For the second exercise, the trunk stretch reverse (see **Figure 15.5**), you will need to lie down on your stomach. This exercise will stretch the back in the opposite direction. You will feel the muscles in both the back and stomach stretch. Place your hands palms down on the floor, one on each side of your face. Slowly raise your upper body until you can rest your elbows on the floor. Hold this position for a count of ten. If this produces no pain, arch your back slowly, moving your head high and back. Hold this position for a count of ten and rest. If this produces no pain, place your palms on the

Figure 15.5 Back Stretch Reverse

floor and continue to raise your upper body until your arms are straight. Go very slowly, and if you feel pain, return to the last position. Hold for a count of ten, and return to the floor and relax. Feel the tension release in your back and stomach. Relax and breathe softly. Repeat the entire sequence five times.

The third exercise is the standing trunk bend (see **Figure 15.6 to 15.8**). Stand with your feet together, legs straight. The first motion will be a side bend. Stretch your arms

Figure 15.6 Standing Trunk Bend (first part)

Figure 15.7
Standing Trunk
Bend (second
part)

over your head. Bend your trunk to the right. Go as far as possible. Try to achieve a right angle to your lower body. Go only as far as you can, and, when there, hold for a count of ten, and return to an erect position. Now repeat to the left. Hold for ten and return. The final move is forward. Bend to a right angle, hold for ten, and return. Move very slowly, feeling the stretch and the contraction. When you have done all three moves, bring your arms down to your side and relax. Sense the feeling of relaxation. Repeat the entire sequence five times.

Figure 15.8
Standing Trunk
Bend (final part)

Wall Reach, Sky Reach, Shoulder Roll, Back Reach, Shoulder Elevation

Chances are you have noticed in yourself or others that, after hours of writing or other deskwork, the natural tendency is to try to stretch out those cramped fingers, elbows, and shoulders. It is a natural reaction, but most people start too late. First of all, they should have prepared themselves better, and second, they should have stopped more frequently and stretched before cramps developed. That is the purpose of this set of exercises. The emphasis is on the relaxation that follows the recoil of the stretch. Sense it, and sense the difference between that feeling and muscle tension.

The first exercise in this group is the wall reach (see **Figure 15.9**), which is done in the standing position. Stand in front of a wall (the wall is not pictured so the arms can be seen) so that your outstretched arms just reach the wall. Place the palms of your hands against the wall. Next, step back about six inches. Extending your arms primarily from the shoulder, reach for the wall. At the same time, spread your fingers and extend them backward. When you make contact with the wall, your shoulder, elbow, wrist, and finger joints should be at full extension and stretch. Hold the stretch for a count of five and return. Repeat five times.

The next one, the sky reach (see **Figure 15.10**), is very similar except that your arms are outstretched over your head. At full reach pause, then with shoulder movement reach a few inches farther, almost as if you were taking something from a shelf just inches out of your reach or as if you were reaching for the sky. The movement is in the

Figure 15.9
Wall Reach

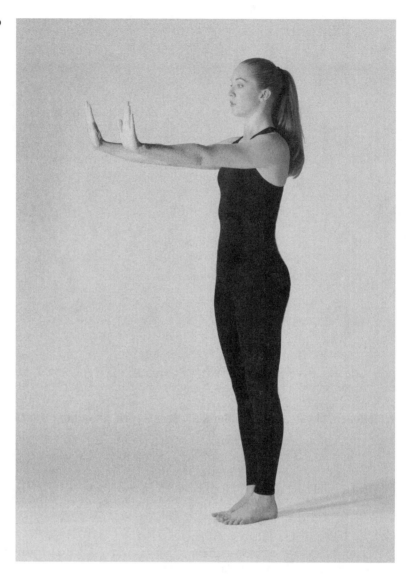

shoulder, so be sure not to rise onto your toes. At maximal extension, hold for a count of five and return to rest. Repeat five times.

While you are standing, do the third exercise, the shoulder roll (see **Figure 15.11**). Clasp your hands behind your back. The objective is to roll your shoulders by first dropping them to the lowest possible point, rolling them back, then up in a shoulder shrug, and then forward before they are lowered once again. Complete five circles and return to rest. Visualize this as a roll to the back as is pictured and then reverse the direction and slowly roll forward to the starting position.

Figure 15.10
Sky Reach

Figure 15.11
Shoulder Roll

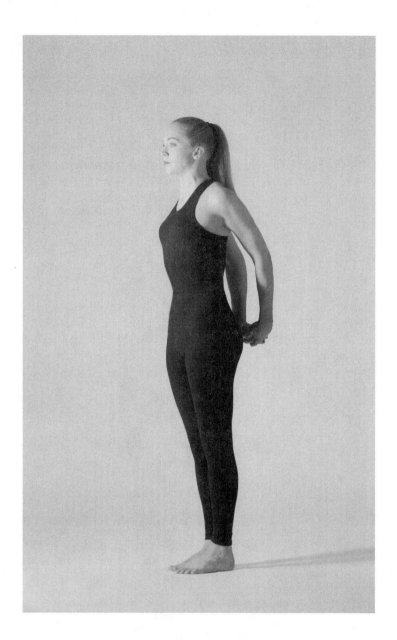

The next exercise, the back reach (see **Figure 15.12**), can be done while stand-ing or while sitting if the back of the chair is not high. Raise your arms above your head and clasp your hands together. Then bend your arms back so that your hands touch the back of your neck. Pause and then stretch so that your hands touch a point farther down your back. Hold the extreme position for a count of five, then rest. Repeat five times.

Figure 15.12
Back Reach

Figure 15.13
Shoulder
Elevation

The last exercise, the shoulder elevation (see **Figure 15.13**), is done while either sitting on the floor or standing. Clasp your hands behind your back, allowing them to rest comfortably against your buttocks. Keeping your back straight, raise your arms as high as possible. Hold in the extreme position for a count of five and return to the resting position, but do not unclasp your hands. Feel the stretch in your shoulders, elbows, and wrists. Feel the relaxation as you return to rest. Repeat five times.

Trunk Bends and Twists

The first exercise in this series is like the standing trunk bend but instead uses the arms for support to allow for more bend at the waist and is commonly called the triangle or deep side bend (see **Figure 15.14**). Stand with your feet shoulder width apart, legs straight.

Figure 15.14 Triangle

The first motion will be a side bend, first to the left. Place your left arm on your thigh or if you can, the left knee. The right arm is up in the air, elbow straight beside your head, and acts as a weight to allow you to bend farther than in the side bend. Bend your trunk to the left. Go as far as possible. Try to achieve a right angle to your lower body. Go only as far as you can, and, when there, hold for a count of ten, then return to an erect position. Now repeat to the right. Hold for a count of ten and return. Feel the stretch in your side about belt level. Feel the relaxation as you return to rest. Repeat five times. This position is usually learned with the bend-side hand on the midthigh and/or knee, and in the more advanced position the bend-side hand can go as low as the midcalf or even the ankle.

Figure 15.15 Spinal Twist

The next exercise is another trunk stretch known as the twist or spinal twist (see **Figure 15.15**). Sit on the floor. Bend your right leg and place your right foot over your left leg on the outside of your left knee. Place your left hand over your right knee and leg to brace yourself against. Now twist your body to the right and look behind you with your head slightly down so as not to get too much upper twist in the neck. Place your right hand on the floor behind you for support as you twist. Feel the stretch in your trunk and lower back. Go only as far as you can, and, when there, hold for a count of ten, and return to a forward-looking position. Now repeat to the left. Hold for a count of ten and return. Move very slowly, feeling the stretch and the contraction. If sitting on the floor is difficult or painful, this exercise can be accomplished while sitting in a straight chair without arms. You can place one leg over the other or not. Either way, use the arm on the opposite leg or knee for leverage. Use the chair version for relief while sitting in class or at your computer.

The third position in this series is another trunk twist, this time using the weight of your leg to allow you to achieve a good trunk stretch. It is called simply the leg over or leg over twist (see **Figure 15.16**). Lie on your back and relax for a minute. Raise your right leg to a bended knee for a second then straight up in air. If you were standing, it would be a high-kick position. Keeping your shoulders on the floor, arms outstretched, move the raised right leg over the left leg, which is still on the floor, as far as you can with the object of trying to touch your right foot on the floor without allowing your

Figure 15.16 Leg Over Twist

right arm and shoulder to rise off the floor. Go only as far as you can without allowing your right shoulder to rise. Hold for a count of ten or fifteen using the weight of your leg to twist your trunk and feel the stretch in your right side and lower back. Return to the central position with both legs on the floor and rest for a few seconds, then repeat to the left side. Move very slowly, feeling the stretch. When you have completed five to each side, lie still for a minute and feel the tension relief in your lower back.

SUMMARY

Strength, flexibility, balance, and reduction of muscle tension are the rewards of stretching. Hatha yoga is an ancient system of body positions and exercises to promote physical and mental harmony. Yoga is also a technique to quiet the mind. Consider the following points:

- Even the beginner can obtain positive results.
- These exercises are called stretch relaxation because the stretch phase eliminates tension and promotes relaxation.

- As with neuromuscular relaxation, learn to feel the tension during the work phase (in this case, the stretch) and then learn to focus on the relaxation that follows.

- Learning to feel the tension serves as a warning system to signal when shortened, tense muscles need attention.

- Set realistic goals, moving along at your own pace to avoid pain and injury.

- As with all the techniques in this book, there are immediate results and long-term benefits.

- The long-term benefits are a result of conditioning the body to be more relaxed, thus making it more difficult to become stressed in the first place.

- With practice the body will become conditioned to the relaxation response, and this will become your "state of being."

SOURCES CITED

Anderson, B., Pearl, B., Burke, B., Galloway, J., and Anderson, J. (2006). Getting back in shape: 32 workout programs for lifelong fitness. Bollnas, CA: Shelter Publications.

Grieco, C. (2002). PNF stretching-training tips. *American Fitness,* July–August.

Muni, S. R. (1994). *Awakening life force.* St. Paul, MN: Llewellyn.

Phillips, K. (2002). *The spirit of yoga.* Hauppauge, NY: Barrons Educational Series.

Sheikh, A. A., ed. (1984). *Imagination and healing.* New York: Wiley.

Trechsel, J. G., and Yee, R. (2002). *A morning cup of yoga.* Birmingham, AL: Crane Hill Publishers.

Weller, S. (1995). *Yoga therapy.* London: Thorsons.

Yee, R. (2002). *Yoga: The poetry of the body.* New York: St. Martin's Press.

Journal Entry 15

Measuring Progress

How do you know you are making progress? Figure out a way to quantify it. We suggest three measures:

1. How close to the advanced position can you attain?

2. How difficult is it for you?

3. How relaxed or tension-free does the muscle of joint feel?

   Pick three or four of the positions or exercises from this chapter or any other book. Write them in the space above the tables below. In the table columns 1, 2, 3, record a number from 1 to 10 that describes the level of attainment of the position and how you felt doing it. Chart your progress for a week.

1. How close to the advanced position can you attain?

   1 = beginning level; 10 = advanced

2. How difficult is it for you?

   1 = very difficult; 10 = easy

3. How relaxed or tension-free does the muscle of joint feel?

   1 = very tense; 10 = very relaxed

Position or exercise:

Day	1	1–10	2	1–10	3	1–10	comments
1							
2							
3							
4							
5							
6							
7							

Position or exercise:

Day	1	1–10	2	1–10	3	1–10	comments
1							
2							
3							
4							
5							
6							
7							

Position or exercise:

Day	1	1–10	2	1–10	3	1–10	comments
1							
2							
3							
4							
5							
6							
7							

Position or exercise:

Day	1	1–10	2	1–10	3	1–10	comments
1							
2							
3							
4							
5							
6							
7							

 Write a positive word or short phrase about sensing the stress within you that will be useful to you in future situations.

CHAPTER 16

Meditation

One of the most important components of a program of stress management is the conditioning of the mind to reduce internal arousal. Meditation is a time-honored technique for going within and moving beyond thoughts and habits to a quiet centeredness.

Meditation teaches us to let go of the past, let go of the future, and just "be" in the present. Our childhood enculturation often conditions us to be "human doings"; we are rewarded for doing things, keeping busy—especially doing things that please others. Rarely do we learn to tap into the deep essence of our personal being. It is as though we are hyperactive children reacting to all stimuli coming in, without the ability to damp out unimportant messages. Like the hyperactive child, the undisciplined mind jumps from worries about yesterday to fears of tomorrow, from desires to demands to planning, all the while judging, complaining, and comparing. Meditation disciplines the mind to tune out the tensions and pressures from others and from ourselves. It tunes us in to our own centeredness, which is the basis of our physical, mental, emotional, and spiritual health.

One of the main benefits of meditation is an increase in one's resistance to negativity, which results in a reduction of one's reactivity to former stressors. Practiced meditators learn to reduce the surface chatter of the mind, the constant thinking, planning, remembering, and fantasizing that occupy the mind's every waking second and keep the mind firmly implanted in the physical matters of living. As mind chatter diminishes, so do one's acquired defenses of physical and psychological survival. Anxiety is reduced, and thus arousal is reduced as both the body and mind achieve the quiet and peace natural to a self-transcendent state of consciousness. Individuals come to meditation for many multilayered reasons—for instance, cultivate ideals such as wisdom and love, to slow down restless minds, to handle problems that have mental or emotional components, to reconnect the body and spirit, to control a mind filled with uncontrollable fear or anger, to better understand behaviors, to meet fellow seekers, to open the heart and awaken the mind, to realize God, and to become enlightened (Das 1999).

The art of meditation is the ability to maintain a state of passive concentration in which alertness and control are maintained but tension is not produced. The meditator is in complete control of the experience.

Brain Waves

In the meditative state, one may become aware of subtle thoughts, energy, and creative intelligence. It is an intended process that takes thought, preparation, and practice. The meditator is thus left with feelings of creativity and accomplishment and a generally positive feeling about the activity.

Meditation can result a more relaxed, quiet mind or in profound reductions in mental and physical arousal. The question everyone asks is: How do you know you are meditating and that something is happening that is different from just sitting there quietly? Biofeedback was previously discussed in relation to reducing muscle tension. Any organ in the body that emits electrical energy can be monitored and examples of the electromyography (muscles) and electrocardiogram (heart) were given. As biofeedback became more popular, researchers and clinicians started using physiological monitoring to verify what was happening in the body as individuals meditated. They found a marked reduction in the activity of most bodily systems governed by the autonomic system. During meditation one usually feels a heaviness or numbness in the extremities and a sense of relaxation and calm. The electromyography (EMG) measured changes in muscle tension and verified that muscles were in fact more relaxed. The electroencephalograph (EEG) measured brain waves and likewise verified changes in mental functioning. Because faster brain waves are generally associated with more active brain functioning and slower brain waves are generally associated with more tranquil states, one would expect meditation to be associated with slower brain waves. EEG studies of experienced students of meditation show that brain waves are slowed during meditation, suggesting that the meditative state and a low-brain-wave state are synonymous.

As one might expect, with millions of cells simultaneously performing thousands of functions, it is impossible for the entire brain to be producing activity at any one frequency at any given time. Thus, the EEG shows a complex pattern of mixed wave-forms occurring at varying frequencies. However, at any given point, there appears to be a dominant frequency emitted from a specific section of the brain, and the analysis of this dominant frequency has become an important area of study as researchers have begun to associate brain-wave patterns with cognitive functioning, emotion, and states of consciousness (see **Figure 16.1**).

The third-slowest brain wave is called the alpha wave. It is a slow, synchronized wave, which means that it occurs in rhythmical fashion indicative of a predictable, non-fluctuating, nonprocessing state. Everyone has alpha waves. When you close your eyes, alpha bursts begin to appear with greater frequency. It is more difficult to remain in alpha for any length of time than to produce it in spurts, but one can be trained to do so.

Subjective reports of the feelings that accompany the alpha state indicate that it is an awake, alert, but calm, restful, and peaceful state. However, most (but certainly not all) authorities in the field agree that alpha waves characterize a state of consciousness free from ongoing personality-involved thought processes. This relative absence of

Brain Wave	Feeling
Beta 14–50 cps	Anticipatory, logical, rational, worried, investigative, challenged, in "flow"
Alpha 8–13 cps	At ease, neutral, sluggish, pleasant, floating
Theta 4–7 cps	Ambiguous, fuzzy, internal, vacillating, unreal, dreamlike, in reverie
Delta 3 cps and below	Sleep

1 Sec.

Figure 16.1 Brain-Wave states and associated feelings

sustained thought pattern is responsible for the relaxed feeling. As has been mentioned many times, a large part of stress is triggered or augmented by personality-involved arousal thoughts; these thoughts are not present during the typical alpha state. Feeding information back to an individual about the general activity of the brain promotes the ability to decrease potentially stress-producing thought patterns.

Another intriguing state of consciousness is associated with theta waves. The dreamlike reverie associated with the production of slowed theta waves has been likened to an advanced meditation experience. This state has been described as being highly creative, producing integrative mental pictures and a low-stress inner awareness that is dissociated from the outside world.

Mind and Life Investigations into Meditation

In Chapter 5 we reported the investigations of the Mind and Life Institute meeting on Destructive Emotions and the exciting possibilities brought to light by leading scientists, the Dalai Lama, and other Buddhist contemplatives. As noted in the Destructive Emotions conference, we now must accept the fact of neuroplasticity—that we have the ability to grow new brain cells, even when we're old and gray. This bit of knowledge holds all kinds of potential, and it has been an interesting research trail that leads us to perhaps the ultimate use of neurogenesis (generating new brain cells): using our minds to change our brains. No one tells this saga better than Sharon Begley (2007), a noted science writer who attended this conference.

Begley presents the case that research as recent as the 1980's and 1990's explained that when experimental subjects constantly used certain fingers to manipulate something (such as a blind person reading Braille with their dominant index finger or a concert violinist pressing the strings time and again), the corresponding part of their brain (motor cortex in charge of fingers) had more neurons. In addition, research found that the areas of the brain that respond with neurogenesis do so due to attention. If you are learning a new skill with your hands and happen to have music playing in the background, your motor cortex area that control the hands will respond with neurogenesis, but your auditory cortex does not. So here is a valuable piece of information—pay attention to what you wish to have happen.

Once the connection between behavior and brain change was thoroughly established, the Dalai Lama proposed a question to science that went something like this, "Is it possible that the mind and brain are different entities? Might the mind work on the brain to change it?" The answer from science at the time was, as you would expect, "No. Everything we do is structure and function. Brain cells respond with neurohormones, the result of which is ultimately directed by cell DNA."

According to Begley, research then found that compassionate meditation, mindful meditation, and certain cognitive behavior techniques (all of which use the mind to alter behavior) could ameliorate conditions such as obsessive-compulsive disorder and depression. Meditation is now a common treatment for stress, pain, and other chronic diseases, and various meditative approaches are being rigorously studied by NIH-supported clinical trials and research projects. A true boon to recent neurophysiological research is the functional magnetic resonance imaging (fMRI) machine that, while entirely non-invasive, can map exactly which areas of the brain are being used or stimulated under various experimental conditions, including meditation.

After putting enough highly-skilled Buddhist meditators (each with hundreds of hours of practice) through the fMRI tube and finding that the left prefrontal cortex of these individuals were more developed than science had ever before seen, it became apparent that they had "built" their brains that way through meditation. Not only was the left prefrontal cortex (PFC) larger than usual, the corresponding right PFC was smaller. Further study found that the left PFC was stimulated when the meditator was enjoying a state of happiness, which diminished the stimulation in the corresponding right brain area. When the right area was stimulated, it evoked feelings of anxiety, fear, and general unhappiness. The balance between these two areas has been dubbed the "happiness quotient."

Bottom line, ready-to-use information: every one of us can increase our happiness quotient by focusing on mindful, compassionate meditation. The work (if that's what you want to call it) could be compared to your cardiovascular fitness—you have to work at it and keep it up as part of your lifestyle.

Types of Meditation

Perhaps the greatest source of our stress problems is our extreme attachment to our senses, thoughts, and imagination. Peace can be greatly enhanced by reducing these attachments, directing our awareness inward, and transcending the incessant bombardment of the consciousness in order to experience a quiet body, a subtle mind, and a unified spirit.

These are the simple goals of meditation, which have motivated millions of seekers for centuries. Although the goals are simple, the fundamentals of meditation are often misunderstood, for meditation itself is difficult to define. Meditation is not a physiological state, nor is it a specific psychological state. Meditation is not East as opposed to West; it is not now as opposed to then; and it is not the domain of any organized religion or prayer. It is a practice universal to all who wish to connect to their quiet mind and their spirit. Meditation is so basic that it has transcended time, culture, races, religions, and ideologies. It is so simple that millions have used it, yet so advanced that to many it represents the highest state of being—the living condition that most closely approximates the tranquil, spiritual state.

Meditation can be best understood as a state of mind, of consciousness, or of spirit. But it is most often defined in terms of an act or a technique. There are numerous meditation techniques embodied in different philosophies. To some people meditation is intended to be a central component in one complete style of living; to others and to us here in this context, a few of its techniques have been successfully extrapolated for the purposes of relaxation and tension reduction.

The philosophical goals of meditation are difficult to achieve without some training. Fortunately, if you are interested, there are groups everywhere. The numerous meditation groups that have arisen throughout the world usually are differentiated more by their subtle differences in technique rather than their overarching philosophies. Goldstein (2003) has written that each discipline can practice with individual integrity and come together in the consideration of their unifying philosophy, which is weaving together the methods of mindfulness, the motivation of compassion, and the liberating wisdom of nonclinging. These three core concepts are not the property of any one group, but are qualities in our own minds.

Concentration

Common to all forms of meditation are concentration and the closely related techniques of contemplation and mental repetition. Concentration here implies attention to one subject and thus control of the mind's usual habit of flipping from one subject to another. A mind discipline through selective attention reduces ego consciousness, and nondirected attention heightens awareness and is thought to release energy. Concentrating on physical processes—for example, the rhythm of one's breathing or internal sensations, such as the mystical "third eye"—is used in several disciplines. One type of yoga, Kundalini yoga, theorizes potential energy coiled up in the nervous system that can be awakened by concentrating on the energy centers (chakras) that progress up the spine. Visual imagery is used in many practices, including focusing the mind's eye on a thousand-petaled lotus. Another popular practice is to concentrate on breathing by counting breaths while working to eliminate all other thoughts and feelings. When ten breaths are counted without losing the count, the mind is more ready to contemplate. Whatever the technique, to the masters, concentration of the mind away from the worries and cares of the personality is the only real freedom a person will ever experience (Dalai Lama and Cuther 1999; Surya Das 1999; Goldstein 1993).

A time-honored vehicle for concentrative meditation is the verbal or mental repetition of a word or sound called a **mantra**, meaning "hymn" or "calming sound." A mantra can be a single word, such as *mu* or *om,* a phrase from Holy Scripture, a name for a god, or specially selected words thought to be calming because of their resonance qualities. Using such words is the core element in the practice of the popular transcendental meditation (TM).

Words with "meaning" tend to elicit many associations. Although the Sanskrit mantras are meaningless for most people, they have deep meaning for Eastern practitioners. For example, *om* ("I am one, we are one") is known in Eastern cultures as the universal mantra that is believed to give cosmic power. In the meditative traditions of Judaism, Christianity, and Islam, the repetition of God's name has mystical meaning. Although the Sanskrit mantras may not be understood literally, they can still have meaning.

Benson (1992) chose the word *one* as the mantra for his "relaxation response" because it is basically neutral and low in association value, but as a connotation of *om*, it can be meaningful for some people.

The "emotionality" of words used for meditation can induce either stress or relaxation depending on the words' associations and the effects they have on the involved individuals. In a physiological and psychological study, on a group given a choice of emotional or unemotional mantras for meditation, most subjects preferred the emotional words (such as *happy, garden, sail,* or *love*) to the neutral words (*om, one*) (Morse 1995). (Mantras will be discussed further in this chapter in the section "How to Meditate.")

Contemplation

Contemplation is closely related to concentration, the primary difference being that the object of contemplation (usually an external object, or mandala) is symbolic, and it is the significance rather than the object that becomes the focus. The Zen Buddhist koan, which is a question, puzzle, or riddle such as "What is the sound of one hand clapping?" has no answer. Rather, it is an artificial instrument to force an open mind and develop in students the Zen consciousness.

The same is true for Christian meditation that uses objects such as the crucifix, a picture or statue of a religious figure, or spiritual passages and prayers as a focus for contemplation as a means to consciousness of Christ. One of the more complete systems of Christian or religious meditation has been outlined by the Association for Research and Enlightenment, made up of the followers of the "Sleeping Prophet," Edgar Cayce. Cayce was adamant in his belief that contemplation should be only a means and not an end, and he quoted Jesus's warning in the Parable of the Displaced Demon, in which the evil spirits that were cast out of an empty mind quickly returned with other devils, leaving the man worse off than before. To Cayce, meditation was attuning the mental and physical body to its spiritual source, seeking to know the relationship to the Maker. There is no emptying in the mind-void sense, only emptying of that which hinders the creative forces from rising along the natural channels or centers. An example of these natural channels are the seven spiritual centers, or chakras, also recognized as being related to the endocrine glands, which in this case provide energy for psychic and religious experiences. Cayce additionally defined meditation as a prayer from within the inner self and made a distinction between prayer and meditation: prayer was external attunement, a pleading, a petition to the Holy Spirit; meditation was an internal attunement, a seeking to know one's relationship with God, an inpouring from the Holy Spirit. Cayce's form of meditation uses the Lord's Prayer as a focus for contemplation.

The contemplation techniques of Christian meditation are similar to those of other types in that they are employed to transcend one's daily cares and worries. The primary difference is in the focus of the contemplation. Contemplative meditation is for the purpose of contemplating what you desire to experience. You become relaxed and think of the spiritual state to which you aspire (Yogi 1995). Whatever the technique, though, the desired outcome is control of consciousness and direction of mind.

Meditation and the Reduction of Stress Arousal

The primary purposes of meditation—peace, enlightenment, and spiritual growth—cannot be obtained as long as the mind is in turmoil and the body is aroused. Thus, most meditative techniques have seemingly elaborate preparatory procedures designed to induce physical relaxation, and meditation itself quiets the mind. Relaxation, an indirect product of meditation, can be therapeutic in the treatment or prevention of stress-related disorders.

Even though meditation is thousands of years old and the physiological feats of meditation masters are legend, the "scientific" study of the body-mind processes of meditation is still quite new. Meditation became scientific when Wallace (1970) published the results of a study showing that the body significantly decreases its consumption of oxygen during meditation, thus producing a hypo-metabolic state (a slowing down of the body's processes). Wallace also found that the skin showed an increased resistance to the passage of an electrical current, which indicates decreased arousal of the autonomic nervous system. Additional findings from this study were a decrease in the lactate/ion concentration, another measure of decreased metabolism; a decrease in heart rate and cardiac output (quantity of blood pumped by the heart per minute), indicating a reduction in the heart's workload; a decrease in respiration rate; and an increase in the amount of time the brain emits slowed brain waves, indicating a more restful state. This restful state physiologically resembled sleep in many ways but was significantly different from it. The meditator was found to be in a restful state but was awake and alert and exhibited increased reaction time, improved coordination, and improved efficiency of perception and auditory ability. While these early studies were not the most rigorous in the literature, they did start the scientific inquiry into the link between meditation and the psychophysical process.

Later research both supported and refuted, at least to a degree, Wallace's early findings. This serves to point out the difficulty of such research, which is largely the result of subject variability and differences in meditation techniques. For example, variations in the length of the meditative session and experience of the meditator are extremely important. Obviously, the more one meditates, the greater should be one's ability to change psycho-physiological states. EEG records of meditation masters show a predominance of alpha and theta brain waves during meditation, which become more marked with years of practice; beginning meditators, on the other hand, show only slight changes in brain-wave patterns.

Another difficulty in research is the difference in the meditative state itself. As mentioned, meditation is not a unitary phenomenon but a series of states including quiet sitting, passive concentration, mental deautomatization or desynchronization, a neutral or mind-void state, and, especially in accomplished meditators, a brain-directed state.

As we have seen, stress arousal is a mind and body response to a particular psychosocial or environmental situation. Each situation produces an immediate stress response but may also leave a residual amount of tension in the body. Response to subsequent stressors is augmented by this leftover tension. As the day wears on, response over activity results from the inability to dissipate residual tension. The physiological relaxation experienced by the meditator is a short-term phenomenon, but the more the relaxation state is induced, the more carryover there is to the nonmeditative state. Meditation helps dissolve tension by quieting the mind's tendency toward "afterthoughts," which prolong the stress response and at least temporarily reduce the physical arousal of the organs. Thus each new stressful situation will produce a reaction sufficient to deal with that particular situation without the added effect of previous stress arousal. The longer one meditates, the more one's general state of arousal resembles the meditative state, and the more ongoing tensions most detrimental to the body are reduced. The accomplished meditator develops the ability to direct thoughts away from physical, mental, and emotional defense, the primary source of stress. The meditator experiences temporary transcendence, but just as the physiological state gradually becomes a stable trait, so can an individual learn to live a life of increased transcendence (Patel 1999).

A review of literature covering twenty five years, 500 scientific studies from 210 different universities in thirty five countries, in summary shows that meditation reduced stress, increased creativity, improved memory, increased energy, increased inner calm, reduced insomnia, increased happiness and self-esteem, reduced anxiety and depression, improved interpersonal relations, improved breathing, and promoted the appearance of younger biological age (Roth 1994).

How to Meditate

There are many types of meditation, each representing a variation in purpose and technique. The type presented in this section is thought to be the best suited for stress reduction, the easiest to learn, and the one most void of cultic, religious, and spiritual overtones. The technique is complete for the purpose of meditation; however, it can also serve as an introduction to more specific types because they all have at least this technique as their core experience. What follows is both explicit instruction and clarifying explanation. Read it through first as an academic discussion, perhaps making a short note next to each numbered item that will serve as your "how to guide" when you later try it for yourself.

1. The first essential element is a quiet environment—both external and internal. A quiet room away from others who are not also meditating is essential, especially while you are learning. Put out the dog, cat, or whatever. Unplug the phone or find a room without one and turn off the cell phone. Generally, do whatever you can to reduce external noise. If you cannot completely eliminate the noise, as is often the case in busy households or in college dorms, use earplugs or, play a CD or tape of soft instrumental sounds or any of the numerous environmental sounds that have been commercially recorded. Many enterprising people take their tape recorders to the woods to record the sound of the wind singing in the trees, a mountain stream, or just the birds at dawn. The sounds of the waves at the seashore also make an excellent background for meditation. In addition to blocking out noise, such sounds help promote relaxation because they usually bring back memories of pleasant feelings.

2. Next, work on quieting your internal environment. One way is to reduce muscle tension. Remember that it is practically impossible to induce a meditative state while the reticular activating system is bombarding the cortex with sensory signals emitted from the muscles. Muscle tension represents one of the largest obstacles to successful

meditation. Spend some time, if needed, relaxing your muscles. You may want to choose one or several of the relaxation exercises from Chapters 12 through 15 and work on the area that is most troublesome for you.

One way to reduce excess muscle tension is to sit comfortably. You may not feel like a real meditator unless you use the cross-legged position; if you desire this position, sit on the floor with a pillow under your buttocks. In this position, the legs are crossed so that the left foot rests on the right thigh and the right foot rests on the left thigh. Unless you have practiced this position or are naturally flexible, you will find this uncomfortable, however. If you really want to sit on the floor, a simple tailor's position (sitting cross-legged) will suffice. If you don't mind being too Western, sit in a straight-backed, comfortable chair, feet on the floor, legs not crossed, hands resting on the thighs, and fingers slightly open, not interlocked.

You should sit still, but remember that meditation is not a trance; if you are uncomfortable or feel too much pressure on any one spot, move. If you itch, scratch. Do not assume a tight, inflexible position or attitude. Relax. Do not lie down or support your head or you will tend to fall asleep. Keep your head, neck, and spine in a straight vertical line. A small but significant amount of muscular effort is needed to maintain this posture, and this effort helps prevent sleep from occurring.

If your shoes, belt, bra, tie, or collar are too tight, loosen them. The goal is to diminish sensory input to the central nervous system. Most people like to have a clock where it can be seen at a glance to reduce the anxiety that arises from the feeling that more time is being spent than was anticipated. Twenty to thirty minutes is the standard amount of time spent per session, although five minutes is better than none. Although not recommended for the first few sessions, occasionally interspersing a one-hour session has been reported to be most profound and relaxing.

3. Before you start, relax and stretch your neck muscles. Move your chin toward your chest, and then back in place. Repeat this three times. Move your head toward your back. Do this three times. Rotate your head clockwise three complete rotations. Repeat these counterclockwise three times. Now relax your neck. Allow your head to drop slightly forward. This is more comfortable than slightly backward.

Sit quietly. *Close your eyes.* Notice immediately how that simple movement quiets the environment. Most of our sensory input enters through the eyes; the simple act of closing the eyes does much to quiet the mind. The ambient noise is reduced, the eyes are closed, muscle tension is reduced, and tactile sensory stimulation is at a minimum. The external and physical environment of the body should now be quiet.

Now concentrate on *quieting the mind.* Foremost in this effort is developing a tranquil or passive attitude. Even if meditation is done for a specific reason, such as to reduce hypertension, cut down on smoking, or increase self-assuredness, you must not dwell on the outcome of meditation or even on how well that particular meditation is proceeding. Such thoughts represent an ongoing competitive type of thought process that the meditation is trying to suppress. The body's external physical environment should now be quiet.

4. Spend ten minutes in "neutral," a period of not controlling or focusing your thoughts. Concentrate on quieting the mind. Foremost in this effort is developing a tranquil or passive attitude. Flow with whatever you may feel, and stay calm with relaxed interest. Touch with your thoughts whatever comes to your mind, and then let it go.

Direct your thoughts away from self, away from the parts you play in the stories of your mind. If you have music or environmental sounds playing, direct your attention to the sound. Float with the sound like a cloud, white and fluffy against a blue sky . . . like a leaf floating down a stream, floating, and twirling around the rocks, over a waterfall. You may notice some warmth or heaviness in your arms or legs. This is an indication of muscles in those areas beginning to relax. You might also notice your head dropping with the relaxation of your neck muscles. Your breathing is probably slower and a bit deeper.

For a moment, concentrate on your breathing. As you breathe in, think "in," then let the air out and think "out." You should breathe in through your nose, thinking "in," and breathe out through your mouth, thinking "out," but do not force the expiration . . . just open your mouth and let the air out. Think in . . . out . . . in . . . out . . . Now each time you breathe out, count the breath. Count ten consecutive breaths without missing a count. If you happen to miss one, start over. When you get to ten, start at one again. Concentrate, anticipate the breath, and block all other thoughts from your mind. Concentrating on breathing is a means of focusing attention inward away from the self in relation to the external world. It is an example of a mental device, a way of directing the mind.

Most meditative techniques utilize some form of mental device to direct consciousness away from logical, cause-and-effect, goal-directed thought processes. The device may be spiritual contemplation, the contemplation of geometric designs, concentration on a body process such as breathing, an internal light, or an external sound, as in biofeedback , but most often the device is a mantra (as described below).

A mantra is used to quiet the mind. Think of the mind as a lake, choppy on the top but calm below. The choppy waters of a lake are caused by the external environment, the wind. Likewise there are reflective thoughts churning around top layer of the brain (the cortex) in response to external stimulation of your senses, your memory, and your thought habits. Concentrating on the mantra directs your attention toward it. But because the word has no denotative or connotative meaning, stories are not formed, memory and imagination are not stimulated, and arousal does not occur. Automatic brain function breaks down, and you drift into an altered state of consciousness. As in the quiet depths of the lake, the quiet, subtler state of mind emerges into consciousness. Gradually, the concentration on the mantra will also disappear and you will remain in a neutral state until a new thought pops into your consciousness, as sporadic thoughts often do. At that point, you can consciously void the thought just by telling yourself, "No, I do not want to think about it," or you can go back to the mantra, or you can direct the thought to a pattern of nonstressful thinking consistent with the particular type of meditation you are practicing.

5. During the concentration part of your meditation period, you may wish to repeat a word, idea, or phrase that depicts peace, beauty, or a spiritual ideal for you. "Om" is the universal mantra. More than just spoken, it is softly chanted aloud on each exhalation (as "aaaaaaooooommmmm") at your individual pitch and tonality. Also during the concentration part of your meditation, you may wish to use a visual focus rather than using sound. A candle flame, a picture that produces serenity for you, or a mandala may be a good eyes-open focus. Whatever visual focus you use, be sure that it does not offer your left hemisphere food for thought, or your mind will be busy analyzing, planning, and evaluating. A mandala (a simple geometric pattern) is used for meditation because the left hemisphere quickly tires of the simple pattern while the rest of the mind continues to focus on it. Circles with a dot in the center, an equilateral triangle, and a square have been used for centuries as meditation aids. Some meditators use visual imagery (eyes closed) as discussed in Chapter 14 as their concentrative focus.

In all cases, you are teaching your mind not to think about or form stories around sporadic thoughts. You are eliminating a bad habit acquired over the course of your life. This method is a form of reeducation of the mind and the central nervous system. We can make an analogy between this practice and dieting. Dieting can help you lose weight, and, you hope, the practice of dieting may help you to develop new eating habits to lessen the chance of becoming overweight again. Similarly, meditation will help make you calm, and the practice of meditation can help develop new thought habits that should diminish stress arousal in the future.

Breathe softly, but now do not concentrate on your breathing. Repeat one of the mantras aloud. Say it over and over. Each time say it more softly until it becomes just a mental thought with no muscular action involved. Pace yourself, gradually lengthening the interval between thoughts of the mantra. Allow the mantra to repeat itself in your mind. Do not force it; just let it flow. Gradually the mantra will fade, and your mind will remain quiet. The quiet will occasionally be broken by sporadic thoughts. Let them come, experience them, go with them until you feel that you are controlling them. Do not allow them to become fantasies or daydreams because daydreams usually involve ego arousal. When this happens, stop the thought process and go back to the mantra.

Remember that meditation is a feeling, a state of mind. It is not simply a technique; it is not saying the mantra. Sit quietly for ten to fifteen minutes and meditate. Keep your movements to a minimum, but if you are uncomfortable, move; if you are worried about time, look at a clock, or the discomfort and anxiety will prevent your full attainment of the meditative state.

6. When you finish meditating, do not be in too much of a hurry to get up. Open your eyes, and stretch a little. Contract your muscles and reactivate yourself slowly. Having at least temporarily altered your emotional reactivity, continue your day with renewed inner capacity for meeting the day's challenges.

One of the greatest obstacles preventing the full attainment of the meditative state is usually the lack of physical and/or mental quietness. Physical quietness is the easier of the two to surmount. Quiet rooms, dim lights, closing the eyes, working to relax the muscles, sitting comfortably, and loosening the clothes all tend to diminish sensory stimulation. You should also eliminate the stimulation that can come from too much food and drugs (including caffeine and nicotine) by abstaining from either before meditating. Meditation is a discipline that necessitates having one's faculties at full command; drugs have no place in the practice.

Mental quietness is more difficult to attain, especially at first. But do not be discouraged. It took many years to develop your current thought processes, and they will not change overnight. Many people are uncomfortable with quietness. They have been so bombarded with stimulation every waking minute since the cradle that they have not learned how to sit still by themselves and simply think of nothing. When one finally does sit down and seek quiet, the mind is filled with: "The car needs a tune-up." "What time will John be home?" "Should I buy that new computer?" But as you learn to disregard these thoughts, they will gradually diminish and finally disappear.

Following is a summary of the six steps in the process of meditation:

1. Quiet your external environment. Put the ringer to the "off" position on your telephone, play some soft classical or other soothing instrumental music (use earphones if you need to), and so on.

2. Quiet your internal environment. Relax your muscles. Sit with your spine straight, hands folded in your lap, then take some deep breaths and relax your muscles.

3. Sit quietly. Close your eyes. Before you open yourself to meditation, extend a protecting envelope of energy around yourself. Some visualize a white-light energy field eight feet in diameter around themselves.

4. Spend ten minutes in a concentrative exercise to clear the mind, to still the active left hemisphere of the brain, and to direct your energy. Open your palms and spend ten minutes in "neutral," a period of not controlling or focusing your thoughts.

5. During the concentration part of your meditation period, you may wish to repeat a word, idea, or phrase that depicts peace, beauty, or a spiritual ideal for you. Flow with whatever you may feel, and stay calm with relaxed interest. Touch whatever comes to you and let it go.

6. When you finish meditating open your eyes, and stretch a little. Contract your muscles and reactivate yourself slowly. Get up and get on with your other activities.

Mental quietness is at the core of meditation. There are numerous books such as *Insight Meditation: A Step-by-Step Course on How to Meditate,* by Salzberg and Goldstein (2002), which cover in-depth various techniques to achieve mental quietness and master the practice of meditation.

Mindfulness and Insight Meditation

The previous meditation exercise is an example of the technique popularized by movements such as transcendental meditation and utilizes concentration or similar practices as a point of focus to stabilize the mind, reduce distractions, and maintain nonstressful attention in an attempt to promote the relaxation response (Benson 1992).

Another school of meditation practice is called **mindfulness** or **insight meditation.** In the practice of mindfulness, you begin by utilizing the concentration meditation to produce calmness and stability, and then you introduce an observing focus as well. When thoughts or feelings come up in your mind, you don't ignore or suppress them, nor do you analyze or judge their content. Rather, you simply note any thoughts as they occur as best you can and observe them intentionally but nonjudgmentally, moment by moment, as events in the field of your awareness (Kabat-Zinn 1993).

Deeply buried in the mind lies a mental mechanism that accepts what the mind perceives as beautiful and pleasant experiences and rejects those experiences that are perceived as painful. This mechanism gives rise to states of mind that cause stress (what we have previously described as sufferings, emotional states such as fear, anger, greed, envy, lust, hatred, aversion, and jealousy). We choose to avoid these hindrances not because they are evil in the normal sense of the word but because they are compulsive and because, once attention is focused on them, it tends to remain fixated in feedback loops that never lead to problem solving, only to stress arousal. Conscious thought has the habit of adding to our experience and of loading us down with concepts and ideas, plans and worries, fears and fantasies. Mindfulness teaches us to see things as they really are. It adds nothing to perception and it subtracts nothing. It distorts nothing. It is bare attention and just looks at whatever comes up.

Paradoxically, noting thoughts that come and go in your mind can lead you to feel less caught up in them and give you a deeper perspective on your reaction to everyday stress and pressures. By observing your thoughts and emotions as if you had taken a step back from them, you can see much more clearly what is actually on your mind and how you react emotionally to those thoughts.

The key to mindfulness meditation is not so much what you choose to focus on but the quality of the awareness that you bring to each moment. It is very important that it be nonjudgmental—more of a silent witnessing, a detached observing. Observing without judging, moment by moment, helps you see what is on your mind without editing or censoring it, without intellectualizing it or getting lost in your own incessant thinking. The goal of mindfulness is for you to be more aware, more in touch with life and with whatever is happening in your own body and mind at the time it is happening—that is, in the present.

The goal is to resist the impulse to try to escape the unpleasantness; instead, you attempt to see it clearly as it is and accept it because it is already present in this moment. It is psychologically impossible for us to objectively observe what is going on within us if we do not at the same time accept the occurrence of our various states of mind. This is especially true with unpleasant states of mind. In order to observe our own fear, we must accept the fact that we are afraid. We can't examine our own depression without accepting it fully. The same is true for irritation, agitation, frustration, and all those other uncomfortable emotional states. You can't examine something fully if you are busy rejecting its existence. Whatever experience we may be having, mindfulness just accepts it. It is simply another of life's occurrences, just another thing to be aware of. Without judging it there is no pride, no shame, no self-deprecation, and nothing personal at stake—what is there, is there.

With this explanation in mind, sit comfortably and quietly. Close your eyes and allow your mind to be quiet, yet alert. As thoughts arise in your consciousness, accept them and concentrate on how your body is responding to the thoughts. Concentrate but don't manipulate the thoughts. Just be aware of your thoughts, your feelings, and your body's reaction. Resist the temptation to judge the experience as pleasant or unpleasant, worthwhile or worthless. Gradually the experience loses its emotional valence, and you begin to break the bond between the thought and the emotion. The training or conditioning has started. Continued practice can result in this detachment becoming your automatic choice for experiencing both the ups and downs of life with a more even keel.

The Need for Practice

Meditation is a skill you must practice if you are to enjoy its benefits. Meditation is not difficult to learn. However, many people are hindered by lack of confidence in their ability to meet their expectation of what meditation is and can do for them. Meditation is not so simple that mere ritual will overcome the hyperactivity of a mind planning, scheming about, thinking about, and reacting to the distractions to which we are all subjected. One cannot go full steam one minute and be tranquil the next. Preparation for quietness is an essential step.

Meditation must be practiced, but one cannot labor at it. You cannot force yourself into transcendence. The key phrase in learning meditation is "let go." Some may be tempted to withdraw from life through meditation. The purpose of meditation, however, is to enhance the experience of life, not to be a vehicle for withdrawing from it. Meditative tranquility trains the mind to allow active participation in an active life without unnecessary stress. Meditation is not a substitute for living.

SUMMARY

Meditation is one of the most powerful tools in the stress management program. It epitomizes the connection between mind and body and requires practice to master the art of mental alertness and passive concentration. Consider the following points:

- Meditation descended from ancient yoga and Zen Buddhism.
- Modern meditative practices represent a mixture of philosophies and techniques.
- Meditative techniques heave two common goals: a quiet body and a quiet mind.
- Meditation reduces the activity of most physical systems as well as emotions.
- Meditation involves the ability to attain a relaxed, passive state of concentration maintaining alertness and control.
- Meditation can relax and reduce immediate tension, but the real value comes from conditioning the mind to "live" in that relaxed state.

SOURCES CITED

Arrien, A. (1987). *Cross-cultural healing practices.* Joy Lake Conference. Reno, NV.

Begley, S. (2007). Train your mind, change your brain. New York: Ballantine.

Benson, H. (1992). *The relaxation response.* New York: Avon.

Dalai Lama, and Cutler, H. (1999). *The art of happiness.* New York: Riverhead.

Das, S. (1999). *Awakening to the sacred.* New York: Broadway Books.

Goldstein, J. (1993). *Insight meditation.* Boston: Shambala.

Goldstein, J. (2003). *One Dharma: The emerging Western Buddhism.* San Francisco: Harper San Francisco.

Kabat-Zinn, H. G. J. (1993). Mindfulness in plain English. In *Mind/Body Medicine,* eds. D. Goleman and J. Gurin, 31–39. New York: Consumer Report Books.

Morse, R. (1995). Love and hate: Their many guises and stressful effects. *Stress Medicine,* 11, 177–97.

Patel, C. (1999). Yoga-based therapy. In *Principles and practice of stress management,* eds. P. M. Lehrer and R. L. Woolfolk, 72–81. New York: Guilford.

Roth, R. (1994). *Transcendental meditation.* New York: Primus.

Salzberg, S., and Goldstein, J. (2002). *Insight meditation: A step-by-step course on how to meditate.* Louisville CO: Sounds True Inc.

Wallace, R. K. (1970). Physiological effects of transcendental meditation. *Science,* 167, 1751–54.

Yogi, M. M. (1995). *The science of being and the art of living: Transcendental Meditation.* New York: Meridian Books.

Journal Entry 16

Meditation

Meditative activities are designed to condition the mind. They aid in general relaxation by reducing stress-inducing thoughts, memories, and anticipations. Meditative practices direct thoughts to produce a peaceful and tranquil state. All the meditative techniques have two common phases: a quiet body and a quiet mind. A primary goal of meditation is to reduce the surface chatter of the mind. If you can reduce the surface chatter, anxiety will be reduced. This in turn reduces general arousal, and the mind can achieve the peace and quiet natural to an ego- or self-transcendent state of consciousness.

The art of meditation is the ability to maintain a relaxed, passive concentration state in which alertness and control are maintained. In the meditative state, one is aware of subtle thoughts, energy, and creative intelligence. It is an intended process that takes thought, preparation, and practice. The mediator is left with the feeling of creativity, accomplishment, and optimism about the activity.

The Process of Meditation in Eight Steps:

1. Quiet your external environment. Put the ringer to the "off" position on your telephone, play some soft classical or other soothing instrumental music (use earphones if you need to), and so on.
2. Sit with your spine straight, hands folded in your lap, then take some deep breaths and relax your muscles.
3. Before you open yourself to meditation, extend a protecting envelope of energy around yourself. Some visualize a white-light energy field eight feet in diameter around themselves.
4. Spend ten minutes in a concentrative exercise (examples are given later) to clear the mind, to still the active left hemisphere of the brain, and to direct your energy.
5. Open your palms and spend ten minutes in "neutral," a period of not controlling or focusing your thoughts. Flow with whatever you may feel, and stay calm with relaxed interest. Touch whatever comes to you and let it go.
6. Once more, close your hands and focus again on a protective envelope of energy about you so that you may remain open to your positive energy, yet be protected from others' negative energy.
7. Wiggle around and let the energy flow throughout your body.
8. Get up and get on with your other activities.

All of the great spiritual leaders promote meditation in some form because it is not only a stress alleviator, but also a way into the understanding of the spiritual self—a way to tap into higher aspects of yourself.

Concentration Methods

Given below are some methods of concentration to try in your meditations. After practicing each of these methods, write down your experience. Did you feel comfortable with the method? Did it keep your mind from wandering? What insights do you have about concentration methods?

1. Sound, Sight, Feeling

In this exercise, you begin with three, four, or five (depending on how active your outside environment is). For this example, we will use five. Close your eyes and listen for five different sounds in your environment. Then, with eyes closed or open, visually focus on five different things. If your eyes are closed, you may see colors, designs, or visions of people, places, or things. You may mix having your eyes open and closed; you are not locked into one mode. Then tune into five different feelings. They may be emotional feelings or actual kinesthetic feelings such as having your hands on your lap. That is round one.

On the second round, you focus on four sounds, sights, and feelings that are different from the ones you heard, saw, and felt before.

On the next round, you focus on three sounds, sights, and feelings that are different from the ones you heard, saw, and felt in the two rounds before this.

On the next round, you focus on two sounds, sights, and feelings that are different from the ones you heard, saw, and felt in the three previous rounds.

On the final round, you focus on one sound, one sight, and one feeling, all of which are different from the ones you experienced before.

If your environment is very quiet, you may wish to begin at four or three and work down.

Write your experience with the sight, sound, feeling meditation. Did any one sense help more than the other two? How did this method work for you?

2. Sky Watching

This exercise may be done in daytime or at night. Experience both. The practice is to sit or lie on your back and stare at the sky, with or without its clouds, stars, satellites, planets, and so on, and breathe in its energy from the edges of the universe. It is not uncommon for mediators to relive wonderful childhood sky-watching experiences.

Write your experience with the sky-watching meditation. Did you experience a calm, meditative state? Were you busy being attached to the stars or clouds? What "cosmic" thoughts did you have?

Write a positive word or short phrase about meditation that will be useful to you in future situations.

CHAPTER 17

Stress Reduction through Physical Activity

Imagine that we offered to give you, free of charge, a major secret to alleviating anxiety of all sorts, enhancing your self-esteem, elevating your overall mood, combating your bouts of depression, and strengthening just about every cell in your body. How much would you pay for it? Well, it might cost as little as a good pair of running or walking or tennis shoes, a physical education class, or rollerblades or a bike. Well, yes, you're right. We're talking about physical activity or exercise. The terms can be synonymous, because all exercise (as we describe it here) is physical activity, but usually exercise is deemed to be a more specific activity designed for its health benefits.

Because this is a study in stress management, we approach the use of exercise as a stress alleviation technique. This chapter is not intended to be a lesson in how to build a sophisticated exercise program, nor is it a treatise on exercise physiology. Rather, we hope to provide motivation and confirmation—motivation for the use of exercise as a stress management strategy for those who are less joyful about exercise; and confirmation for those who already participate in sports, go to the gym regularly, or otherwise make exercise a part of their lifestyle. The evidence here supports the use of exercise for a healthy lifestyle.

In the plethora of good things that happen with an exercise regimen, we include not just the physical health that you might be more familiar with, but also those things that enhance the mental and emotional parts of your lives (see **Table 17.1**). Although it is impossible to separate the effects of stress on body and mind, we've categorized the benefits of exercise into two parts: alleviation of mental/emotional stress, and prevention and treatment of physical stress and disease.

Exercise and Mental/Emotional Stress Alleviation

As Table 17.1 points out, "Most people report that they feel good after exercising, less stressed, anxious or depressed." Their mood is elevated and they either feel more equipped to handle the stressors in life or realize that what they were stressing about is

Table 17.1   Some Important Ways That Exercise Helps Alleviate Emotional, Psychological, and Physical Stress

- Most people report that they feel good after exercising, as well as less stressed, anxious, or depressed.
- Exercise triggers feelings of calmness or happiness from a few minutes to hours afterward.
- Regular exercise increases cardiovascular fitness, muscular strength, and flexibility.
- It helps control weight, which positively affects self-esteem.
- It helps regulate sleep cycles; you sleep better and wake up more rested.
- It actually increases energy levels, better preparing you to seize the day.
- People who exercise usually make healthier nutrition choices.
- Exercise can help increase concentration and mental alertness.
- It can give you a sense of accomplishment.
- It can help take your mind off your worries.
- It provides a way to release pent-up stress, tension, and frustration.
- It promotes a sense of well-being long after the exercise is over.
- It decreases skeletal muscle tension, thus increasing relaxation and decreasing continuous muscle feedback that keeps you tensed.
- It uses up excess adrenaline (the presence of which in the bloodstream keeps you in a state of arousal and vigilance).
- It improves circulation, digestion, utilization of food, and elimination processes.
- It decreases bad cholesterol, increases good cholesterol, and decreases blood pressure.

not really all that bad. What follows is some of the research that supports the use of exercise to combat depression, anxiety, and negative moods, and to enhance self-esteem.

Depression

Depression and anxiety are the leading mental health concerns of college students and it appears that college mental health woes are on the rise (DeNoon 2003). Because most students feel lethargic, fatigued, and unmotivated when they are depressed, it seems apparent that exercise would be a good antidote for many mental health symptoms. Research is lending its support to physical exercise (Callaghan 2004; Mather 2002; Salmon 2001) by pointing out that:

- Physically active people are less likely to develop depression.
- Both aerobic and resistance exercise may be used to treat moderate and more severe depression, usually alongside standard treatment.
- The antidepressant effect of exercise can be equal to that of psychotherapy.
- No negative side effects of exercise in the treatment of depression have been noted.

It appears that the antidepressant effects of exercise begin as early as the first session of exercise and persist beyond the end of the exercise program. These effects are not dependent on age, gender, exercise group size, or the type of depression inventory used—subjective or objective. It does not appear that an increase in physical fitness level is necessary to achieve a reduction in depression symptoms.

It has also been found that breast cancer survivors who regularly work up a light to moderate sweat in aerobic activity (such as on a treadmill, stepper, or exercise bike) not only physically condition themselves but also feel significantly less depressed and anxious. In addition, the sooner they start exercising after they recover from surgery, the greater the beneficial impact on their mental health (Kolden 2002).

Anxiety

The vast majority of the qualitative reviews and all of the meta-analytic reviews (reports that analyze and summarize a number of research studies on the same subject, allowing for a summary of results across studies) support the conclusion that in studies published between 1960 and 1995 there is definitely a relationship showing that both short-term and long-term exercise reduce anxiety (Landers 1999).

Gosselin and Taylor (1999) report that both single and multiple sessions of exercise appear to have an anxiety-reducing effect. These studies have used subjective self-report measures of anxiety as well as objective measures of physiological arousal. Both measures show that physically active individuals suffer less from stress and stress-associated illnesses than do the nonactive. Research also shows that there is improvement in various psychological parameters such as reduction in anxiety and depression and better mental function after yogic practices and dynamic tae kwon do exercise (Ray 2001; Toskovic 2001).

Landers (1999) reports that to reduce anxiety with exercise, the best results for anxious subjects occur after weeks of regular aerobic exercise, and the benefits are greater in those who have high anxiety and who are not particularly physically fit to begin with.

Self-Esteem

As an important aspect of self-concept, your level of self-esteem (described in Chapter 6) is based on your ability to succeed at any particular task, which could include an exercise program or learning a specific sport. Self-esteem is an indicator of well-being and can be used as a mental health marker. Schafer (1996) noted that self-esteem is often found to be low in those suffering from stress, and individuals with high self-esteem appear to be less prone to stress.

Bandura's theory of self-efficacy (Bandura 1997) states that when people master a task they perceive to be difficult, they increase their feelings of self-efficacy and thus feel better about themselves. In this way, exercise can improve one's physical self-worth and other important self-perceptions such as body image. Increase in physical self-worth may be accompanied by improvement in general self-concept (again, as described in Chapter 6). Gosselin and Taylor (1999) and Morgan (1997) note that:

- Positive effects are likely to be greater for those with initially low self-esteem, and for children and middle-aged adults.
- Aerobic exercise and resistance training are the most effective activities for changing self-perceptions, and resistance training shows greatest effectiveness in the short term.
- Positive physical self-worth contributes to mental well-being in its own right and should be considered a valuable goal in an exercise program.

- Improvements in self-esteem do not appear to be dependent on fitness gains and may last up to twelve months posttreatment.

Exercise and Emotional Energy or Mood

At least 70 percent of our total energy is emotional, manifesting as motivation, passion, and enthusiasm. Emotional energy is the font from which flows everything we care about, and everything worth doing, especially if it is difficult. Failure to reach our goals comes from a lack of emotional energy to do the "right" thing. Physical energy may droop as we exhaust ourselves at work or play, but emotional energy keeps us alive and ready to tackle things again and again.

The underlying cause of elevated mood is unlikely to be a function of any individual factor, but instead is a complex intermingling of factors that feed on each other to produce positive results. Some of the important points noted by scholars in this area (Hansen 2001; Hassmen, Koivula, and Uutela 2000; Lee 2001) include:

- Aerobic exercise has a small-to-moderate effect on aspects of mood.
- There is a positive relationship between moderate physical activity and feelings of well-being.
- Having exercise goals that relate to personal improvement is associated with moderate-to-high positive emotion.
- A group exercise environment in which people feel a sense of personal mastery is associated with greater motivation and well-being than an environment in which competition is stressed.
- Exercise helps reduce negative mood states and increase positive mood states, with best results achieved with moderate-intensity exercise.
- Mental health benefits often occur before fitness levels have improved.
- The underlying cause of elevated mood is likely to be a combination of the factors mentioned above (e.g., increased self-esteem, decreased anxiety and depression).

The Benefits of Exercise in Preventing and Alleviating Physical Stress and Disease

In addition to the stress management benefits to mental and emotional health, there are many physical benefits that impact our stress levels, at either a treatment, alleviation, or prevention level. Any good fitness or exercise physiology book provides deeper understanding of these benefits; we summarize these benefits here.

Neuroplasticity

We have mentioned neuroplasticity several times in this book—as it relates to stress management and emotions and also meditation. Now we find it is pertinent to physical exercise, too. Begley (2007) reports that physical exercise results in neurogenesis (the generation of neurons) in the motor areas of the brain that control the parts of the body that are being exercised. However, neurogenesis occurs only if the exercise is not forced. It is also interesting that leisure or sport-related exercise—exercise that is done for fun—is a more effective weight loss activity than is work-related exercise. It appears that if exercise is stressful, the hormones of stress negate the beneficial neurological aspects of the activity. This might be an added motivator for everyone to choose a leisure sport that is enjoyable, and engage in that activity regularly to enjoy both body and brain benefits throughout life.

Weight Loss and Maintenance

With the obesity crisis occurring in America, not enough can be said about the use of exercise to reduce fat stores in the body. Weight loss is key to reduced illness from diabetes, high blood pressure, and a multitude of other health conditions (in Chapter 8, we delineated the health dangers of overweight and obesity). At least as important as the physical benefits of being at optimum weight is the mental and emotional lift one gets from using exercise as a means to attaining a healthy weight (Kiernan 2001).

As an individual becomes involved in an aerobic program, the body begins to use up adipose (fat) tissue and develop more muscle tissue. Fat pads diminish, and muscular curves develop and become more apparent. An aerobic exercise program is a must for weight management (Sharkey 2001).

To prevent the gradual accumulation of excess weight in adulthood, up to thirty additional minutes per day may be required over the thirty minutes for reduction of chronic disease risk and other health benefits. That is, about sixty minutes of moderate to vigorous physical activity on most days may be needed to prevent unhealthy weight gain (USDHHS 2005).

Increased Muscle Strength and Endurance

Exercise involving the large-muscle groups helps develop the size and fluid capacity of the muscles through greater capillarization (blood supply), increased muscle-fiber mass, and greater efficiency of contraction (Shephard and Astrand 2000). A weight management program should involve gaining muscular strength because the more muscle mass, the more tissue there is to consume fat for energy.

Because muscles act as pumps to help blood return to the heart, they develop a positive-feedback cycle; they send more blood back to the heart, and the heart pumps out more nutrients and oxygen to the muscles. Without the help of the muscles to send blood back to the heart, the heart takes on the full load of pumping blood throughout the system. This is why it is physiologically preferable to cool down slowly rather than just stop after vigorous activity.

Stronger Heart and Better "Tuning" of the Heartbeat

The heart is a muscle that increases in size and strength with use. It is the prime mover of the blood, which provides the tissues with oxygen and nutrients. Regular aerobic activity puts overload demands on the myocardial tissue, which responds by becoming stronger. As the heart becomes stronger, it can pump out more blood per beat, resulting in a slower resting heart rate. Aerobic training also changes the timing of the heart so that the heart spends less time in contraction and more time at rest. During the rest portion of the heart cycle, blood flows into the emptied cavities and also through the coronary arteries (the arteries that feed the heart muscle itself). This leaves more time for unrestricted blood flow to the myocardium, which in turn allows better nutrient flow and removal of wastes (Wilmore and Costell 1999).

Research has definitively shown the benefits of exercise in cardiac rehabilitation for decades, and exercise is now a standard component of postcardiac treatment. Historically, the prevalence of heart attacks in men was greater; thus the data were generated on men. Even a short-term exercise program for only one week started as soon as possible after myocardial infarction was shown by Greif (1995) to have beneficial effects for male patients.

It has also been shown that women realize the same benefits. After a cardiac-rehabilitation exercise program, women showed significant improvements in percentage of body fat, exercise capacity, and most components of behavior and quality of life (Buchner et al. 2005). In addition to the use of exercise for the cardiovascular health of both men and women, it is used for treatment in many other diseases as well (Crandell 2006; Redford 2007).

Increased Lung Capacity

Just as in other deep-breathing relaxation exercises, vigorous aerobic activity demands that the lungs expand and the diaphragm drop, which helps squeeze blood from the trunk back to the heart. In addition, intercostal muscles are strengthened and greater oxygenation of the blood occurs (Housh, Housh, and Devries 2002).

Stronger Bones

When the long bones of the body are stressed with exercise, they respond by becoming denser and thus stronger (Turner and Robling 2003). Many older women we have met in workout gyms have told us they are lifting weights to combat bone loss. Weight-bearing exercise has been shown to prevent osteoporosis at any age.

Improved Serum-Cholesterol Level and HDL/LDL Ratio

Chronic aerobic exercisers have higher HDL (high-density lipoprotein) as opposed to low-density lipoprotein (LDL) levels than do nonexercisers. HDLs (sometimes called "good cholesterol") are blood constituents that carry cholesterol to storage, getting it out of the bloodstream so that it is not as likely to be involved in atherosclerotic plaquing of the smooth arterial walls (Wilmore and Costell 1999).

Increased Range of Motion

As a safety measure, part of every exercise program involves stretching exercises. Without this kind of exercise, the muscles become organized at the semicontracted length and may create muscle cramps, soreness, and chronic pain. The exerciser should be able to enjoy a full range of motion in all muscles. As discussed in Chapter 15, yoga and stretching exercises also stimulate the relaxation response (Ray 2001).

Greater Efficiency, Attention, and Economy of Movement

Another safety factor and stress management benefit of a regular physical activity program is that the body becomes more efficient, cutting down on useless expenditure of energy. It is the difference between the beginning swimmer who thrashes around in the pool, expending great amounts of energy, and the trained swimmer who uses only the necessary energy to get from one end of the pool to the other. Because an activity program contributes to the alleviation of fatigue and anxiety, less meaningless activity is generated in this way.

Greater Alertness

Aerobic fitness improves nerve transactions throughout the body. All electrochemical transactions become more efficient, resulting in greater overall alertness and awareness.

Diminished Effects of Aging

Many of the characteristics that we attribute to the aging process are those that characterize the unfit individual. If we were to state the opposing side of each of the nine items just listed, we would get a picture of a debilitating process: inflexibility, low endurance, brittle bones, low respiratory capacity, creeping obesity, less alertness and awareness, and so on. When comparing our senior citizens, those who have been more physically active throughout their lives and continue to engage in vigorous activity appear to be younger and healthier than their nonactive counterparts (Crandell 2006; Redford 2007).

It has been reported that chronic stress appears to accelerate the aging process by shortening the life span of cells, opening the door to disease (Le Beau 2005). In an experimental group of mothers, scientists measured three factors of immune system cells: *telomeres,* which cap the ends of chromosomes and become shorter as cells reproduce; *telomerase,* an enzyme that replenishes telomeres; and *oxidative stress,* which damages DNA. They found that the higher the stress level, the more severe the cellular decline. The cells of people under a lot of stress aged the equivalent of nine to seventeen years more than the cells of people under little stress. And it wasn't just the stress itself—it was also how stressed out people *thought* they were. If the link between stress and premature aging is confirmed, telomere length could help health professionals prescribe life-extending therapies that could slow down cell aging—therapies such as exercise, meditation, prayer, or other forms of stress reduction, proving that health can indeed be a matter of mind over body.

The benefits outlined here, along with the specific stress management benefits discussed earlier, are compelling evidence that everyone should conduct a personal exercise program.

Why Do People Exercise?

Have you ever watched the so-called Xtreme Games on television? These are races where individuals and/or teams compete in arduous (to say the least) physical activities, such as running fifty miles through mountainous territory, then kayaking down tortuous rapids, then trekking across a desert, and so on. Do you ever wonder, "Why are they doing that?" On a smaller scale, you may even wonder why someone would quit a nice comfortable couch, enjoyable video or TV show, and nice snack in order to go to the gym and work out. Perhaps a short study of exercise motivational theory will give you some answers to the question of why people exercise. The theories overlap because the physical, emotional, social, psychological, and spiritual aspects of our lives cannot be neatly categorized. Again, though, for the sake of study, we point out several different theories: the social interaction theory; the self-efficacy theory of Bandura (1997, 2001); the distraction theory as explained by Gosselin and Taylor (1999); the fitness theory explained by Brown (1991) and Cox (1998); and the authors' meta-reward theory.

- If you do not enjoy exercising by yourself, yet find pleasure in a bout of frisbee or a friendly game of softball or touch football, you may recognize the inherent truth in the social interaction theory. According to this theory, people participate in activities that present pleasurable socializing with friends and/or colleagues (Turner and Robling 2003).

- Recall Bandura's self-efficacy theory from Chapters 6 and 7. Briefly, the theory states that when individuals master a new task or goal, they create for themselves positive feelings and thoughts, feelings of self-efficacy, and enhanced self-confidence and self-worth, all of which in turn reduce their stress. In the realm of conquering new skills or advanced goals in exercise, it is important that the newcomer is carefully coached and supported or the reverse effect may occur—he or she may shun exercise because of a bad experience.

- The distraction theory is exactly what you would suppose—that people use exercise to get their mind off their worries. Gosselin and Taylor (1999) state that although researchers have found that meditation and rest are as effective as exercise for reducing stress, they conclude that chronic or habitual exercise is more powerful and effective for reducing negative emotional energy than either relaxation or other distracting but enjoyable activities. They also note that distraction may provide an explanation for a short-term reduction in depression and anxiety, but not for a long-term reduction.

- The fitness theory suggests that by increasing their cardiovascular and muscular (both strength and flexibility) fitness, individuals improve their mood state (Housh et al. 2002; McArdle, Katch, and Katch 2001; Sharkey 2001).

In light of the numerous physical benefits of exercise that were stated earlier (enhanced immune system, decreased weight, improved physical stature, and so on), it is easy to make the connection between these benefits and enhanced mood and self-concept that improve one's life quality and reduce the worry, fear, and anxiety associated with poor health.

The unifying feature of achieving fitness is that (1) during activity, the body reacts in an ergotropic manner, with all systems stimulated for action, and (2) after physical activity, the systems are slowed down in a trophotropic manner, dominated by the parasympathetic nervous system, causing tranquility. If you are a consistent exerciser, you know the feeling of postexercise relaxation and perhaps are aware of its lasting effects throughout the day. The relaxation that comes after exercise brings with it a certain imperturbability (a lowered resting reactivity to the environment), which helps the regular exerciser react more appropriately to stimuli. Physiologically, exercise gives the body a chance to practice dealing with stress, forcing the body's systems to communicate much more closely than usual. This demand on the body's communication systems may be one of the true values of exercise.

- The meta-reward theory of exercise states that perhaps the highest purpose of physical exercise is to gain a sense of well-being—you participate because it feels right (and, conversely, it feels wrong when you don't), because it enhances positive feelings toward yourself that bounce off others as positive energy, and because it helps make your life complete. The "runner's high," the tranquility state, the oneness, the internal calm experienced by those who become deeply involved in their activity make the prospect of a regular exercise program intriguing.

- Exercise is a natural form of expression. We were made to move. And when we are motivated to exercise, if social sanctions do not prevent our psychological acceptance of the activity, we rediscover the original unifying thread of mind and body. It makes us feel naturally healthy, just as we feel when we know that we're eating the right foods and dealing with social problems in a self-enhancing manner.

Some Guidelines and Principles of Exercise

At this point, you should be able to determine that there are many benefits of exercising. To maximize its effect for enhancing moods, decreasing stress, and increasing fitness, an exercise program should strive to achieve the following objectives.

The Most Beneficial Exercise Is Regular Exercise

In 2002, the National Academy of Sciences (NAS) stated that thirty minutes per day of regular activity was insufficient to maintain body weight in adults in the recommended body mass index (BMI) range of 18–24 (see **Table 17.2** to find your body mass index). In order to prevent weight gain as well as to achieve additional, weight-independent health benefits of physical activity, the NAS now recommends **sixty** minutes of daily moderate intensity physical activity (e.g., walking/jogging at 4–5 mph) in addition to the activities required in a sedentary lifestyle (National Academy of Sciences 2002). In qualitative terms, the NAS defines exercise as activity sufficiently vigorous to raise breathing to a level where conversation is labored and sweating is noticeable on temperate days. Their recommendation reflects physical activity habits equivalent to walking 5–7 miles/day at 3–4 mph in addition to daily activities. Therefore, to increase physical activity and thereby facilitate fitness and weight control, recreational activities and physical training programs need to be added to (not substituted for) other physical activities of daily life.

The American College of Sports Medicine *Guidelines for Exercise Testing and Prescription* (American College of Sports Medicine 2004) is recommended reading for someone starting a fitness program. It delineates guidelines for the frequency, intensity, and/or duration of various types of fitness programs. In addition, there are a number of Web sites that help individuals design a customized fitness program free of charge (e.g., www.feel-better-with-exercise.com and www.reeboku.com). Also, any search engine will find appropriate sites for you.

Table 17.2 Body Mass Index (BMI) Chart

BMI =	19	20	21	22	23	24	25	26	27	28	29	30	31	32	33	34	35–39.9
							Body Weight (pounds)										
Height Inches			NORMAL						OVERWEIGHT					OBESE I			OBESE II
58	91	96	100	105	110	115	119	124	129	134	138	143	148	153	158	162	167
59	94	99	104	109	114	119	124	128	133	138	143	148	153	158	163	168	173
60	97	102	107	112	118	123	128	133	138	143	148	153	158	163	168	174	179
61	100	106	111	116	122	127	132	137	143	148	153	158	164	169	174	180	185
62	104	109	115	120	126	131	136	142	147	153	158	164	169	175	180	186	191
63	107	113	118	124	130	135	141	146	152	158	163	169	175	180	186	191	197
64	110	116	122	128	134	140	145	151	157	163	169	174	180	186	192	197	204
65	114	120	126	132	138	144	150	156	162	168	174	180	186	192	198	204	210
66	118	124	130	136	142	148	155	161	167	173	179	186	192	198	204	210	216
67	121	127	134	140	146	153	159	166	172	178	185	191	198	204	211	217	223
68	125	131	138	144	151	158	164	171	177	184	190	197	203	210	216	223	230
69	128	135	142	149	155	162	169	176	182	189	196	203	209	216	223	230	236
70	132	139	146	153	160	167	174	181	188	195	202	209	216	222	229	236	243
71	136	143	150	157	165	172	179	186	193	200	208	215	222	229	236	243	250
72	140	147	154	162	169	177	184	191	199	206	213	221	228	235	242	250	258
73	144	151	159	166	174	182	189	197	204	212	219	227	235	242	250	257	265
74	148	155	163	171	179	186	194	202	210	218	225	233	241	249	256	264	272
75	152	160	168	176	184	192	200	208	216	224	232	240	248	256	264	272	279
76	156	164	172	180	189	197	204	213	221	230	238	246	254	263	271	279	287

What Is Your Body Mass Index (BMI)?

What is obesity? Being overweight? The body mass index (BMI) is a current and widely used means of determining your weight category: normal, overweight, and three levels of obesity. Table 17.2 presents a body mass index chart for a quick check of your BMI. BMI scores are read across the top.

Source: National Institutes of Health (2002).

Choose a Variety of Activities

A total fitness program includes:

- aerobic training for cardiovascular fitness and fat loss
- a muscular strength and endurance program
- a flexibility program (an excellent program is presented in Chapter 15)

Within each of these programs, variety not only helps keep you interested but also provides cross-training. The body tends to become efficient when you do the same exercise day after day, so optimal gains may not be seen. Mix running, walking, rollerblading, biking, swimming, or other enjoyable aerobic activity in that part of your program. (**Table 17.3** provides an activity chart that shows the advantages and disadvantages of various kinds of exercise activities.) A strength program might mix weightlifting with calisthenics with honest-to-goodness work like digging fence-post holes, cutting wood, or loading boxes on a truck. Yoga, pilates, various commercial workout tapes, and gymnastics all offer stretching activities.

Table 17.3 Activity Chart

Activity	Advantages	Possible Disadvantages*
Walking	No cost, no equipment, no special facilities. Everyone can participate. Year-round activity.	Time commitment, must walk fast for conditioning effect.
Jogging (less than 5 mph)	Promotes weight loss, leg strength, cardiovascular endurance. No special facilities.	May be hard on knees and other joints. Must have physical checkup, proper shoes.
Running (more than 5 mph) Stair climbing Step training	Promotes weight loss, cardiovascular conditioning, and well-being.	Must have physical checkup, good shoes. Can be hard on joints.
Dancing (folk, rock, aerobic, and other vigorous fast dances)	Promotes weight control, total-body conditioning, especially aerobic dancing (doing cardiovascular exercises to music). Year-round activity.	Must be brisk for conditioning. Requires coordination, rhythm for set dance patterns. May be hard on joints.
Biking	Good cardiovascular conditioning, promotes weight control, easier on joints than walking, jogging, running. Energy-saving transportation.	Danger from autos, cost of bike, requires learned skill.
Alpine skiing	Promotes total-body conditioning, especially legs. Enjoyable, apt to promote well-being.	Requires learned skill, expensive equipment. Can be dangerous (especially if not in condition) from falls, cold weather, and altitude. Seasonal.
Cross-country skiing	Excellent for cardiovascular conditioning, total-body fitness. Little jarring to body joints. Apt to promote well-being.	Requires some learned skill, special equipment. Cold and altitude may be a negative factor. Seasonal.
Swimming	Excellent for cardiovascular conditioning and muscle toning. No jarring to joints.	Requires some skill, pool, minimum cost of swimsuit.

(Table 17.3 continues)

Table 17.3   Activity Chart (*Continued*)

Activity	Advantages	Possible Disadvantages*
Racket sports (tennis, squash, racketball)	Excellent total-body conditioner if fast game is played. Promotes weight loss.	Requires learned skill, special equipment, and facilities. Must play at high level for conditioning effect.
Golf (walk, carry own clubs)	Enjoyable and relaxing if not self-critical. Some of the same benefits of walking.	Requires learned skill, special equipment. Walking briskly without intermittent stops is a better conditioner.
Bowling	Relaxing and enjoyable if not self-critical. Better than just sitting.	Almost no conditioning effect. Requires learned skill and special equipment. Not recommended as treatment or preventative relaxation technique.
Slow, low-impact aerobic dance	Brisk, total-body exercises have conditioning value, especially muscle toning. No cost, little or no equipment. Year-round activity.	May exacerbate existing muscle problems. Tendency to overdo initially.
Weightlifting	Increases strength, improves physique, and may improve self-image. Can improve cardiovascular efficiency by lifting lighter weights for greater reptitions or by circuit training.	Requires special equipment. Some risk of muscular injury unless properly trained and prudently utilized.

*Another possible disadvantage in most of these activities is high-level, ego-involved competition.

Exercise Precautions

Although it is difficult to draw a line between "young" and "old," it is important to note that the aging process is generally related to decreased muscular strength, flexibility, and cardiovascular endurance. Much of this decrease does not have to happen. For those who stay in good physical shape through exercise, the precautions here may not apply until much later in life. However, many who are overweight and out of shape should heed the following precautions, even if they don't consider themselves "elderly":

1. Always spend a short time (five to ten minutes) warming up your muscles before engaging in strength or cardiovascular exercise.

2. Always spend a short time (five to ten minutes) cooling down after a workout.

3. In weightlifting, use light weights with slow motions.

4. Breathe throughout the exercise. Do not hold your breath.

5. If you have arthritis or other joint problems, swim or bicycle rather than jog or run.

6. Do body-twisting exercises slowly and in a seated position.

7. Use slow, smooth movements of the head up and down and to the right and left rather than doing head or neck rolls with 360-degree rotation.

8. Always do slow, steady stretching. Do not bounce or jerk.

9. Do not put your body weight against stiff or locked joints.

10. Avoid straight-leg sit-ups or leg lifts.

11. Perform knee bends with no more than half a contraction.

12. Take a warm shower or bath after a workout.

13. Training heart rate may be as low as 110 to 120 beats per minute.

14. If in doubt about certain exercises or activities, ask a health professional.

15. Get a physical checkup and a medical approval to start a physical activity program. (Dusek 2004)

The more fun the activity, the more likely it will facilitate a lifestyle change.

The Overload Principle

In order to increase physical strength and endurance, you must push yourself beyond what you can easily do. For example, if you can walk at a brisk pace without being out of breath, you must move faster—at a jog or run—in order to improve your aerobic capacity. If you can easily lift and use a 10-pound weight, then a heavier one is necessary to develop your arm muscles beyond their present state. Throughout a fitness program, work with greater resistance until it feels comfortable, and then increase the resistance again. When you get to the level of fitness at which you are aiming, level off with a maintenance program (that is, one designed to help you maintain a strength and endurance level).

In order for exercise to contribute to a stress management program, it is not necessary to strive for marathon endurance or the strength of an Olympic weightlifter. However, the greatest benefits to all-around health demand that the program increases your fitness level rather than just giving you sporadic exercise (McArdle 1999).

Aerobics Program

Most of the benefits of physical fitness come from a program of aerobic exercise, that is, activities that are vigorous, rhythmic, and involve the large-muscle groups of the body. Cardiorespiratory fitness is effectively enhanced when an individual works at 60 percent of maximum capacity or more (capacity being measured according to heart rate).

Heart Rate

Your heart rate tells you two important things about aerobic exercise: (1) how vigorous the activity must be for you to benefit from the exercise and (2) how your system is responding to the exercise program, as reflected by your resting heart rate.

To find out how strenuous your workouts should be, you must have several items of information. One is your resting heart rate. Take your pulse for sixty seconds while lying in bed after just waking up. Your pulse is located on the thumb side of your wrist, on the outer side of the tendon that goes down to your hand. It is also located at your temples and other pressure points on your body, including the neck. However, when pressure is applied to the neck to find a pulse rate, the heart responds to the pressure, and you might not obtain a true reading.

Take your pulse several mornings in a row, and average the three readings. Enter your resting heart rate here:

Date _____ Resting heart rate _____

A second item of information you need to have is your maximal heart rate. The formula to determine this is 226 (for females) or 220 (for males) minus your age. Your maximal heart rate tells you how fast your heart can beat under a strenuous workload. The figures for men and women are slightly different because women apparently have a slightly higher maximal capacity (Althoff, Svoboda, and Girdano 1996). Enter your maximal heart rate here:

Women: 226 – _____ (age) = _____ (beats per minute)

Men: 220 – _____ (age) = _____ (beats per minute)

When you begin an aerobic or maintenance program, you must determine your starting abilities. If you are minimally fit (that is, if even minor exertion is exhausting for you), you should begin your aerobic program at 50 to 60 percent of your maximal capacity. As your program gets easier for you, you can increase the load to 60 to 70 percent and higher. If you already engage in vigorous activity, begin your program at 70 to 80 percent maximal. If you are highly trained and very physically fit, you will want to use a range of 80 to 90 percent.

The last item of information that you must have is how to calculate your training heart rate. To do this, take 60, 70, 80, and 90 percent of your maximal heart rate. For example, a twenty-year-old male would have a maximal heart rate of 200. Sixty percent of that is 120 beats per minute. Seventy percent of 200 is 140. If this individual is beginning a program at a 60 to 70 percent range of maximal, he should keep his heart rate between 120 and 140 beats per minute during his workout. As he becomes conditioned during his program, he will move up to a 70 to 80 percent range, which then demands that he keep his heart rate between 140 and 160 beats per minute.

When you are doing aerobic exercise, it is important to keep moving slowly as you take your heart rate so that you do not let blood pool in the lower extremities with only the heart beat to pump the blood back up the body. When you move, your legs work as muscle pumps to continually squeeze blood back up to the heart. For this reason, rather than taking the pulse for sixty seconds, you should take it for six seconds and multiply by ten.

To easily determine whether you are working within your target heart rate range, divide the top and bottom figures of the range by ten to identify what a six-second reading should be. In the previous example, when working at a 60 to 70 percent range, this man's six-second pulse should be between 12 and 14. When taking a six-second pulse, always count the first pulse as zero in case you just missed a beat. It is better to err on the low side than on the high side.

To determine how intensely you must exercise to get to your training heart rate range, you must experiment. Begin walking at a slow pace for two minutes, and then take your six-second pulse. If your heart rate is too slow, pick up the pace and repeat. Repeat this process until you find an intensity that will lift you into your range and keep you there. Take your pulse immediately after you exercise because your heart rate starts to slow down as soon as you slow down. It is extremely important that you adhere to your beginning heart rate range to avoid burnout. Many people who start an exercise program are so highly motivated that they try to get all the benefits in just one day. They exercise too strenuously for too long a time, end up with aching muscles, joints, and bones, and decide that exercise is not for them.

Intensity and Duration

An aerobic program will not maximally benefit you unless its intensity is at your training heart rate and its duration is at least fifteen minutes. However, there is an inverse relationship between intensity and duration that enables you to gain training effects at lower intensity levels if the duration is longer. This means that even a low-intensity walking program will give you training effects if you walk for a long period of time. Performing an exercise for three hours at a heart rate of 110 beats per minute will give you the same training effect as performing one for twenty minutes at a rate of 140 beats per minute (Cooper 1994).

The American College of Sports Medicine and the Centers for Disease Control and Prevention recommend that every U.S. adult should accumulate thirty minutes or more of moderate-intensity exercise (comparable to a brisk walk) on most, preferably all, days of the week (American College of Sports Medicine 2004).

When beginning a program, the duration of exercise should be low, perhaps as little as five to ten minutes per day (especially if one's fitness level is very low). Duration should then increase progressively.

For developing and maintaining cardiorespiratory fitness, perform large-muscle, rhythmic exercise three to five days a week, fifteen to sixty minutes per workout, at 60 to 90 percent of your maximal heart rate.

When you choose an activity, keep your interests, abilities, and objectives in mind. Make sure the activities you choose are compatible with your lifestyle.

Set realistic short- and long-term goals for yourself, and chart your progress. This helps with motivation and adherence to the program.

Get assistance in starting your program if you need more information or even motivation. It may be helpful to work out with others.

Always warm up and cool down.

Aerobic exercises include running, jogging, walking, cycling, rowing, cross-country skiing, aerobic dance, rope skipping, hiking, swimming, and stair climbing. Depending on how they are played, many games, such as handball, racquetball, soccer, tennis, and basketball, may be aerobic.

Intermittent activity or activity of low energy output has some effect on increasing cardiovascular fitness, but more vigorous exercise gives greater increase in fitness.

Flexibility Program

Stretching exercises are essential to any fitness program. Exercises such as the ones discussed in Chapter 15 should be performed for your relaxation program as well as for a part of your aerobic activity. The key to safe, effective stretching is slow, constant pressure. Do not bounce—it may cause harm.

Muscular Strength and Endurance Programs

Two kinds of programs to develop muscular strength and endurance are available. One is a weightlifting program in which dumbbells, barbells, or machines are used for resistance. These programs are becoming very popular with both men and women and are available in schools, recreation centers, and workout studios. The second program involves using yourself as the resistance. Whichever program you choose, follow the safety guidelines that apply to the kinds of exercises you will be doing. Some possible benefits of a muscular strength and endurance program include:

- Improvement of overall body contour—your shape will improve.
- More muscle mass helps eat up calories, making weight loss easier.
- Loss of inches because toning the muscle takes out the "sag."
- A stronger appearance; you move in a more controlled manner with more poise and balance.
- Regular weight-bearing exercise promotes bone formation and may prevent many forms of bone loss.
- Strength is the basis of balance; thus, it especially helps older people prevent disastrous falls.
- All physical movement is easier and more purposefully controlled—this translates to everything from driving a car to walking your dog.

SUMMARY

Exercise is an excellent stress management tool for many reasons. Its mental, emotional, social, and physical benefits interact in a way that may be used for the treatment, prevention, and alleviation of stress. Consider the following points:

- Exercise utilizes stress by-products, thereby shortening the time the body is exposed to damaging levels of nervous system and endocrine secretions.
- Exercise is known to help alleviate depression and anxiety.
- Exercise is known to help enhance self-esteem and positive emotional mood states.

- Motivations to exercise include the desire for social interaction, to increase self-efficacy, as a distraction from stress and anxiety, to feel better due to physical fitness, and to induce a tranquil state.

- Exercise enhances all physical systems (heart, lungs, muscles, blood chemistry, and so on) when performed in a safely prescribed manner.

- Exercise programs should include aerobic, muscular strength and endurance, and flexibility aspects.

- Exercise programs should be varied, graduated in intensity and duration, performed regularly, and have continued motivational aspects.

SOURCES CITED

Althoff, S. A., Svoboda, M., and Girdano, D. A. (1996). *Choices in health and fitness.* Scottsdale, AZ: Gorsuch and Scarisbrick.

American College of Sports Medicine. (2004). *American College of Sports Medicine guidelines for exercise testing and prescription.* Baltimore: Lippincott, Williams and Wilkins.

Bandura, A. (1997). *Self-efficacy: The exercise of control.* New York: W. H. Freeman.

Bandura, A. (2001). Social cognitive theory: An agentic perspective. *Annual Review of Psychology,* 52, 1–26.

Begley, S. (2007). Train your mind, change your brain. New York: Ballentine Books.

Brown, J. (1991). Staying fit and staying well: Physical fitness as a moderator of life stress. *Journal of Personality and Social Psychology,* 60 no. 4, 555–61.

Buchner, B., et al. (2005). Stress and heart disease in women. *Herz,* 30, 416–28.

Callaghan, P. (2004). Exercise: A neglected intervention in mental health care? *Journal of Psychiatric and Mental Health Nursing,* 114, 476–83.

Cooper, K. H. (1994). *The antioxidant revolution.* Nashville, TN: Nelson.

Cox, R. (1998). *Sport psychology: Concepts and applications,* 4th ed. New York: WCB/McGraw-Hill.

Crandell, S. (2006). Living longer. *AARP Bulletin,* September/October, 90–93.

DeNoon, D. J. (2003). College mental health woes on the rise. *Professional Psychology: Research and Practice,* 34, 10.

Gosselin, C., and Taylor, A. (1999, October). Exercise as a stress management tool. *Stress News,* 11 no. 4, 3.

Greif, M. A. (1995). The effects of short-term exercise on the cognitive orientation for health and adjustment in myocardial infarction patients. *Behavioral Medicine,* 21, no. 2, 75–85.

Hansen, C. J., Stevens, L. C., & Coast, J. R. (2001). Exercise duration and mood state: How much is enough to feel better? *Health Psychology,* 20, no. 4, 267–75.

Hassmen, P., Koivula, N., and Uutela, A. (2000). Physical exercise and psychological wellbeing. *Preventive Medicine,* 30, no. 1, 17–25.

Housh, T. J., Housh, D. J. and Devries, H. A. (2002). *Applied exercise and sport physiology.* Scottsdale, AZ: Holcomb Hathaway Publishers.

Kiernan, M., et al. (2001). Men gain additional psychological benefits by adding exercise to a weight-loss program. *Obesity Research,* 9, no. 12, 770–7.

Kolden, G. G., et al. (2002). Group exercise training for women with primary breast cancer. *Psycho-Oncology, 39,* 939–50.

Landers, D. M. (1999). The influence of exercise on mental health. In C. B. Corbin and R. P. Pangrazi (eds.), *Toward a better understanding of physical fitness and activity.* Scottsdale, AZ: Holcomb Hathaway Publishers.

LeBeau, C. (2005). Stress. *AARP Bulletin,* January, 3–4.

Lee, R. E., et al. (2001). A prospective analysis of the relationship between walking and mood in sedentary ethnic minority women. *Women Health, 32,* no. 4, 1–15

Mather, A. S. (2002). Effects of exercise on depressive symptoms. *British Journal of Psychiatry, 180,* 411–15.

McArdle, W. D., Katch, F. I., and Katch, V. L. (2001). *Exercise physiology.* Hagerstown, MD: Lippincott, Williams and Wilkins.

Morgan, W. P. (1997). *Physical activity and mental health.* Dallas, TX: Taylor & Francis.

National Academy of Sciences. (2002). *Dietary reference intakes for energy, carbohydrate, fiber, fat, fatty acids, cholesterol, protein, and amino acids.* Washington, DC: Food and Nutrition Board (FNB), Institute of Medicine (IOM).

National Institutes of Health. (2002). *Do you know the health risks of being overweight?* Bethesda, MD: Author.

Ray, U. S., et al. (2001). Effect of yogic exercises on physical and mental health of young fellow-ship course trainees. *Indian Journal of Physiological Pharmacology, 45,* no. 1, 37–53.

Redford, G. (2007). Get stronger, live longer. *AARP Bulletin,* May/June, 22–24.

Salmon, P. (2001). Effects of physical exercise on anxiety, depression, and sensitivity to stress: A unifying theory. *Clinical Psychology Review, 21,* no. 1, 33–61.

Schafer, W. (1996). *Stress management for wellness.* San Diego, CA.: Harcourt Brace.

Sharkey, B. (2001). *Fitness and health.* Champaign, IL: Human Kinetics.

Shephard, R. J., and Astrand, P-O., eds. (2000). *Endurance in sport.* Champaign, IL: Human Kinetics.

Toskovic, N. N. (2001). Alternations in selected measures of mood with a single bout of dynamic taekwondo exercise in college-age students. *Perceptive Motor Skills, 92,* no. 3, Pt. 2, 1031–8.

Turner, C. H., and Robling, A. G. (2003). Designing exercise regimens to increase bone strength. *Exercise and Sport Science Reviews, 31,* 45–50.

USDHHS. (2005). *Dietary guidelines for Americans.* Washington, DC: U. S. Government Printing Office.

Wilmore, J., and Costell, D. (1999). *Physiology of sport and exercise.* Champaign, IL: Human Kinetics.

Journal Entry 17

Exercise, Exercise

It is important to know that the human stress response is intended to end in physical activity. The outpouring of sugar and fats into the blood is meant to feed the muscles and the brain so that they can actively contend with the provoking stressor; the heart and respiration rates speed up to meet the demand. This is not the time to sit and feel all of these sensations tearing away at the body's systems. This is the time to move, use up the products, and relieve the body of the destructive forces of stress on a sedentary system. The right thing to do is total-body exercise.

How Much Exercise Do You Get?

Use the following assessment to see how much activity you usually get in a day. A number of different activities that are a part of many people's daily routine are listed. If you engage in an activity other than that listed, try to approximate that activity with one given here, and use the points accorded to it. After completing the exercise, you will have twenty-four hours of activity listed. For each hour or partial hour, multiply the weighted score given for the activity, then total the points. This is your physical activity score. Use a different color for one weekend day and one week day. Compare the two.

List the number of hours per day you spend.

Sleeping	_____ hours	@.85 points/hour _____
Sitting		@ 1.5 points/hour _____
Riding/driving	_____ hours	
Studying/deskwork	_____ hours	
Meals	_____ hours	
Watching TV	_____ hours	
Reading	_____ hours	
Other	_____ hours	
	_____ hours	
	_____ hours	(total sitting × 1.5) _____
Standing		@ 2 points/hour
Standing	_____ hours	
Dressing	_____ hours	
Showering	_____ hours	
Other	_____ hours	
	_____ hours	
	_____ hours	(total standing × 2) _____

Walking

Slow walk	_____ hours	@ 3 points/hour	_____
Moderate walk speed	_____ hours	@ 4 points/hour	_____
Very fast walk	_____ hours	@ 5 points/hour	_____

Occupational

Housework and/or light physical work	_____ hours	@ 3 points/hour	_____
Heavy physical labor	_____ hours	@ 4 points/hour	_____

Heavy total-body physical exertion

Rapid calisthentics	_____ hours	@ 4 points/hour	_____
Slow run (jog)	_____ hours	@ 6 points/hour	_____
Fast run	_____ hours	@ 7 points/hour	_____

Recreational

Racket sports	_____ hours	@ 8 points/hour	_____
Team sports (e.g., basketball)	_____ hours	@ 9–10 points/hour	_____
Stair climbing	_____ hours	@ 8 points/hour	_____

Total hours   24   Total Points _____

If you have **40 total points or less,** what will you be willing to change to get your activity level to **45?** to **50?**

Do you have an exercise outlet for stress buildup? What is it? How well does it work for you?

What is your motivation to exercise? If you do not exercise regularly and/or are not physically fit, why?

Write a brief motivational message for yourself that you will use to help you increase your activity or fitness level.

It has been emphasized in almost every chapter in this book that every stress management technique offered has two benefits. The first is to do the activity to reduce the stress immediately. The second is to continue to do the activity on a regular basis to condition the system to resist stress in the future (this is the stress prevention plan). The same advice is offered for exercise: do it now, and do it regularly.

CHAPTER 18

Your Personal Stress Management Plan

Up to this point, we have discussed what stress is and what can be done to avoid excessive stress and burnout. However, knowledge alone is usually insufficient for initiating a lasting behavior change. Most people require a plan of attack. This chapter is designed to help you develop an individualized plan for personal stress management. This approach to developing a plan involves some introspection and some diligence in record keeping. Many people do not want to bother with the specifics; they would just rather deal in generalities and try a few comfortable exercises. That is understandable because there are a lot more fun and pressing things to do with your time. However, we have found that attention to the details produces results. The highest predictor of failure in smoking cessation programs was unwillingness to fill in the forms about smoking habits. Likewise, in weight management, the highest predictor of failure was unwillingness to fill out diet recall forms and track calories. Stress management research yields the same results; failure is associated with noncompliance with doing the exercises. Pure and simple, compliance signifies commitment and motivation equals success.

In an overwhelming majority of cases, people experience stress because they have a stressful lifestyle and have learned through years of conditioning to react in a stressful manner. With regard to health and illness, a stressed person is one who exhibits physical arousal in response to social-emotional conditions. This exaggerated arousal is usually unnecessary for dealing effectively with the situation. A vicious cycle develops to the point where minor happenings are met with major arousal, and the individual never really relaxes.

The stressed person experiences what can be termed mind-body arousal because both psychological and physiological systems are activated. Usually various physical, mental, and emotional arousals occur together, but the precise way that individuals manifest the stress reaction varies greatly. Because stress reactions are so complex and varied, it follows that no two individuals will react in exactly the same manner to a similar stressor. The type of stimulus that causes the stress response in individuals is highly variable; what causes one person excessive stress may cause less stress or even no stress for another individual. This is because stress is a reaction based on an individual's perception of the circumstances or situation, and it is safe to say that no two individuals perceive any given stimulus in exactly the same manner.

By understanding the concepts and nature of stress, it becomes evident that the management of stress is best achieved by an intervention plan that is custom made for an individual. You will recall from an earlier section of this book that personal stress management is best when holistic, that is,

- individualized
- practically designed to suit personal preferences
- multidimensional
- flexible

Readiness

Before we get into the development of your own stress management program, we would like to elaborate on the final journal entry, which concludes this book, because it utilizes the concept of readiness, which is essential to your success.

Readiness is the state of being that precedes change; it makes change happen. Readiness might be defined as motivation, or potential energy that builds inside until it bursts forth as behavior. Readiness is the possession of behaviors, attitudes, skills, and concomitant resources that make it possible for individuals to incorporate a new health behavior into a permanent lifestyle. Unlike many learning experiences in which motivation is needed on a one-shot basis, readiness denotes a continuum that reflects minimal to maximal motivation to change an old behavior or institute an entirely new one.

The Readiness Scale

The observable steps along the readiness continuum are shown in the final journal entry. On the low end of the readiness scale is the defensive avoidance of a behavior change—the person who "can't" adhere to an exercise or eating plan in order to get to a lower weight, or the stressed person who "can't" find the time to practice a relaxation program. Somewhere in the middle of the scale is the person who has conflicted adherence to the behavior change during the program, then allows the change to become extinguished after the program is over. This is the person who will participate in the recommended exercise, diet, or relaxation program while supervised, but finds it difficult to continue the behavior with internal support only. At the high end of the readiness scale is the person who is committed to an unconflicted change progression and incorporates the new behavior readily into his or her daily lifestyle.

As behavior change counselors, we have successfully incorporated readiness theory, readiness testing, and readiness activities into every behavior change program we have developed. These include smoking cessation (Girdano and Dusek 1975, 1987), weight management (Dusek 1982, 1989, 2004), stress management, exercise, changing careers, dealing with love relationships (Girdano 1981), and those treating low back pain, irritable bowel syndrome, and insomnia (Girdano and Dusek 1987). What do all these programs have in common? They all include the progression through the stages that the literature shows are essential for eventual success in the change of any health behavior (Prochaska and DiClimente 1994).

Readiness Stages

1. Knowledge—the factual material about stress and stress management.

2. Valuing—What you want to do and be, and how will this new behavior make you and your life better? This is the "Why be healthy?" question.

3. Feeling—involves both (1) emotions and (2) the physiological state of the body. Feelings can be evaluated as positive, such as the feelings of comfort, joy, or being at peace; or they can be evaluated as negative, such as anxiety, fear, or anger in relation to a particular behavior or thought. Feelings that describe a physiological state encompass identifying the depth of breathing, the degree of muscle tension, or the difference between tension and relaxation. These are essential dimensions that are necessary in order to learn skills.

4. Skills—define the ability to do a particular behavior, that is, what you can do or know how to do.

5. Behavior—the actual living or doing of an act, combining knowledge, skills, feelings, and values.

The progression toward a behavior change usually proceeds through a hierarchy of stages. The steps on the readiness scale show a progression from knowledge gathering and understanding to complete adoption of the new behavior into the lifestyle without misgivings or second thoughts. Each stage is outlined below.

Stage 1. Understanding the concepts. The readiness continuum begins with knowledge. Sometimes you are so ready to change that just reading about the prospective behavior, learning of its benefits and dangers, and understanding its ease of incorporation will be enough to catapult you from the knowledge end of the continuum to the complete adoption of the new behavior into a new lifestyle in a very short period of time. When asked how this change occurred so quickly and easily, the usual answer is "I guess I was just ready." However, this is not the usual case. For instance, we know that nearly all cigarette smokers understand the grave dangers of smoking, and that people who continually try to reduce their weight know a great deal about nutrition and the dangers of obesity. Educational theory now readily accepts that knowledge alone, although an essential first step, is not enough of a motivator to change behavior.

Stage 2. Valuing the new behavior. As you progress up the readiness continuum, you will move from knowledge acquisition to a stage where you value the behavior and will tell others that this new or changed behavior is good and right. Behavior is not yet incorporated, but you see the value of the behavior.

Stage 3. Believing that the new behavior is possible. This next stage involves an internalization that the behavior is possible to achieve and that the behavior, once learned, will result in a new or different and better lifestyle. You begin to personally want or desire to have that behavior. If there is no motivation to progress on the readiness scale at this time, the desire for such a change will lie dormant or perhaps one small change will be tried. What often happens at this stage is that someone near to you has tried meditation or some other relaxation technique and has been successful using it.

At this stage, you must be able to see yourself with the new behavior. This is an internalization of the view, which means you must be able to be inside the new behavior looking out and seeing how the world looks and feels from the perspective of the new behavior. This is both an emotion—the joy of feeling good about acquiring the new behavior—and the feeling of actually moving and performing the new activity.

Stage 4. Believing in ability to change behavior.   To continue the readiness for lifetime change, it is important that you feel the availability of internal resources that will support continuance of the new behavior. Resources may be classified as primary and secondary. Primary resources are those that are specific to solving the problem at hand or acquiring the new behavior such as motivation and skills. Secondary resources are more general behaviors or personality traits that allow you to better utilize primary resources. Self-esteem is the basis for this step—success is easier if you can find positive resources from the past that can be applied to present situations.

Stage 5. Utilizing internal and external resources.   Stage 5 utilizes internal and external resources to keep getting positive feedback about the behavior change. At this stage, you are willing to tackle whatever has blocked that behavior change from occurring in the past. In the great majority of cases, those previously unclaimed or undiscovered blocks are anger and hostility, anxiety, fear, and/or some secondary gain you receive by hanging on to the old behavior.

Stage 6. Seeing proof of attainment.   At this rung of the readiness ladder, you look around for proofs that the targeted change in behavior does, in fact, make a change in your life. When those proofs are concrete enough in your mind, readiness moves up another step to trial behavior. You who have been trying some of the exercises presented in this book are at this stage. The remainder of this chapter is dedicated to helping you move beyond this stage and toward incorporation of the skills you have learned into your lifestyle.

Stage 7. Possessing necessary skills and practices on a regular basis.   Stress management involves learning new skills. These may be skills of recognizing tension, doing relaxed breathing, lowering muscle tension, being assertive, nurturing oneself, or using positive resource states. One theme in this book has been the teaching of the right combination of skills to get the job done.

By this stage, you should be practicing the new skills on a regular schedule. The skills must be overlearned before they are put into service in actual situations. After that, move to practicing the skills in real-life situations. Soon you will be practicing the skills almost without thinking about them or at least not regretting the time and energy spent in practice. Essential at this stage is receiving feedback from the changes you have made. Do you feel and act differently? Do you or others see the change in you? Added support from positive resources in conjunction with additional work to diminish the negative impact of blocks gives you a high probability of a truly successful change.

Stage 8. Adopting new behaviors into your lifestyle.   Any time you have a choice between the old behavior and the new behavior, there is no hesitation to choose the new behavior because the action is reflexive rather than reflective.

Review the stages. Stages 1 and 2 are mainly based on knowledge, whereas feeling and valuing heavily drive Stages 2 through 5. Skills are important in Stages 6 through 8, when the new behavior becomes quite automatic. The skills you learn may be somewhat reliant on the targeted behavior change and could range from assertiveness to journaling, diary keeping, or actual physical skills such as meditation or exercise.

Remember that the reason for the readiness concept is that success occurs on a continuum, and because it does, behavior change and readiness change along this continuum become criteria for success.

Developing the Plan

A good starting point is to address your stress reaction. Summarize what you feel are your serious or obvious symptoms of stress. Give them serious thought. Try this visualization exercise.

Step 1. What Do You Want to Accomplish?

Goals   Find a comfortable sitting position. Kick off your shoes, lean back, and relax. Sit quietly. Tell yourself that you are going to use the next five minutes to focus on yourself and to relax. Gently close your eyes. As you inhale, feel the air filling and expanding your chest, your stomach area, and your abdomen. When your lungs feel full, hold the breath for five seconds, and then begin to slowly exhale, controlling the air as your abdomen begins to contract. Push all of the air out of your body at the end of your exhalation. Repeat three times.

After practicing the full breathing part of the exercise, shift your attention to your body. Scan your face, shoulders, upper back, lower back, abdomen, legs, knees, and ankles. Ask yourself, "How do I experience the stress in my life?" "Which sections of my body are affected when I am stressed?" "What happens to those body parts?" Scan your body, becoming more and more aware of it as you go inside yourself to gather this information. Remember this information for further use. Focus on your breathing again, and, when you are ready, open your eyes. Slowly stretch your hands, feet, arms, and legs as you become active again. The preceding exercise is an opportunity to get in touch with yourself and to discover the ways in which you internalize stress. Use the following space to write what you felt during this first body-scanning exercise.

To further your insights about how stress affects you and to begin developing that awareness, complete Exercise 2. Your responses to this exercise may indicate which systems in your body are likely to be subjected to stress arousal and become weakened. This exercise lists some of the potential arousal signs. Check the symptoms you usually experience, then describe (in the space provided) additional symptoms you may also experience.

Signs and Symptoms   Check the items that you often experience.

_____ stiffness in neck

_____ fingers and hands tremble or shake

_____ twitch in muscles (specific muscle:)

_____

_____ difficulty standing still or sitting quietly

_____ stuttering or stammering speech

_____ frequent headaches (location on head:)

_____

_____ muscle tension (specific muscles:)

_____

_____ voice quivers

_____ nervous mannerisms; for example, biting nails, twisting hair, tapping feet, and so on

_____ heart pounding

_____ feeling lightheaded or faint

_____ cold chills

_____ cold hands

_____ cold feet

_____ dry mouth

_____ profuse sweating (location:) _____

_____ upset stomach

_____ sinking feeling in stomach

_____ frequent digestive disturbance

_____ moist or sweaty palms

_____ flushed or hot face

_____ preoccupied

_____ frequent insomnia

_____ uneasy or uncomfortable

_____ nervous or shaky

_____ confused

_____ forgetful

_____ insecure

_____ overexcited

_____ angry

_____ irritated

_____ worried

_____ anxious

_____ exhausted

_____ heart beats faster and harder

_____ backache

_____ shaky hands

_____ shallow, rapid breathing

_____ increased blood pressure

_____ stomachaches

_____ frequent diarrhea

_____ frequent constipation

_____ frequent indigestion

_____ hyperventilation

_____ skin rashes

_____ teeth grinding

_____ tension in the jaw (TMJ)

_____ chronic exhaustion

_____ inability to concentrate

_____ forgetfulness

_____ inability to concentrate

What does this tell you about your stress response in general?

Have you seen this exercise before? Look back to Journal Exercise 3. Did you check the same items, more of fewer items? What does this say to about how thing are going in your life since Chapter 3?

Stress and Stressors   After you get a picture of your stress reaction, next concentrate on your usual triggers of the stress reaction. For this exercise, close your eyes to let visualization help you picture your stress and stressors. Think about each question, then open your eyes and write your thoughts in the space provided.

1. Close your eyes, but in your mind picture a tense person. Scan your picture of this stressed person. What does the person look like when stressed? What is the person doing with his or her legs . . . arms . . . face? How is this person sitting or standing? Also picture the people and activities surrounding this individual in the stressful situation.

2. How are you like the image of the stressed person? How are you different?

3. Can you recall a stressful environment or situation in your life? How is this environment like your image, and how is it different?

Generally, what are the major ongoing stressors in your life? To better understand these stressors and to add to your picture of your stress reaction, do the following exercise.

1. Go to your stressor profile (Appendix A), and examine each of the stressor self-assessments.

2. Identify the stressors to which you feel vulnerable. Your self-assessment scores will reveal your current degree of stress for each stressor.

3. List your top three stressors in descending order.

My most significant stressors are

a. (score: _____)

b. (score: _____)

c. (score: _____)

Pick one of these three to work on first and write it here:

Write a short statement about why you have chosen this stressor over the other possibilities.

Write a short list of ways you can prove to yourself that you have achieved your stated outcome.

These are proofs:

Step 4. What Are Your Useful Resources?

This is an enjoyable part of the program because it helps build self-esteem by recalling resources and successes. When you feel confident about your ability to succeed in obtaining your outcomes, almost nothing will hold you back. Resources are both internal (personal characteristics) and external (environmental, social, or economic). Examples of internal resources are integrity, tenacity, willpower, energy, a sense of humor, self-love, and other self-concept issues. External resources may be the money to buy a good set of running shoes, the availability of certain facilities, or a devoted partner who will give support during the program. Resources may be general (as the suggestions given earlier) or specific to a situation (such as the *Cool Hand Luke* example). Both are very useful, but the best resources are those that use a specific skill that has been programmed in a certain situation.

Finding a Resource State   The intent of finding a resource state is to give you access to positive feeling states within yourself. The process itself builds self-esteem, promotes good feelings at the time, and can be "anchored" into the mind and body for retrieval of these positive feelings at later times.

Resources   Scan through your experiences and choose a time when you felt very fulfilled, confident, joyful, or peaceful—a state that felt very good to you. There have probably been many, many experiences in the past that would be appropriate, but choose one specific time and experience.

The resource state exercise gives the very best results when you can take yourself back to relive a specific experience. Generalities do not work as well because they are not as powerful as a singularly wonderful experience or feeling state. When finding a resource state, you should be able to vividly recall that experience. You can almost smell the flowers and look down and re-create all the details from the color of your shoes to the things you were saying to yourself and command the very same feeling you felt at the time of the original experience. Get back into the original experience, create a detailed picture, "hear" all the sounds in the experience, and re-create the feeling you had at the time. You might want to select a colorful name that will have special meaning and help you recall the feeling. Some of the effective names people have chosen have been Strawberry Blond, Cool Hand Luke, Smart Lady, Eagle Wings, and Hot Shot. Others have come up with words such as *confident* or *strong,* which describe their resource state, or words such as *rock* or *soaring,* which depict location or action at the time. The colorful and specific names elicit greater response than the generic names, perhaps because words such as *strong, confident,* or *rock* can conjure up many other meanings for many people.

Coping Skills

_____ 1. Give yourself 10 points if you feel that you have a supportive family.

_____ 2. Give yourself 10 points if you actively pursue a hobby.

_____ 3. Give yourself 10 points if you belong to a social or activity group that meets at least once a month (other than your family).

_____ 4. Give yourself 15 points if you are within five pounds of your "ideal" body weight, considering your height and bone structure.

_____ 5. Give yourself 15 points if you practice some form of deep relaxation at least three times a week. Deep-relaxation exercises include meditation, imagery, yoga, and so forth.

_____ 6. Give yourself 5 points for each time you exercise thirty minutes or longer during the course of an average week.

_____ 7. Give yourself 5 points for each nutritionally balanced and wholesome meal you consume in an average day.

_____ 8. Give yourself 5 points for each time you do something that you really enjoy, "just for yourself," in an average week.

_____ 9. Give yourself 10 points if you have some place in your home that you can go to relax and/or be by yourself.

_____ 10. Give yourself 10 points if you practice time management in your daily life.

_____ 11. Subtract 10 points for each pack of cigarettes you smoke in an average day.

_____ 12. Subtract 5 points for each evening during the course of an average week that you take any form of medication or chemical substance (including alcohol) to help you sleep.

_____ 13. Subtract 10 points for each day in an average week that you consume any form of medication or chemical substance (including alcohol) to reduce your anxiety or just calm you down.

_____ 14. Subtract 5 points for each evening during the course of an average week that you bring work home, if it is work that was meant to be done at your place of employment.

_____ Total Score

If you have not calculated your total score, do so now. A "perfect" score would be 115 points. If you scored in the 50 to 60 range, you probably have an adequate collection of coping strategies for most common sources of stress. However, you should keep in mind that the higher your score, the greater your ability to cope with stress in an effective and healthful manner. Also pay particular attention to the adaptive-versus-maladaptive coping dichotomy. Items 1–10 are all adaptive, health-promoting coping tools, but Items 11–14 are all maladaptive, health-eroding ways of coping with stress. How did you do? Ideally, you would limit your coping strategies to only adaptive techniques.

How do you cope with stress? What techniques do you employ to give yourself a sense of mastery (or self-efficacy) over the environment, and how do you handle the stress it can elicit? Exercise 6 was designed to help you see how you cope with the stress in your life. Coping can be defined as action-oriented and intrapsychic efforts to manage external and internal demands that tax or exceed a person's resources. Coping can occur prior to a stressful confrontation, in which case it is called anticipatory coping, as well as in reaction to a present or past confrontation. As was discussed earlier, coping behavior may be considered adaptive or maladaptive. Adaptive coping tactics are those that can be successfully employed to reduce stress and promote long-term health.

1. Look at your coping assessment. Items 1–10 help you manage stress and avoid burnout when practiced on a consistent basis. Items 11–14 may help you cope with stress in the short run, but they can erode your health in the long run.

2. List your three most commonly practiced coping tactics:

   a. _____

   b. _____

   c. _____

(Are they adaptive, as in Items 1–10? Or are they maladaptive, as in Items 11–14?)

Write one or two statements describing a personal resource that will help you achieve your goal. Write them in the form of affirmative statements, as if you already have the resource—because you do. Example: "I am organized and I always obtain my goals."

Affirmation 1.

Affirmation 2.

Everyone possesses the skills for achievement of outcomes—they usually have not associated their positive resources with the problem situations, or they have blocked their use

for some reason. The following is an outline of the procedure used for maximizing the use of resources in obtaining outcomes:

1. List your resources.

2. If each resource is valid, you will feel good about it and be excited to use it.

3. Decide what you will accept as proof that you have use of the resource. Look for measurable behaviors.

4. You should be able to create a resource state. Going to your resource state should make you feel better.

5. Think of specific ways to recall and use each resource in getting your desired outcome.

6. If the resource is one of high energy, but you remain "down," either the resource is not a positive, well-anchored one, or you are choosing to be "down." When you choose to remain in the problem state, it is time to suspect a secondary gain, which, as mentioned, is a hidden benefit of being "down."

7. You should be seeking support in your environment for the use and reinforcement of stated resources.

Step 5. What Are Your Blocks to Success?

Within each individual who has ambiguous feelings about behavior change, there is a part that would like to achieve the outcome, but there is another part that is afraid to try or to succeed. Feelings and actions that prevent a person from achieving his or her outcomes are called blocks to success. Blocks may be exaggerated parts of the stress problem itself (for example, excessive anxiety; lack of skills such as assertiveness; behaviors such as excessive anger; or secondary gains, including fear of failure).

Fear of Failure   If a person with stressful behavior fails to adopt the new outcome behavior or fails to change the problem behavior, conditions are no better or no worse. The negative behavior has simply been kept a while longer (which would have happened if the person had not attempted the program in the first place). Many people see this as no harm done. Others see that some harm has been done because failure at an attempted program diminishes self-esteem and self-efficacy. Individuals who "fail" at a program are likely to think less of themselves, and, more important, the program is associated with negative feelings. It will take more motivation to try again. An individual may say, "I tried that once and it didn't work, so why bother?" Many people would rather not try than risk failure, so they simply do not go beyond finding out what the problem is, or they rationalize the situation away. If the activities in Step 2 did not result in a clear picture of how life will be better, you will need to work on activities to increase the probability of program success.

Health behaviors are developed to fulfill a need; they all have a positive intention behind them. Unfortunately, sometimes the behavior turns out to be unhealthy. Nevertheless, it did something positive, or it would have spontaneously extinguished itself. When a certain behavior is eliminated (for example, a stressful lifestyle), the need for

that behavior (recognition or sympathy from others for being a hard worker) will go unfulfilled unless a substitute behavior is adopted to fulfill the old need, or the old need is eliminated. When you find that the thought of being without that behavior or lifestyle is often too much to face, you "fail" to change. If you are not making progress at the expected rate, or if you are not practicing relaxation techniques or completing homework assignments, chances are that you are not ready to give up the old behavior.

Step 6. Devise an Action Plan

Review the earlier chapters and journal entries that presented stress management techniques. As you do, your task will be to identify two or three of the techniques discussed there that you are not currently using. As you review the numerous options, remember to consider your personal preferences and be practical.

Techniques and Times

Write down some techniques or action plans that would help you accomplish your outcomes.

Set a timetable for achieving this goal.

1. Break the total time into smaller intervals (for example, one month into four weeks).
2. Make a calendar of specific day-to-day activities, and place it where you can see it. An example is provided (see **Table 18.1**). Specific exercises and techniques are abbreviated. A blank calendar is also provided to get you started (see **Table 18.2**). A large month-by-month appointment calendar is preferable for your ongoing program.

For each week, write outcome and resource statements.

This week's outcomes:

Table 18.1 Example of Monthly Stress Management Calendar

SUNDAY	MONDAY	TUESDAY	WEDNESDAY	THURSDAY	FRIDAY	SATURDAY
		31	**1** AM Breathing exercise PM Breathing exercise D.D. ✓✓	**2** AM Breathing exercise PM Breathing exercise D.D. ✓✓	**3** AM Breathing exercise PM Breathing exercise D.D. ✓✓	**4** AM Breathing exercise PM Breathing exercise Physical activity D.D. ✓
5 AM Breathing exercise PM Meditation D.D. ✓✓	**6** AM Breathing exercise PM Muscle relaxation D.D. ✓✓	**7** AM Breathing exercise PM Visual imagery D.D. ✓✓	**8** AM Breathing exercise Resource statement PM Stretch relaxation D.D. ✓✓	**9** AM Breathing exercise Resource statement PM Stretch relaxation D.D. ✓	**10** AM Breathing exercise Resource statement PM Muscle relaxation D.D. ✓	**11** AM Stretch relaxation Resource statement PM Physical activity D.D. ✓
12 NEW Resource statement AM Visual imagery PM Muscle relaxation Resource statement D.D. ✓✓	**13** AM Stretch relaxation Resource statement PM Meditation Resource statement D.D. ✓✓	**14** AM Breathing exercise Resource statement PM Physical activity D.D. ✓	**15** AM Breathing exercise PM Meditation D.D.	**16** AM Breathing exercise Resource statement PM Breathing exercise Resource statement Physical activity D.D.	**17** AM Breathing meditation Resource statement PM Breathing exercise Stretch relaxation Resource statement D.D. ✓	**18** D.D. ✓✓
19 NEW Resource statement Meditation Resource statement D.D. ✓	**20** AM Your choice PM Physical activity D.D. ✓✓	**21** AM Visual imagery Resource statement PM Resource statement Stretch relaxation D.D. ✓✓	**22** AM Meditation PM Physical activity Resource statement D.D.	**23** AM Visual imagery Resource statement PM Muscle relaxation D.D. ✓	**24** AM Meditation Resource statement PM Your choice D.D. ✓✓	**25** AM Physical activity Resource statement PM Your choice D.D. ✓✓
26 AM Meditation Resource statement PM stretch relaxation D.D. ✓✓	**27** AM Your choice PM breathing exercise Resource statement D.D. ✓	**28** AM Visual imagery PM physical activity D.D.	**29** AM Your choice PM relaxation Recall + resource statement D.D. ✓✓	**30** AM Relaxation Recall + resource statement D.D. ✓		You are on your own

Table 18.2 Your Monthly Stress Management Calendar

Sunday	Monday	Tuesday	Wednesday	Thursday	Friday	Saturday

This week's resource statements:

Establish a program of activities. Get help from a health professional if needed. Design a practical plan in order to implement the new stress management techniques you've just selected. In the space that follows, describe how you will integrate these new techniques into your daily and/or weekly habits. Use the contract method that follows. Many participants have found it an effective method for organizing their activities and for helping with their motivation.

Example

Technique 1   *Yoga*

How I will use it:

Every morning before breakfast when I feel excessive tightness in muscles

My Plan

I have decided to begin to use the following new stress management techniques:

Technique 1

How I will use it:

Technique 2

How I will use it:

Technique 3

How I will use it:

Remember, stay flexible, reevaluate your plan in two to four weeks, and if you need to change this personal plan, use the next section to indicate the revised plan. Don't forget activities such as the Daily Feeling Diary, the Daily Stress Response Diary, or the Monthly Stress-Management Calendar.

Revised Plan

Technique 1

How I will use it:

Technique 2

How I will use it:

Technique 3

How I will use it:

List these tools:

Using material from earlier chapters, choose one or more exercises provided in those chapters to create a monthly stress management plan as shown on the Example of Monthly Stress Management Calendar (Table 18.1). Also, complete the two daily diaries, and record their completion with a checkmark each day.

A Sample Practice Plan

A total plan is more than just a promise to use certain techniques. It includes keeping a list of carefully selected techniques, records of the times used, feedback on your progress, and evaluation of success. Here is a sample plan.

A. Techniques
   1. Breathing and centering
   2. Resource statements
   3. Technique 1: Goal Path Model or other cognitive activity
   4. Technique 2: Muscle relaxation
   5. Technique 3: Meditation
B. Practice Plan
   1. Practice each daily sequence twice a day.
   2. Ponder or repeat the resource statements you have made.
C. Record Keeping
   1. Record times and make some notes about your experience with the practice.
   2. Complete the daily diary as a monitor of your progress (see **Tables 18.3** and **18.4**).

Most athletic coaches agree that good practice leads to good performance on game day. The same philosophy applies to stress management. Good practice of relaxation techniques will lead to good application of the skills when needed. Take time to fill out the practice feedback sheets. If your practice is not going well, do something about it now!

Have you ever taken steps to reduce this stressor before?

_____ Yes _____ No

If yes, what were the results?

If no, why not?

Write a brief but specific outcome statement.

I want to

Rate on a scale of 1 to 10 how ready you are to alleviate this stressor.

1   10

Low   High

Rate your ability to do it now.

1   10

Low   High

If you did not give yourself at least an "8" on both scales, your chances of success will be decreased. In that case, you may wish to reconsider your other major stressors and focus on your second choice.

Step 2. How Will Things Be Different or Better in Your Life?

This question is often overlooked in stress management programs. It is the motivation question. Everyone is committed to some degree, and everyone undertaking a stress management program would like to be more in control, but only the very committed will finish the program and change the behaviors necessary to be successful. The committed will be able to visualize the new behavior and clearly see how life will be different or better than it was with the old behavior. To strengthen that picture in your mind, try the following visualization exercise.

Outcome Visualization Outcome visualization is used for programming or imprinting a new thought about behavior or belief about oneself. The technique involves seeing, hearing, and feeling yourself doing the new behavior. By mentally practicing the desired new behavior, a potentially stressful situation that would have previously triggered the old behavior instead triggers the new behavior because it has been rehearsed in the mind. Try this now.

Visualization Close your eyes, and visualize yourself having accomplished the new behavior. Visualize yourself without the stressor or as a more relaxed person in the old stressful situation.

If you have difficulty in this exercise, it may mean that you are ambivalent about giving up the stressful behavior because, on some level, that behavior has served a very useful purpose, possibly for many years. Sometimes individuals cling to stressful behaviors because of some conscious or subconscious gain or benefit. Most stress behaviors are done for a positive reason, regardless of whether that purpose is consciously known. When an individual experiences difficulty in or ambiguity about giving up an old behavior, it is time to explore the cause of this reluctance. The phenomenon of continuing a negative behavior because it fulfills some need is called secondary gain, and the exact nature of the secondary gain is often not realized on a conscious level. For example, some commonly observed secondary gains accompanying stress are the following:

1. Maintaining control of life—many people fear becoming lazy and feel that keeping their "nose to the grindstone" protects them.

2. A strong need to please others and gain recognition often pushes people to take on more than they can handle. Again, it provides external motivation for those who cannot do it for themselves.

3. Control of others through manipulation or to give oneself permission to rest or quit—this occurs when people overwork themselves to the point of fatigue, illness, or accident.

Step 3. How Do You Know When You Have Achieved an Outcome?

What Will You Accept as Proof?   As with Step 2, this critical phase of the program is often forgotten or omitted. It is easy to accept vague statements such as "I will feel better," "I will look better," or "I will have more energy." However, you must have definite, measurable proofs. How will you know that you feel better, look better, or have more energy? What will you accept as proof of these outcomes? The important word in this step is *measurable*. If your outcome is being more relaxed, how will you measure that outcome?

If you are having difficulty setting behavioral proofs, think of how you would observe this behavior in someone else. For example, how would you know if a person was energetic; what behavior would be proof or evidence of that to you? You might make a list of the behaviors and apply them to your situation. If you are still experiencing difficulty, choose a personal friend or someone in the movies or on TV who exhibits the behavior you desire. What would you accept as proof or evidence that the other person has the behavior? Can you make a similar observation in your life? If the answer is yes, it can be accepted as proof, and the process continues.

One of our students who was working on a stress management program with an outcome of self-confidence had difficulty with Step 3 until he identified the character Luke from the movie *Cool Hand Luke* as the model for his behavior. *Cool Hand Luke* not only provided him with a model for his targeted behavior, but the name also became a reminder or "anchor" of a time when he was self-confident.

Journal Entry 18

Readiness

People change when they are ready. Usually change happens in small increments, however. If you are motivated to become less stressed and are committed to putting thought and effort into the entries in this journal, this is a commitment to change. The degree of change that you do depends on (1) where you are now and (2) where you intend to go. Success is measured in how many steps you take from no readiness at all to finally reaching your goal. On the next page, you will find a model of the readiness concept. Use this model to determine just how ready you are to change stressful behaviors in your life and then where you want to go from there.

Behavior change is a scary thing to most people. We become accustomed to being the way we are, thinking the way we do, and saying the things we and others like to hear. Doing things in a different way, however, is like stepping into a cold river—it's not very comforting and it's easier to step back out rather than go through it to the other side. But, like all endeavors, the only way to get to the other side is by going through it (not backing out or trying to get around it). You've probably found in your life that you can change, and if you go about the change with small steps (like little stepping stones in that cold river), you get to the other side in good order. And once there, you feel good about your progress.

On the Readiness Scale, locate where you are regarding your readiness to live a less stressful life. Rather than working with the concept of a "less stressful life," first identify your top three stressors and/or worries. What are the things that you do that cause stress/worry in your life? Take the responsibility here—don't say that it's your roommate, boss, or teacher that stresses you.

1.

2.

3.

The Readiness Scale*

8. I have met my goal. I have adopted this in my everyday life and get constant, positive feedback.
7. I practice this regularly, when I think about it, and get good feedback.
6. I have had positive feedback that proves to me that I can do this and feel good about it.
5. I have done this at least once before but did not continue.
4. I believe in my ability to do this.
3. I think this is valuable for me to know and do.
2. I believe that it is possible for people to do this.
1. I think I understand what this concept is about.

*Source: Girdano and Dusek, *Changing Health Behavior.* ©1987. Reprinted by permission from the authors.

With each of these three identified stressors, make a statement of intent to change (assuming that you would like to change the impact of these stressors in your life). If you have chosen a stressor that you definitely do not want to work to change, choose another one that you are willing to change.

1.

2.

3.

Now consider your readiness to make the changes that you intend. Locate where you are with Level 1 on the Readiness Model, Level 2, and so on.

Here's an example:

#1 Stressor	Commuting thirty minutes every day
Intent	I intend to leave earlier before the traffic gets heavy, play a relaxing or inspiring tape while I drive, and treat other drivers courteously.
Place on the Readiness Scale	Between Levels 3 and 4. I really do know that I have to do something about this, that it will be a good thing, and that others do it successfully.

Write the level for each of your choices and verify that in words (as in the example).

1.

2.

3.

 Now journal your insights and feelings about the process of change in general, and your ability to effect positive change related to your stressors/worries.

 Write a positive word or short phrase about your desire and ability to change (such as "I can do this") that will be useful to you in future situations.

Final Note

You will never live a life of no stress. Nor would you want to—it would be boring without challenge, and you would never know how good you really are. When we are young, we feel the endless bounds of energy and we are at our closest point to optimal health, at least physically. However, it is so easy for life to overwhelm us and for stress to get the upper hand. We only need to look around us to see the devastating effects that poor lifestyle choices have on our health. Our health care system is near collapse under the pressure of excess use resulting from chronic diseases stemming from lifestyle choices. Problems such as smoking, obesity, and lack of exercise and emotional difficulties, to mention a few, at their core are all related to our stressful lifestyle. Life is neither easy nor fair. We all have our successes and failures. You will be presented with a million chances to decide one path or another. One of the paths with a million choices will concern your health. One health choice is stress. Hopefully, after reading this book you have a better understanding of stress and have learned some stress-management techniques.

Several decades ago, we envisioned an academic approach to behavior change programs that would not just teach about stress management, but would also teach how to manage stress. We were so sure that students could and would learn the skills that we adopted a performance-based evaluation philosophy that measured success on how well students reduced their stress (Girdano and Dusek 1977). After working with students and clients for thirty years, we remain convinced that one can learn these skills and, if properly motivated to use them, can develop a lifestyle that diminishes the harmful effects of excess stress and tension. You now have these skills. Your stress and your health are your choice. The most important factor is motivation. How much do you value it? What are you willing to do to be healthy? That, of course, is up to you.

Final Journal Entry

The Toolbox

At the end of each of the previous Journal Entries, you have been asked to write a word or brief phrase that would remind you to use the information, journaling, and insights that came from that exercise. These written reminders are your tools for stress management.

We ask you now to rewrite your tools in the space below opposite the number of the Exercise. Take this opportunity to shorten your response (where possible) into a "quick hitter," something short and meaningful that that will immediately remind you of that lesson.

The final exercise in this journal is to apply your tools to the stress problems you experience every day. From now on, when you recognize that you are feeling stressed, use your journaling skills to quickly write down how you are feeling about the problem, then choose which of your tools will help you resolve the stressful feelings you are having.

Here are a couple of examples of the combined use of journaling and stress-management tools. Each is written by someone who is experiencing a current problem. The situation is described, then the journalist has chosen several of his or her tools to help in the management of the current stressor.

April 25

What is going on here?? This is the third time this week I've been crying after my father called! He calls and says something nice to me or we just chat, and before I know it he has turned the whole conversation around to my grades, the money he spends for my education, and how I am on the edge of being cut off. He gets me talking about fun things I do and in a flash he turns it into I'm the bad guy. It's kind of like he sets me up. I'm so dumb I never see it coming. I end up feeling like the ungrateful scum of the earth, crying, depressed, and then I can't study. I have got to be ready for him next time.

Tools:

People don't plan to fail; they fail to plan.

I deserve and demand respect.

I am in control of my emotions.

I can't be stressed when I'm breathing relaxed.

People see what they want to see.

I can get what I want easier if I give something the other person wants.

March 20

Well, that's the straw that's going to do in this relationship. Count on it. Just talked to Carol and she tells me that she has a new roommate. I knew she had to share expenses with somebody in order to stay in school and she really wants to do that. And I want her to do that. Being fifty miles away isn't bad enough though. No! She has to go out and find a male roommate!! Is this some kind of message to me? I can just hear it. "Come on, roomie, let's eat breakfast together. Come on, roomie, let's study together. Come on roomie, let's get real chummy with each other." What do I do now?

Tools:

Remember to breathe!

Everything turns out OK, or at least for the best.

There's nothing to be afraid of; don't make more out of it than there is.

Love is unconditional.

In the space below, write two of your stressful experiences. You may first wish to photocopy the page and use it as your journaling format in the future.

Experience 1

_____

_____

_____

_____

_____

_____

_____

_____

Experience 2

_____

_____

_____

_____

_____

_____

Take time now to reflect about this total journaling experience. Do you feel that you have more tools to control the stress and tension in your life? Are you more committed to doing so? Do you have more periods of time now in which you are calm, or at least react in a calmer way than previous to this journal experience? Write your insights.

_____

_____

_____

Personal Stressor Profile Summary

This Appendix gives you a chance to get a total picture of your own stress vulnerability by transferring each of your scores from the eleven self-assessment exercises to the Personal Stressor Profile Sheet on the following page. After you have filled in your scores on each of the scales, connect all of the points. You have now plotted a graph of your stressor profile. Although there is no linear relationship between the self-assessment exercises, the line will help you visually assimilate your total profile and will be most helpful when you compare results from retests at some later date. Knowing the source of your stress is vital to managing that stress.

A final note: You may be quite vulnerable to stress from a specific determinant even though your score was low on the assessment test in which it occurred. The reason for this is simply that several of the exercises consisted of two or three aspects under the same general heading. For example, you may be a "catastrophizer" of the greatest magnitude, and this may cause your life to be a very stressful one. However, it is possible that your score on the anxiety scale was low because you didn't suffer from the other feedback mechanisms. Therefore, it is important that you carefully consider each question in which you score poorly and determine how significantly this aspect of stress affects your life.

On the other hand, remember that although these eleven scales are extremely useful tools for beginning to assess the sources of stress in your life, they are not clinically validated psychological tests and should not be treated as such.

At some later dates, you will probably want to come back and retake the self-assessment exercises, formulating a second, third, or fourth profile as a record of your progress. Using the same profile, simply use different colors to indicate different dates.

Table Appendix 1   Personal Stressor Profile Summary Sheet

Exercise	1	2	3	4	5	6	7	8	9	10	11
	Emotion	Self-Perception	Type-A Behavior	Anxiety	Control	Change	Frustration	Overload	Boredom, Loneliness	Nutrition	Occupational Stressors
Scores Indicative of:	45	40	40	40	40	400	40	40	40	40	40
High Vulnerability to Stressors	40	35	35	35	35	350	35	35	35	35	35
	35	30	30	30	30	300	30	30	30	30	30
Moderate Vulnerability to Stressors	30	25	25	25	25	250	25	25	25	25	25
	25	20	20	20	20	200	20	20	20	20	20
Low Vulnerability to Stressors	20	15	15	15	15	150	15	15	15	15	15
	15	10	10	10	10	100	10	10	10	10	10

This profile is an educational tool and was designed to promote basic health education. It is in no way designed to be a substitute for the diagnostic procedures used by physicians or psychologists. Any concerns about your physical or mental health should be directed to your family physician, your local medical society, or your local psychological society.

Glossary

acetylcholine a neurotransmitter substance of the parasympathetic nervous system.

ACTH adrenocortical stimulating hormone, involved in releasing total-body stress hormones.

acute stress intense, short-duration stress.

adaptation the tendency of the body to fight to restore homeostasis in the face of forces that upset the natural bodily balance.

adaptive stress the stress imposed on the body during attempts to cope with or adapt to stressful situations.

adipose tissue tissue in which fat is stored.

adrenal gland a small gland on the top of the kidney that secretes stress hormones.

aerobic the production of energy within exercising muscles with the use of oxygen. To be considered aerobic, exercise must be rhythmic, lasting more than twenty minutes.

affirmation positive self-talk in the form of behavior-specific, present-tense "I" statements written/spoken to affirm and remind ourselves of what we want to become.

aggressive (communication) a demanding, bossy, patronizing, or demeaning style that insists that someone obey your wishes.

aldosterone a mineralocorticoid hormone that increases water retention.

alveoli air sacs in the lungs where oxygen and carbon dioxide exchange takes place.

amino acids chief components of proteins.

angina pectoris chest pain associated with narrowed coronary arteries and lack of oxygen to heart muscle during exertion.

antigens foreign agents that stimulate the immune response.

anxiety acute or chronic arousal, usually fear, but often undirected.

anxious reactivity the body reacting to feelings of anxiety with more anxiety and more arousal, making resolution difficult.

arrhythmia irregular heart beat.

arteriosclerosis the hardening and narrowing of artery walls.

arthritis inflammation of joint tissue, often causing pain and swelling and ultimately permanent joint damage.

assertiveness saying what is liked or disliked about someone or something without using degradation; getting what is wanted, but not at the expense of someone else.

atherosclerosis the gradual accumulation of fat on blood vessel walls; the most common form of arteriosclerosis.

autogenic self-generating; the body responding to self-talk or visual imagery.

autonomic nervous system part of the central nervous system, consisting of sympathetic and parasympathetic components, that requires no conscious thought.

behavior therapy a system of record keeping and motivation designed to help change a behavior (e.g., stress).

biofeedback a change technique that uses electrical instrumentation to magnify the subtle signals from the body so they become more noticeable and thus more controllable. Electrical impulses from muscles, brain waves, and/or skin temperature are most commonly used.

biological rhythms naturally recurring cycles of biological activity governed by the nervous and hormonal systems.

body mass index (BMI) index commonly used to determine normal weight, overweightness, and obesity; based on height and weight.

bronchiole small branch of airway; sometimes undergoes spasm, making breathing difficult, as in exercise-induced asthma.

burnout a state of mental and/or physical exhaustion caused by excessive stress.

calisthenics exercises in which your body weight serves as the resistance.

calorie the amount of heat required to raise 1 kilogram of water 1 degree Centigrade in temperature. In common usage, a "calorie" is the same as a "kilocalorie" in scientific literature.

cancer a large number of diseases characterized by development, uncontrolled growth, and spread (metastasis) of abnormal cells.

carbohydrate a nutrient compound consisting of molecules of sugar linked together in large complexes (called complex carbohydrate or starch) or in pairs or existing as single molecules.

carcinogens cancer-producing substances.

cardiac output volume of blood pumped by the heart each minute; product of heart rate and stroke volume.

cardiovascular disease (CVD) diseases of the heart and blood vessels including heart attack, stroke, and hypertension.

cardiovascular fitness the combined abilities of the respiratory and circulatory systems to provide adequate oxygen to large- and small-muscle groups while they engage in continuous, rhythmic exercise for extended periods of time.

central nervous system (CNS) the brain and spinal cord.

cerebral cortex the large outside layer of the brain that is responsible for conscious movement, awareness, logic, and higher forms of thought.

chakras major energy centers traversing the spine from the coccyx to the crown of the head.

cholesterol a form of fat found in every animal cell and a major constituent of human bile and sex hormones; the liver makes all the cholesterol the body needs; high levels in the blood are associated with increased risk of cardiovascular disease.

chronic conditions diseases and conditions that tend to take a long time to develop and usually require continuing treatment.

cognitive restructuring a coping technique whereby one changes thoughts from threatening to nonthreatening, negative to positive.

competent coping meeting demands while managing stress levels.

coping behavior that neutralizes stress arousal.

cool-down a period of continued activity (e.g., walking or stretching) following vigorous exercise, done to avoid blood pooling and dizziness, and to promote recovery.

coronary arteries the first blood vessels that originate from the aorta and supply oxygen and fuels to the heart muscle itself.

coronary prone having risk factors related to the development of heart disease.

coronary thrombosis a clot that blocks an artery in the heart.

corticosteroids stress hormones released by the adrenal cortex.

cortisol a corticosteroid.

defense mechanism thought pattern used to decrease pain.

deprivational stress the psychophysiological stress response caused by states of boredom or loneliness.

diabetes a metabolic disease that diminishes the body's ability to metabolize glucose, by either inadequate production of insulin (Type I diabetes, usually occurring in children and young adults) or inability to utilize available insulin (Type II diabetes, usually occurring in adults, many times related to overweight and obesity).

diaphragmatic breathing deep, but not exaggerated, breathing in which air is taken to the bottom lobes of the lungs, during which you can feel the diaphragm move up and down with each breath.

diastolic pressure the lowest blood pressure level that occurs when the heart is resting between beats.

distress debilitating or harmful stress with which the individual is not coping well; also referred to as negative stress.

duration of exercise how long one engages in activity.

electrocardiogram (ECG) a graphic recording of the electrical activity of the heart.

electrolytes solution of ions (sodium, potassium) that conducts electric current in the body.

emotion a subjective feeling that is closely interwoven with cognitive and physiological processes. Emotions call for action.

emotional intelligence the ability to control emotions and express them appropriately and comfortably.

endorphins endogenous mood changers.

energy balance a state in which the caloric intake equals the caloric expenditure over time.

environmental stress stimuli arising out of the environment that produce a stress response in most individuals.

enzyme an organic catalyst that accelerates the rate of chemical reactions.

epinephrine one of two hormones (the other is norepinephrine) secreted by the body under conditions of stress, including vigorous exercise; also termed *adrenaline*.

ergotropic an excited or work phase where systems are stimulated for action.

eustress positive, action-enhancing stress.

exercise regular physical activity engaged in for health and fitness.

fight or flight Walter Cannon's term for the stress response that prepares the body to either fight or run.

flexibility the ability of body segments to move through a range of motion.

frequency how often one engages in activity.

frustration excessive stress that occurs when we are blocked from doing what we want to do.

General Adaptation Syndrome (GAS) the theory of stress arousal developed by Hans Selye, involving three stages: (1) the alarm reaction, (2) the stage of resistance, and (3) the stage of exhaustion.

glucocorticoids adrenal cortex hormones that help control glucose level.

gluconeogenesis the formation of glucose from available glycogen and amino acids.

glycemic index a measure of how rapidly a carbohydrate is digested and absorbed into the blood.

hardy personality combination of personality traits consisting of control, commitment, and challenge, which help a person combat stress.

hatha yoga a form of yoga that uses breathing, body positions, and exercises to promote physical and mental harmony.

health conceptual term referring to overall level of functioning at any particular point in time, including the physical, emotional, social, mental, and spiritual dimensions of life.

homeostasis the state of the body in which exists stable equilibrium of internal functions.

hypertension (high blood pressure) blood pressure levels chronically higher than 140 systolic and 90 diastolic.

hypoglycemia low blood sugar.

hypothalamus an inner brain structure involved with subconscious processing.

hypothermia life-threatening heat loss brought on by rapid cooling, energy depletion, and exhaustion.

imperturbability a lowered resting reactivity threshold to stressors.

inhibition opposite of excitation in the nervous system.

insulin pancreatic hormone responsible for getting blood sugar into cells.

intensity how hard one engages in an activity.

internal environment the "world" within the body; as discussed in stress management, the term usually refers to the nervous system. Quieting the internal environment is a goal of relaxation activities.

ischemia lack of oxygen-carrying blood to a specific area such as the heart muscle.

journaling a stress management technique involving insights gained from written thoughts, feelings, emotions, and behavior.

lifestyle how one lives in the sociocultural environment; the events of one's life as well as daily work and play activities; often mentioned as the most important determinant of stress.

ligand amino acid molecule.

limbic system portion of the brain related to emotional memories and behavior.

lipoprotein a fat-protein complex that serves as a carrier in the blood.

mantra a vehicle (word, phrase, picture) used to aid concentration during meditation.

massage therapy the manipulation of body tissue for the purpose of releasing tension.

maximum heart rate the highest heart rate value one can attain; usually measured during heavy exercise.

meditation exercises, postures, and other rituals developed in an attempt to slow body activities to a point at which the mind would also be allowed to become quiet.

mental health the ability to learn and to use intellectual capabilities.

mindfulness conscious direction of thoughts.

mindfulness meditation (also *insight meditation*) using directed thoughts to gain insight as you remain in the meditative state.

mineralocorticoids adrenal cortex hormones that govern water balance in the body.

myocardium heart muscle.

neuromuscular relaxation training systematic exercises that train not only the muscles but also the nervous system components that control muscle activity. The objective is to reduce the tension.

neuron nerve cell that conducts an impulse; basic unit of the nervous system.

neuropeptides neurotransmitter-like proteins that travel via blood and cerebrospinal fluid to deliver information throughout the body (include ligands, steroids, and peptides).

neuroplasticity the concept that the brain continually changes as a result of experience.

neurotransmitters biochemicals (such as acetylcholine, epinephrine, dopamine, and norepinephrine) that transmit neural responses at nerve synapses.

norepinephrine see *epinephrine*.

obesity excess body fat above a level that most experts consider as healthy.

optimal stress a point between eustress and distress that promotes a maximal level of performance.

osteoporosis weakening of the bones via the loss of bone minerals.

overload a state in which the demands of life exceed one's capacity to meet them.

overload principle the training maxim that describes the body's adaptive response to physical stress applied regularly.

overweight excess weight relative to the average person of the same gender and stature. Persons who are overweight often, but not always, have excess body fat.

passive behavior nonassertive action, lacking skill to ask for what is wanted; mode of operation is to manipulate.

peptides amino acid molecules (see *neurotransmitters*).

personality may be thought of as the summation of personal characteristics, attitudes, values, and behavior patterns that individuals manifest in interactions with the environment. The dynamics of an individual's self-perception and characteristic attitudes and behaviors that may somehow contribute to excessive stress are called *personality stressors*.

physical fitness the capacity to meet the demands of modern-day life with relatively little strain.

physical health the ability to carry out daily tasks with energy remaining for unforeseen circumstances; biological integrity.

pituitary gland inner brain structure below the hypothalamus that stimulates the stress hormone process.

plaque a growth of cellular debris and low-density lipoprotein cholesterol that impedes blood flow in arteries.

protein basic structural substance of the human body, composed of carbon, hydrogen, oxygen, and nitrogen arranged into amino acid strands.

psychoneuroimmunology (PNI) a branch of science that studies the relationship between thoughts, emotions, and the immune system.

psychosocial stressors a function of the complex interaction between social behavior and the way our senses and our minds interpret those behaviors.

psychosomatic disease any condition thought to be the result of excess emotional arousal, maladaptive coping, and chronic distress.

readiness s state of being open to movement (mental, emotional, physical).

recruitment incorporation of additional physiological systems or psychological defenses to aid in coping.

resistance exercise an exercise, such as weightlifting, that demands an increased effort from the muscle(s).

reticular formation (also RAS) network of nerve cells extending from the spinal cord up to the thalamus that links sensory and motor impulses.

reward system area of the brain that reinforces behaviors.

risk factors factors associated with a higher risk for a certain disease.

secondary gain a hidden motivation for behavior.

self-actualization the process of being and becoming the most one can be; developing one's fullest potential.

self-concept a combination of core personality traits including self-love, self-esteem, self-respect, self-confidence, self-awareness, and self-worth. These aspects are important determinants of how one reacts to stress.

self-contract a motivational device in the form of a written promise to yourself to try a specific plan of action for a designated time period.

self-efficacy a concept popularized by Albert Bandura that states that when people believe they can do something, they increase their chances of success.

self-talk internal dialogue with oneself; can be positive or negative.

spiritual health the belief in some unifying force such as nature, scientific laws, or a godlike entity.

stress the body's reaction to outside pressures manifested by mental and physical arousal, increased blood pressure, and muscle tension, which can fatigue body systems to the point of malfunction and disease.

stress management a pattern of behavior that involves understanding the stress response, recognizing stressors, developing stress reduction skills, and regularly incorporating these into one's lifestyle.

stressor any condition or event that causes a stress response; may be physical, social, or psychological, including imaginary.

sympathetic response the stress response of the nervous system that prepares the body for stress.

sympathomimetic agents chemical substances that mimic the sympathetic stress response.

synapse junction between neurons.

systolic pressure the highest blood pressure level that occurs when the heart is contracting.

target heart rate a heart rate value during exercise which falls within your training-sensitive zone.

target organ an organ or tissue that is the target of excess stimulation.

thought stopping a technique whereby the stressed person intentionally breaks the anxious cycle by abruptly leaving the obsessional thoughts.

time-urgency personality trait extensively studied as part of the famous cardiovascular Type A–prone personality construct describing individuals who tend to be impatient, driven by an excessive time and task orientation, and more often prone to excessive feelings of anger and hostility.

tone a conditioning or predisposition.

trophotropic domination of the parasympathetic nervous system that promotes tranquility (rest phase).

type A behavior see time-urgency personality trait.

visual imagery a relaxation technique involving self-directed mental mages of relaxed states.

vitamin an organic compound that is necessary for growth and for proper body functioning, but provides no calories for energy.

warm-up a process of gradually preparing the body for more vigorous exercise by beginning with gentle activities that emphasize range of motion at slow to moderate speeds.

Index